AN HISTORICAL INTRODUCTION TO MODERN PSYCHOLOGY

Founded by C. K. Ogden

The International Library of Psychology

GENERAL PSYCHOLOGY
In 38 Volumes

AN HISTORICAL
INTRODUCTION TO
MODERN PSYCHOLOGY

GARDNER MURPHY

With a Supplement by Heinrich Klüver

First published in 1928 by
Routledge and Kegan Paul Ltd

Reprinted in 1999 by
Routledge
2 Park Square, Milton Park, Abingdon, Oxfordshire OX14 4RN
711 Third Avenue, New York, NY 10017
First issued in paperback 2014

Routledge is an imprint of the Taylor and Francis Group, an informa company

Transferred to Digital Printing 2006

© 1928 Gardner Murphy

The publishers have made every effort to contact authors/copyright holders
of the works reprinted in the *International Library of Psychology*.
This has not been possible in every case, however, and we would
welcome correspondence from those individuals/companies
we have been unable to trace.

These reprints are taken from original copies of each book. In many cases
the condition of these originals is not perfect. The publisher has gone to
great lengths to ensure the quality of these reprints, but wishes to point
out that certain characteristics of the original copies will, of necessity, be
apparent in reprints thereof.

British Library Cataloguing in Publication Data
A CIP catalogue record for this book
is available from the British Library

An Historical Introduction to Modern Psychology
ISBN 978-0-415-21034-8 (hbk)
ISBN 978-0-415-75799-7 (pbk)
General Psychology: 38 Volumes
ISBN 978-0-415-21129-1
The International Library of Psychology: 204 Volumes
ISBN 978-0-415-19132-6

TO MY MOTHER

CONTENTS

PART II

FROM WEBER'S EXPERIMENTS TO THE AGE OF
WUNDT

PART III

CONTEMPORARY PSYCHOLOGY

PREFACE

PSYCHOLOGY, in the sense of reflection upon the nature and activities of mind, is a very ancient discipline, one which reached great heights in ancient Greece and has continued (in intimate relation with philosophy) with every phase of European civilization. During the nineteenth century this literary and philosophic psychology underwent profound changes, chiefly as a result of the progress of biology, from which both concepts and methods were freely borrowed. Many of its greatest students began to rely upon experimental and mathematical method, believing that psychology could become a science akin to other biological sciences. It is the purpose of this volume to trace the course of those changes in the nineteenth and twentieth centuries which have thus tended to transform psychology and to give it its present character.

To see our contemporary psychology in perspective becomes each year more difficult. A sketch of the development of the science since the beginning of the nineteenth century should help to some extent to give such a perspective. No purpose would be served, however, in seeking to duplicate the existing historical studies of psychology. Brett's three-volume *History of Psychology* presents a comprehensive and eminently readable account of psychology from the time of the ancients through the nineteenth century; the third volume of this work has proved of immense value in the present study. But, simply because our purposes have been different, the duplication of material is not great. Brett's work shows the interconnections of nineteenth-century psychology with that of earlier periods, with emphasis upon many problems which have not as yet been found amenable to just that experimental approach which chiefly concerns the present work. Moreover, about half of the material in the present volume belongs to the twentieth century, material excluded by the chronological limits which Brett imposed on his own work (Preface, vol. II, page 5). The nearer a decade is to our own time, the more attention I have given it ; the plan might remind one of Mercator's Projection.

I have, indeed, attempted a brief account of certain phases of psychological history from the seventeenth century to the beginning of the nineteenth century, in order to make the psychology of the early nineteenth century intelligible. No one could be more keenly aware than I am of the complete inadequacy of this sketch. Its purpose is not to present a unified picture of psychology during the seventeenth and eighteenth centuries, but to throw into relief a few movements whose influence was still strong at the opening of the nineteenth century. With the nineteenth century, and especially with the beginnings of experimental psychology, the quantity of psychological writing becomes so vast that a panoramic survey rather than a minute inspection of individuals and movements is all that can well be attempted. Even so, I have doubtless failed at many points ; I shall be very grateful to readers who will call my attention to errors, whether great or small.

The scope of " psychology " has enlarged so much in the past few generations, and the present usage of the term varies so much with individual points of view, that the limits of our present work need to be defined. The reader will find an apparent over-emphasis upon the results of research work as opposed to the progress of psychological theory. This is due, in part, to an attempt to reflect adequately the trend towards empirical, especially experimental, method. I have, however, another reason for the relative neglect of psychological theory within the period of contemporary psychology. A survey of psychological literature within any decade since the founding of Wundt's laboratory would show that very little of the speculative material has survived. Here and there a striking exception appears ; a man of great magnitude impresses his outlook upon a whole generation, while some experimentalists weave their findings and their interpretations into a vital unity which stimulates and directs further research. But in general the framework of the science is constituted by its empirical methods and results ; and though I trust I have not unduly neglected the thought of the builders, it is upon the character of the building that I would lay emphasis.

The central purpose which I have kept before me in the treatment of the more recent phases of psychology is to show the constantly widening range of experimental and quantitative method, to include ever more complicated problems. As each new field is conquered, and as methods become standardized and research titles numbered by the hundreds, it ceases to be capable of treatment in a general volume such as this. The reader will find, for example, practically nothing about studies of sensation since the work of Helmholtz; nothing about psychophysics since Fullerton and Cattell; nothing about association-tests since Jung's first work. In part I have imposed these limitations on the work because it was the only way in which justice could be done to the many fields of psychology; in part I have done so simply because good historical treatment is already available for each thoroughly established special field.

My intention, then, is to present in rough chronological order the conquest by scientific method of one research field after another. In accordance with this line of attack it is quite impossible to afford any just treatment to the philosophical forms of psychology, or to the problems of epistemology and theory of value. Much significant work ordinarily regarded as psychological must quite arbitrarily be excluded, if any sort of unified purpose is to be achieved. A single illustration will show where I have tried to set the boundary. In *The Analysis of Mind* Russell clearly indicates his purpose: " I am interested in psychology not so much for its own sake, as for the light that it may throw on the problem of knowledge " (p. 15). This does not prevent his making valuable psychological observations; but it is natural that a man's chief interest should determine the field of his chief contribution. This holds good of much contemporary philosophical work in which psychology is a tool rather than an end. And on the other hand, the *philosophy* of mind bears a relation to the history of psychology very similar to the relation which the philosophy of physical sciences bears to the history of these sciences; *i.e.*, wherever such philosophical contributions *shape the course* of the science, they may be regarded as a part of its history. The line of exclusion is, of course, an arbitrary one; some sort of line must nevertheless be drawn.

But whereas contemporary British, French, and American

psychology can be portrayed in some degree of detachment from prevalent philosophic systems, no such separation is possible in relation to contemporary German psychology. Germany is witnessing in many quarters a widespread revolt against experimentalism, and a recourse to methods which are as fully philosophical as they are psychological. In the two concluding chapters, Dr. Heinrich Klüver describes the outlook and methods of a number of schools of contemporary German psychology, which are more or less interwoven with contemporary philosophy.

It will not be possible to treat of the *applications* of psychology. Such applications do, of course, yield at times new psychological principles. It is only when they do so that they can be considered here.

Some years ago, I was puzzled by the reflection that there existed no historical approach to that contemporary psychology which arose in the nineteenth century as a result of the interaction of experimental physiology, psychiatry, the theory of evolution, and the social sciences, constantly working upon certain materials from the history of philosophy, and guided by progress in the physical sciences and statistical method. Now, having made the attempt, I am no longer puzzled. Probably no one who had mastered the vast materials necessary for such an undertaking would have the courage to make a beginning. Perhaps it is just as well that the first venture in this direction should be made by one who, because he sees but few paths, trudges the more cheerfully on the way. For the strange silences and vast lacunæ which mark these pages I may therefore make no apology. For the sins of deliberate omission, however, I cannot so easily be comforted. The sins become more and more grievous as the work approaches present-day psychology. When one considers that the *Psychological Index* carries thousands of titles annually, one may well ask by what right a mere handful of these are mentioned. I can but mention three factors influencing my decisions. First, where a movement is represented by many titles I have preferred to quote one individual's research, making his methods and results clear, rather than to indulge in generalizations which the reader would find difficult to verify. Secondly, I have chosen as best I could in terms of the importance which attaches to each problem ; an elaborate investigation extending a known principle might well be omitted, while a brief and inadequate treatment of a significant new problem might receive attention. Thirdly, and perhaps most important of all, I have chosen in accordance with my own conception of psychology and my own personal interests. When beginning to prepare the volume I fondly dreamed of an absolutely impersonal and objective record of modern psychological history. Fairness in presenting the work and opinions of others I have hoped to attain ; but I am convinced that the tasks of selection and emphasis make a purely objective record, at least for the present author, quite impossible.

Much as I am indebted to Brett's volumes, I am even more deeply grateful for his generous aid in reading the present volume in manuscript, in rectifying errors and in giving valuable suggestions. The same generous gift of time and counsel has been given by Professors Margaret Floy Washburn, K. S. Lashley, Horace B. English, Harry L. Hollingworth, Albert T. Poffenberger, and Robert S. Woodworth. I cannot adequately express the degree of my indebtedness to each of them. To my students for whom this material was first prepared I owe constant inspiration ; especially to Shailer Lawton and George Schoonhoven. For assistance in preparing the manuscript I wish to thank Dr. Georgene Hoffman Seward, Miss H. A. Dandy, Miss Louise Sobye, and Mrs. Enrica Tunnell ; Harvey W. Culp, Donald W. Eckley, Walter A. Hall, and Sam Rubinson ; and, most of all, my wife and my mother.

G.M.

October, 1928.

B

PREFACE TO THE THIRD EDITION

THE principal changes made in the Second Edition (April, 1929) and in the present edition consist in corrections of errors and in additional references to recent work. The chapters most affected are those on " Child Psychology " and on " Psychoanalysis." Among the many regrets relating to the book's limitations, perhaps the most disturbing lies in the impossibility of doing justice, in limited space, to contemporary psychoanalysis ; the reader will find a more adequate account in R. S. Woodworth's *Contemporary Schools of Psychology* (1931).

Since the First Edition of this book, the task of the historian has been completely altered by the appearance of E. G. Boring's *History of Experimental Psychology* (1929). A host of important subjects which I have either left untouched or handled only in the most sketchy fashion are treated by Boring with vigour, clarity, and completeness. I therefore see no sound reason why I should struggle to round out my book at these points ; it is sufficient to refer the reader to Boring.

It appears that my earlier preface has not made entirely clear the reasons underlying the order of the chapters in Part III. The order is roughly chronological, each chapter being " identified " by an event (or a movement) which occurs a little after the event which marks the beginning of the preceding chapter. Thus, William James is wedged in between Ebbinghaus and Titchener for no subtle reason, but simply because 1890 is between 1885 and 1892. Each chapter, however, has to go on until it makes a whole or until it has prepared the reader for the next one. I hold no brief for this plan as against others ; I merely wish to explain a point which seems to have been obscure to many readers.

My failure to give initials of authors seems to have caused

confusion in some cases.   Initials are now added in the name index.

For helpful suggestions I am indebted to many, especially to G. S. Brett and Hulsey Cason.

I wish to thank Messrs. Kegan Paul, Trench, Trubner and Company and also Messrs. Harcourt, Brace and Company for kind compliance with a number of unseasonable requests.

G.M.

January, 1932.

An Historical Introduction to Modern Psychology

PART I

The Pre-Experimental Period

CHAPTER I

THE INTELLECTUAL BACKGROUND OF SEVENTEENTH-CENTURY
PSYCHOLOGY

" Their fine ways of explaining Nature mechanically charmed me."
—Leibnitz

FROM colour-theories to defence-mechanisms, from the functions of a white rat's vibrissæ to the mystic's sense of unutterable revelation, from imaginary playmates to partial correlations—wherein lies that unity of subject matter which leads us to speak, compactly enough, of " contemporary psychology "? From behaviourism or *Gestalt* psychology to psychoanalysis or the objective measurement of character, the eye wanders over an interminable range of experiments, measurements, hypotheses, dogmas, disconnected facts, and systematic theories. In a sense it is true to say that through all this vast mélange the very birth-cry of the infant science is still resounding. In another sense psychology is as old as occidental civilization, and all these seething multitudes of investigations and opinions spring from an inconceivably rich and variegated history. The complexity of contemporary psychology suggests that its understanding may well require the use of that *genetic* method which it has itself repeatedly demanded in recent years. Whatever difficulties there may be in finding unity in the various psychological disciplines, there is at least one unity to which we may cling for orientation and perspective, for appreciation and synthesis ; and this is the tranquil unity of history.

The centuries since Descartes and Hobbes have woven together the psychology of antiquity and the physical science of the Renaissance, the nineteenth-century triumphs of biological science and the twentieth-century genius for measurement, while a multitude of social forces, as well as strokes of individual genius, have shown unities of method and conception underlying all the problems of psychology, and indeed of life itself. For what is experimental psychology if not an embodiment of the notion of a fundamental unity between psychology and physiology, and what is behaviourism if not an attempt to make that unity more complete ; what is psychoanalysis if not an insistence on the fundamental unity of normal and abnormal, and of conscious and unconscious motives ; what is the *Gestalt* psychology if not an emphasis upon those Aristotelian " forms " which contribute the patterns both of the things of the physical world and of the data of immediate experience ?

Yet each of these movements towards unity is itself but a more complete and systematic expression of movements that have been with us at least since the seventeenth century : behaviourism, for example, a refinement of Descartes' automatism and Hobbes's mechanism ; the emphasis on the unconscious a reminiscence of Leibnitz's idea of perceptions of which we are not aware ; experimental psychology itself an application of that experimental and quantitative conception of nature which Galileo and Newton so brilliantly set forth.

And the venerable antiquity of psychology shows through the gloss of its newness, and makes the finality of each new emphasis seem, perhaps, a little less final. Not indeed that there is very great usefulness in that cheerful modern dogma which asserts that each achievement of science gives but a new name to the discovery of some Hellenic thinker. But psychology has made its recent rapid advances only because of the richness of its own history, and because of the centuries of general scientific progress which lie immediately behind us.

An historical approach to contemporary psychology necessitates at the outset a clear picture of the psychology of the early nineteenth century. But the early nineteenth century will be intelligible only if we first give brief attention to some tendencies at work several centuries earlier, and largely outside of the special field of psychology. We must attempt a brief sketch of some phases of the Renaissance, and of some psychological schools which grew out of it.

The revival of learning and the Renaissance were, of course, vastly complicated social and intellectual movements, the origin and nature of which are not, at least in our own day, to be stated in any clear and final terms. But the following facts seem to be reasonably well established. The Crusaders of the twelfth and thirteenth centuries had discovered and carried back to Europe much of the civilization of the Near East, in which many elements of classical culture had been embedded. New phases of culture showed themselves ; the new universities of the thirteenth century promoted the study of the Classics, and a great artistic revival, the Proto-Renaissance, spread over southern Europe. The true Renaissance began, roughly speaking, even as early as the fourteenth century, and reached its greatest height in the sixteenth.

It gloried in explorations of all kinds, not only physical but intellectual. But perhaps the realm of geographical discovery is as representative and enlightening as any. A beautiful epitome of the whole movement is found in the coinage of the Spanish empire, changing as a result of the explorations of Columbus. In the days before the discovery of America, some of the coins of Spain bore the words *Ne Plus Ultra*. Spain and the Pillars of Hercules were the edge of the world. Then came Columbus and the age of the explorers. The inscription was changed. *Ne* was removed ; and the words read *Plus Ultra*. There *was* " more beyond."

Everywhere men sought for the new, both in the new appreciation of the culture of antiquity, and in the search for new knowledge and new possessions, material and immaterial. Among the more obvious expressions of the movement was the search for new routes to the East, and the beginning of the building of empires to include the " New World," the colonization of which was one of the great achievements of the sixteenth and seventeenth centuries. As the Holy Roman Empire slowly decayed, France, Great Britain, and the Netherlands played their parts, each looking for lands and wealth beyond anything dreamed of in the past.   In the economic sphere an equally novel change was appearing.   During this period went on apace the " Commercial Revolution " which followed upon the growth of towns and the development of trade by land and sea, deriving from new routes to the East and from the general improvement in means of travel and communication.   The political revolution in which Cromwell was the leader and Charles I was executed, and even more definitely, the Revolution of 1688, in which the House of Orange was called to the throne, marked the emancipation of the commercial classes in Great Britain. They meant the end of the traditional " divine right of kings," and the beginning of the self-assertion of a middle class, the great trading class which grew up as these economic changes occurred.

Such tremendous unrest and activity were bound to show themselves in the intellectual world, as everywhere else ; they were apparent in the interests, spirit, and modes of thought of those who devoted themselves to art, to letters, to philosophy, and to practical affairs.   In science a revival had begun as early as the twelfth century.   The first great achievement was that of Copernicus (1543).   His doctrine that the earth and the planets moved in circles about the sun (the revival of a theory dating from the third century B.C.) was the beginning of modern astronomy.   But inductive methods were not yet understood.   Copernicus was far from being a bold investigator ; his method was almost purely deductive, having as its purpose the substitution of a simple conception for the complicated Ptolemaic system.   His views seem, moreover, to have been inspired by Greek philosophy.

After Copernicus came Tycho Brahe, who spent his life making and recording with scrupulous exactness such observations on the motions of the heavenly bodies as the best instruments of his time permitted.   He found the Copernican system unacceptable.   It did not agree with his observations, and he did not guess that the reason for the inconsistency lay in the fact that the orbit of the earth's motion about the sun is not a circle but an ellipse.   Even Tycho, the observer, believed that heavenly bodies must of necessity move in perfect curves, and to him the perfect curve was the circle.   Nevertheless, in the hands of Tycho and his immediate successors, science was beginning to take on a definitely empirical cast, the spirit of indifference to the perfection of theory, and eagerness for accurate data as the first step toward a sound hypothesis. In the work of Kepler there was a combination of the work of these two predecessors. Through close study and the most brilliant mathematical genius, he succeeded in showing that Copernicus was essentially correct, but that the figures accumulated by Tycho necessitated the assumption of elliptical rather than circular orbits. With Kepler came into being the first great fusion of inductive with mathematical method.

A similar step was being taken by Gilbert in England in the study of magnetism. For him direct observation was the basic method; he varied the conditions of observation in a way genuinely deserving the modern term "experimental." The foundation was then very speedily laid for the development of experimental science; and in many branches of physical science such investigations were soon under way. The work done by Gilbert was admired by Galileo, who in the first half of the seventeenth century extended the experimental method and went far beyond Gilbert both in the range and in the importance of his observations. Galileo and his followers concerned themselves primarily with the fundamental problems of mechanics and optics.

In all this group we can distinguish the leaders and the trumpeters, those collecting data and those blaring forth to the world what had been and what was to be done. Francis Bacon was the herald of the new empirical spirit as it fought its way among the many forces of the Renaissance. He was, in fact, given credit for the invention of the inductive method; but he was so far from originating such a method that he did not even recognize the significance of the work of Gilbert (nor the immensely important discoveries of Harvey). Nevertheless, as a systematizer and interpreter, he contributed much to the rapid spread of enthusiasm for empirical methods.

The greatest combination of mathematical with empirical method in the seventeenth century was that effected by the genius of Sir Isaac Newton. Newton's work consisted both in the development of new mathematical method and in the continuation of the work of Kepler in the elaborate logical use of empirical results. He was adept in using the empirical data of others as well as his own.   He contributed important original experiments, such as those relating to the composition of white light.   Newton contributed much also to the philosophy of science.   He gave expression to a system of thought which could be used coherently in the advancement of knowledge.   He not only made observations and employed mathematical ways of generalizing from data, but occupied himself also with the fundamental conceptions with which, as he conceived it, science must deal : mass, motion, force, etc.

We need to keep in mind these three different kinds of scientific progress in the seventeenth century : the use of mathematical method ; the desire to vary conditions, *i.e.*, to experiment ; and the interest in the philosophical significance of the new acquisitions.

A few words about the organization of science.   The only country which had organized a definite means of scientific co-operation by the second half of the seventeenth century was France ; its work was confined chiefly to the city of Paris.   The French Academy of Sciences began to receive royal support in 1671, which furthered the collaboration of investigators.   The new impetus to scientific work given by the French Crown is in striking contrast to the situation in Britain.   Newton worked practically alone.   There was indeed a Royal Society, which was intended to give better means of co-operation, but he remained far greater than his own circle ; and pitifully inadequate funds were granted by the Crown.   The same condition existed in the German States.   Germany, of course, was not a political unit, and naturally enough there was even less co-operation among its scattered men of science than in France and Great Britain, although the German university system was destined in the eighteenth century to serve as a centre for the awakening interest in scientific effort.   Galileo, in Italy, had worked alone, and under the suspicion of Church and State.   The energies of Spain and Portugal were being expended in explorations and conquests in the New World.   So, if we are inclined to ask why a given " discovery " was announced when the facts were already known to contemporary investigators, the answer is that almost until the beginning of the nineteenth century scientific progress throughout western Europe was, with few exceptions, the fruit of the efforts of individuals, frequently working without knowledge of kindred efforts in their own and other lands, and destined to be forgotten until some scientist or scholar of a later day stumbled upon their work.

This holds strikingly true in the biological sciences. The revival of classical medicine, particularly in the Italian universities, was actively proceeding in the sixteenth century. If vague notions of "humours," "vital principles," etc., persisted, they were scarcely more conspicuous than the similar conceptions of force, attraction, and the like, in physical science. The desire to describe, to understand in terms of observation, rather than by speculative and deductive methods, was just as marked in biological science as in other fields, though generalizations were more difficult. The empirical movement was active generally, and in the Netherlands it led in the seventeenth century to the inauguration of epoch-making clinical and post-mortem studies in anatomy. The reader will remember, for instance, Rembrandt's painting, the *Anatomy Lesson*, a representation of the then novel and amazing art of dissecting the human body. The same clinical spirit was manifested in the study of mental diseases ; Burton's *Anatomy of Melancholy* (1621) gave descriptions of familiar types of insanity. In 1692 appeared Sydenham's *Processus Integri*, with a description of the varieties of mental disease, the empirical spirit and accuracy of which have been very generally recognized. But the most epoch-making discovery in the field of medicine was Harvey's demonstration in 1628 of the circulation of the blood. Before the time of Harvey the prevalent doctrine was Galen's theory of red and blue blood, each type of blood being supposed to pulsate backwards and forwards. Harvey demonstrated by actual experimentation that the blue blood became red in the course of circulation. And, almost at the same time, this discovery was paralleled in the field of instrumentation by great improvement of the microscope in the hands of the Dutchman, Leeuwenhoek, opening new fields to biological science.

CHAPTER II

THE PSYCHOLOGY OF THE SEVENTEENTH AND EIGHTEENTH
CENTURIES

Heraclitus . . . says . . that it is by something in motion that
what is in motion is known ; for he, like most philosophers, conceived
all that exists to be in motion.—*Aristotle*.

THE scientific movement of the seventeenth century may
then be summarized in the statement that its spirit was
empirical, and that its appeal was to direct observation
rather than to reason or authority. Its most fruitful concepts
were mechanical, that is to say, they dealt with the movement
of bodies in space.

The development of objective observation had immediate
and definite effects on psychology. Much of the psychology
which resulted from this new spirit of inquiry was, of course,
the restatement or the reinterpretation of the psychology of
antiquity.[1] A very considerable amount of original psychological work was, however, done in the seventeenth and
eighteenth centuries. The psychology of these centuries,
though influenced by specific discoveries, especially those
pertaining to mechanics, was not so much guided by *specific*
scientific developments as by the general trend towards
empiricism, and the desire to understand man in those aspects
of his nature which are open to direct observation.

The first great name in the psychology of the Renaissance
was that of Descartes.[2] He was an international figure
whose contributions ranged from mathematics to physiology.
He was indeed one of the greatest of mathematicians, and the
discoverer of " analytical geometry," which shows the fundamental spatial relations subsisting between variables when-

[1] The scope and purpose of this volume do not permit any sort of
consideration of the psychology of the ancient nor of the mediæval
world. The reader who would grasp the psychology of the Renaissance
in its relation to the previous history of psychology should read a
comprehensive history of philosophy, and, in conjunction with it, vols.
I and II of Brett's *History of Psychology*.
[2] *The Passions of the Soul* (1650).

ever the latter are represented in two-dimensional form. He concerned himself with the rapidly developing science of physiology, and enthusiastically applauded Harvey's discovery. The study of the nervous system had begun, after a long period of inactivity, to make new strides. In fact, during the sixteenth century important discoveries concerning the topography of the brain had been made. Descartes was interested in the sensory and motor functions of nerves and in the significance of these functions for psychological theory. He was the first to attempt a detailed description of the relation of nervous functions to mental processes and behaviour.

Descartes utilized the current notion of " animal spirits," which by motion within the nerve substance bring about the movements of the body. He sought to show how such conduction within the body could account for automatic and habitual acts. But some acts required the intervention of the soul. Now, if man was a free agent, as he was asserted to be, and determined his own conduct, how could his freedom operate in a mechanical universe ? Descartes solved the problem by postulating a fundamental difference between animals and men. Animals were machines ; their bodies were controlled by physical laws. If this were true, then there must be specific mechanisms provided for these acts. Nervous and muscular reactions followed predictably from the stimulation of the sense organs ; incoming and outgoing pathways provided fixed channels for the arousal of the animal's whole repertory of acts. This conception of the *reflex* is the groundwork which psychologists of a physiological turn of mind have used ever since, on which to build up an explanation of the more complicated activities of life. Modern mechanistic psychology grew out of this seventeenth-century conception, greatly stimulated, of course, by progress in the science of mechanics in the hands of Newton and his followers.

But the explanation of human acts seemed to require a new hypothesis. Descartes divided these acts into two groups,. those of a mechanical nature and those of a rational nature. The rational acts were utterly distinct from the merely mechanical, and made possible judgment, choice, and will. This theory involved a sharp cleavage between animal and intellectual functions. Descartes retained the soul as an entity outside the spatial order ("unextended"). The lucidity of his treatment helped to make clear the opposition between strict dualists who accepted his distinction, and monists, like Spinoza,[1] who stated that soul and body are ultimately one.

Descartes himself recognized serious difficulties in this position. If mind and matter were totally different things, how could there be a working relation between the two ? How could the body act upon the soul, and *vice versa* ? This question caused much trouble. Descartes had to look about for the point of interaction, the " seat of the soul." Some of the ancients had placed the soul in one place, some in another. But medical studies had begun to point clearly to the import- ance of the brain. The trouble with the brain for Descartes' purposes was that it is " paired," right and left, and divided more finely into smaller structures which are arranged symmetrically on either side. But the pineal gland, the functions of which were unknown, is deeply embedded in the centre of the brain. There is only one pineal gland ; and it necessarily follows, thought Descartes, that it is the seat of the soul. This gland acted to transmit physical stimuli to the soul, and to transmit impulses from the soul to the body. The soul's control of the body was through simple mechanical regulation of the connections between sensory and motor impulses in the nerves ; the connection between the different sensory and motor nerves was directly affected by the move- ments of the pineal gland. " This gland is variously affected by the soul. . . . it impels the spirits which surround it toward the pores of the brain, which discharge them by means of the nerves upon the muscles."[2] This assumption reduced the problem of the action of the soul directly to the move- ments of the pineal gland, but no theory was vouchsafed as to the way in which an immaterial entity could exercise such mechanical effects. This dualism, or fundamental distinc- tion between soul and body, so emphatically outlined by Descartes, has been the centre of many psychological systems ever since. There had been dualism before, notably among the Church fathers, but the acuteness of the difficulty was not apparent until Descartes' bold selection of the organ through which interaction was effected.

[1] *Ethics* (1677).
[2] *Op. cit.*, Part I, Article XXXIV.

One other feature of Descartes' work, significant for later psychology, is the analysis of the emotions. The " passions " are treated almost like mechanical events ; they are explained through motion in the brain, the blood, the " spirits," and the vital organs. Descartes' account of the " passions of the soul " reduces the complexity of emotional life to six elementary passions : wonder, love, hate, desire, joy, sadness. The process of dissecting human nature into elemental emotional experiences or impulses, which in their combination give all possible modes of emotion, is so fascinating that it has never ceased to occupy psychologists.[1]

But the emotions listed by Descartes were described as though they were intellectual functions. Love, he believed, depends upon one's calculation of the pleasure an object may bring, and hate depends upon expected evil. The non-rational was translated into terms of the rational. The nine-teenth-century " economic man," who avoided pain and sought pleasure, grew slowly and inevitably from this type of rationalism.

Shortly after Descartes worked out this application of physics and its methods to psychology, a somewhat similar approach was made by another mathematical genius, Leibnitz.[2] He sought, as had Descartes, an answer to the problem of the relation of mind to body. Leibnitz held that it was impossible to accept the doctrine of an immaterial soul acting upon a material body. For real interaction either the soul must be material, or the body must be spiritual, or the two identical, made of the same substance. It is true that Spinoza had seen the difficulty and had chosen the third of these alternatives, making body and mind merely two *ways* in which the same reality is known ; but despite his position in philosophy, he had strangely little influence upon psychologists.

The relation of mind and body was stated by Leibnitz in terms nearly as dualistic as those of Descartes, but dispensing altogether with the troublesome concept of interaction.

[1] Among the better known attempts are those of Hobbes, Cabanis, Gall, Lotze, James, McDougall, and Watson.
[2] *A New System of Nature* (1695).

There is, Leibnitz taught, a body which follows its own laws ; that is, the laws of mechanics. The acts of a human body are just as mechanical as those of an animal. Leibnitz insisted that we must explain *all* acts of the human body in terms of known physical causes. Mental acts and sequences must on the other hand be explained in terms of mental causes. The soul carries on its acts without any direct reaction upon the body. Mental life displays an orderly sequence of events, while bodily life does the same, but these two never interact. His famous analogy was that of two clocks[1] so constructed that they always agreed perfectly, without either one acting upon the other. Thus if we know what time it is by one clock, we know what time it is by the other. Mind and body *seem* to interact simply because of a " pre-established harmony " between them. We can understand mental changes only by understanding the preceding mental changes, and we can understand physical changes only by understanding the preceding physical changes ; there is no causal connection between mental and physical. This doctrine made irrelevant the whole conception of interaction between mind and body, and sought to do away with all those apparent contradictions involved in asking how a mental event occurs in consequence of a physical event. We have in Leibnitz's system a " parallelism " of mind and body to which many shades of contemporary parallelism bear close resemblance. Through Descartes' interactionism, Spinoza's monism, and Leibnitz's parallelism, the seventeenth century outlined three of the major psychophysical theories which dominated eighteenth and nineteenth-century thought.

Mental events were themselves classified and graded according to their degree of clearness, ranging from the most definitely conscious to those which were most vague and obscure. This led to a further distinction which remained prominent in German psychology, a distinction which is now current in treatments of attention. We might, Leibnitz held, be quite unconscious of our obscure perceptions. There may be perceptions of which we are not aware, while others are clearly grasped or apperceived.[2] *Perception* is an

---

[1] *Second Explanation of the System of the Communication between Substances* (1696).
[2] Aristotle had distinguished between " having " and " observing " an experience.

internal condition "representing external things," and *apperception* is "*consciousness* or the reflective knowledge of this internal state."[1]

Continental psychological work in the latter half of the seventeenth century was dominated chiefly by the school of Descartes. With the exception of Leibnitz there was no figure on the continent comparable in magnitude to Descartes; in fact, it was he himself rather than his followers who inspired, nearly one hundred and fifty years later, the use of the theory of reflex action in the brilliant work of the French physiological psychologists.

But significant as were the psychological systems of these two men, probably the most important stream of tradition for us to consider in order to understand the psychology of the eighteenth and early nineteenth centuries is the English "empiricism" of Hobbes and his successors.

The starting point for Hobbes, even more obviously than for the other thinkers we have considered, was the social and intellectual environment in which he lived. He was, in particular, engaged in the study of the great political upheaval going on about him, that surging forward of the commercial classes which weakened the grip of the nobility upon its exclusive power and prerogatives. Charles I was executed in 1649; and Hobbes published his *Leviathan* in 1651. It was, in a sense, an "heroic" age, characterized by charges of cavalry, the leader sleeping in his armour, the lyrics of Lovelace, and the echo of wars across the channel. But Hobbes bitterly hated both the commercial and the political revolution; for he was a royalist, and his conception of life aristocratic. The organization of society was for him based upon the authority of some individuals over others. The "natural" state of man (without organized society) would be "solitary, poor, nasty, brutish, and short."[2]

Nevertheless, he was an observer who in spite of his prejudices was singularly detached; and this in a hyper-political age in which every thinking Englishman was startled

---

[1] *The Principles of Nature and of Grace* (1714), 4. Perception is a condition of a *monad*, a psychic individuality or soul. Monads are irreducible psychic entities.

[2] *Leviathan*, Part I, Chapter 13.

C

to witness the disruption of the time-honoured order.[1]
Though he was in a sense a part of this upheaval, he was still
a spectator rather than a participant.[2] He observed in a
spirit in which few before him had observed ; even Machiavelli and Sir Thomas More, his great predecessors in political
theory during the Renaissance, had had a case to prove and
a practical goal to win. He sought to understand the
revolution and the human nature which lies behind both
war and peace. He was the first " social psychologist "
among the moderns, and the principles which he laid down
were epoch-making both for social and for individual psychology.

Hobbes drew the distinction between original nature and
the products of experience.[3] Some human acts he attributed
to innate constitution ; but most specific activities he
regarded as acquired. Hobbes started out to catalogue the
inherited tendencies, but he quickly lost interest. Hunger,
thirst, and sex impulses were but mentioned and passed over
in a moment, being such obvious things that their psychology
did not interest him. But in relation to social life, he gives
a much fuller exposition of the principles of motivation, an
exposition based chiefly on Aristotle's *Rhetoric*.[4] These he
described not as purely impulsive forces, but as strivings based
on expectation of pleasure and pain.[5] First and foremost
came fear, fear conceived not as a blind impulse but as
perception of pain inherent in an object, causing withdrawal
from it. Fear is dependent upon calculation of evil results.
The desire for honour is another dominant motive ; it is
based on the recognition of pleasure which must accrue from
standing well with one's fellows. Now these elements of
human nature (hunger, thirst, sex tendencies, fear, desire for
honour, and, through all, the search for pleasure and the
avoidance of pain) are the mainsprings of social conduct,
and the basis for social organization. Each individual in

---

[1] Milton, for example, attached greater importance to his political
writings than to his poetry ; it was his great regret that he was snatched
away from politics by his blindness. The political intensity and bitter-
ness of the age reverberates even in Gray's stately rhythms three generations later.

[2] He took refuge in France during some of the stormiest years.

[3] *Op. cit.*, Part I, Chapter 6.

[4] *I.e.*, the list of motives which the orator must sway.

[5] This simple hedonism was not particularly original. Many of the
ancients assumed it ; its elements were present also in More's *Utopia*.

human society was conceived by Hobbes to have proclivities which he wished to satisfy, and pains which he wished to avoid. Without society, each individual, alone, would directly seek pleasure and avoid pain. He would be obliged to engage in warfare with his neighbours in order to take from them the things he wished for himself, and to ward off the attacks which they in turn levied upon him. Man is competitive, and if alone in his self-defence is necessarily miserable through the constant seizure of his possessions or the ceaseless task of self-defence. The only hope for men lies in the organization of commonwealths in which each man agrees to forego the pleasures of robbery in order to avoid attack from others.[1] In social groups each one is prevented by the community from carrying out any attack on his neighbour. A rational social organization prevents the selfishness of original nature from making for general chaos— a conception of statecraft which borrowed freely from Machiavelli. Hobbes, like Machiavelli, insisted that the mainsprings of human conduct were self-interested, and that the most important was fear. Moralists had pointed out the essential baseness of humanity, and Augustine's and Calvin's emphasis on man's sinfulness was an expression rather than a cause of the age-long grudge which Western thought has cherished against man's moral nature. And this conception has been acceptable to penologists and to practical statesmen for centuries. Fear is the central note of deterrent punishment, as of international politics and diplomacy.

Another mechanism of social control lay in the establishment of a nobility and of other special groups to whom honour was given in greater or less degree. Hobbes believed that gratification derived from high station, as well as from approval of one's acts, was a necessary part of the social order. But royalty is a very special form of noble rank, for the sovereign personalizes or represents society as a whole. The revolt against the sovereign is a contradiction in terms. The sovereign is the representative of all ; by receiving supreme power he protects society against marauders. The king therefore rules, not only by " divine right," but by the collective values which he holds within himself as represent-

[1] A similar conception of the Commonwealth was traced (by Glaucon) in Plato's *Republic*.

ative of the Commonwealth. Hobbes believed the over-throw of the sovereign to be vicious as well as ultimately futile. Subsequent events, especially the expulsion of the Stuarts, were not such as his scheme of society demanded, and the fact tended in some measure to discredit his theory of the State.

But there was here a system of ideas of immense import-ance, ideas rooted in the thought of antiquity and now revived in opposition to the doctrines of the Middle Ages. There was first the idea that human acts result from an objectively knowable human nature ; that man is made in such a way that analysis may make possible prediction and control. Society can so organize itself as to control individ-uals and create for itself a complex but reasonably stable system of social relations. We shall see later how the "political economists," especially Bentham, continued another branch of Hobbes's thought, namely, "psychological hedonism," the doctrine that self-interest is the basis of conduct.

This description of social life, however, was supplemented by a keen analysis of certain principles of general psychology, as well as by a systematic philosophical inquiry. Philosophi-cally, Hobbes was captivated by the desire to reduce everything to *motion*. He was delighted by Galileo's mechan-ical experiments, and believed that through such methods the ultimate nature of "things natural" was to be discerned. This systematic (and dogmatic) emphasis on motion, even where motion could not be demonstrated, perhaps justifies the question whether Hobbes really was as purely "empir-ical" as is alleged. "He attempted a task which no other adherent of the new 'mechanical philosophy' conceived—nothing less than such a universal construction of human knowledge as would bring Society and Man ... within the same principles of scientific explanation as were found applicable to the world of Nature."[1] With the mechanical viewpoint, the notion of bodies as bits of matter moving in space and time, Hobbes built up the scheme of human nature as a purely mechanical thing, avoiding altogether the inter-actionism of Descartes. It is no exaggeration to say that Hobbes took the whole fabric of the seventeenth-century

[1] C. Robertson in *Encyc. Brit.*, 11th ed., XIII, p. 552.

physical view of the world and fashioned from it a conception of human nature. Every thought, feeling, and purpose was simply internal *motion*.

His psychology is nevertheless in large part an empirical psychology. He uses the principle of motion chiefly in relation to motion as supposed to occur in the *brain*, an assumption which was supported by some evidence ; and whatever may be thought of his metaphysics, his psychological observations have both a matter-of-fact empirical spirit and a richness of content very far indeed from the formalism which had characterized most psychological systems. His psychology is in large part Aristotelian. Aristotle gave him a " naturalism " which he could set in opposition to the " supernaturalism " of the Scholastics. But, though Aristotle taught him where to look, much of his material evidently came from his own keen analysis. His work as a psychologist centres in close observation of his own mental processes, with the request that the reader " consider, if he also find not the same in himself."[1]

All experience, Hobbes held, was some special form of motion. He made, for example, no distinction between the *will* to do a thing and the doing it.[2] Appetites and fears were internal motions which led to action, and will was simply the last appetite or the last fear which in the course of deliberation precipitated overt movement.[3] The difference between act and impulse was merely a difference in the locus and extent of movement. Similarly, sensation was continuation of that motion which had impinged upon the sense-organs, transmitting its motion through the nerves to the brain. Descartes had taught that in higher mental functions the soul, by means of the pineal gland, controlled the passage of an impulse from one nerve to another ; but Hobbes did not require the intervention of the soul. Motion in the brain was sufficient. The motion occurring within the brain substance constituted the basis for all qualities of sensation. He proceeded to attack the popular conception that the qualities

---

[1] *Op. cit.*, Introduction.

[2] A protest against a Scholastic teaching that the internal motion was merely metaphorical.

[3] *Humane Nature* (1651), XII, 2.

of experience are *inherent in* the objects we perceive.[1]
" There is nothing *without us* (really) which we call an *image*
or colour . . . the said image or colour is but an *apparition*
unto us of the *motion*, agitation, or alteration, which the
object worketh in the *brain*, or spirits, or some internal substance of the head."[2] Moreover, after the external object
has ceased to act upon the sense-organ, the motion in the
brain may continue. Such residual or " decaying " sensation constitutes the material of memory and imagination.[3]

There remains, however, the problem as to the *order of
events*, the " trains " of imagination and thought. All
thought follows the same sequence as the experiences caused
by the world about us. " Those motions that immediately
succeeded one another in the sense, continue also together
after sense : insomuch as the former coming again to take
place, and be predominant, the latter followeth."[4] This
simple and epoch-making doctrine is basic for the associationist teaching which flourished for two centuries thereafter.

But we cannot predict from a given thought which one of a
variety of other thoughts may follow. A thought may have
been followed, in different situations, by a variety of different
thoughts. There may be many competitors, each one of
which has a definite claim upon the next position in a mental
series. A passage in his *Humane Nature* may perhaps mean
that he believed the factor of primacy to be of paramount
importance. " The *cause* of the *coherence* or consequence of
one conception to another, is their first *coherence* or consequence at that *time* when they are produced by sense : as for
example, from St. Andrew the mind runneth to St. Peter,
because their names are read together ; from St. Peter to a
stone, for the same cause."[5] But in the *Leviathan* we read :

---

[1] The astronomer Kepler had clearly distinguished a half-century
earlier between such objective reality as motion, and such subjective
phenomena as colour. For the history of these concepts from Kepler
to Berkeley, see Burtt, *Metaphysical Foundations of Modern Physical
Science* (1925).

[2] *Ibid.*, II, 4. Hobbes constantly emphasizes the brain, as had some
of the Greeks ; but he is a good enough Aristotelian to emphasize motion
from the brain to the heart, and to give the latter a position of importance in mental life.

[3] Again an Aristotelian doctrine.

[4] *Leviathan*, Part I, Chapter 3.

[5] *Humane Nature*, IV, 2.

" In the imagining of anything, there is no certainty what we shall imagine next ; only this is certain, it shall be something that succeeded the same before, at one time or another."[1] He failed to work out his position. Neither he nor his immediate successors realized the possibility of attaining a more adequate statement of the varieties of association. It was not, in fact, until the work of Thomas Brown, in the beginning of the nineteenth century, that this problem was fairly faced, reducing the problem of mental sequence to a large number of specific laws of association, taking into account the *competition* among experiences.

But Hobbes did take account of the vital distinction between such free or uncontrolled association, on the one hand, and directed or purposive thinking, on the other hand. " Mental discourse is of two sorts. The first is *unguided*, *without design* and inconstant . . . The second is more constant ; as being *regulated* by some desire, and design."[2] He devoted much attention to the " regulated " type, taking account of the " desire " which guides the process, and of the tendency to seek causes for consequences and *vice versa*. He proceeds to give illustrations of the familiar (Platonic and Aristotelian) principles of association by contiguity and similarity. Association by similarity had, curiously enough, been omitted in the discussion of unregulated thought.

Hobbes had, then, outlined an empirical psychology in which sensation was emphasized as the source of our ideas, and had given a rough sketch of association which served to explain the interconnections between the elements of experience.

The first great follower of Hobbes had an immense advantage over him as an intellectual leader. Locke[3] was one to attract not only the attention but the allegiance of the intellectuals of his age. He was gentle and delightful in his exposition, clear and easy to read. Whereas Hobbes had wanted to fight, to argue, and to make fun, Locke was winsome and approachable.

Locke devoted himself primarily to the study of perception

[1] *Leviathan*, Part I, Chapter 3.
[2] *Ibid.*, Part I, Chapter 3.
[3] *An Essay Concerning Human Understanding* (1690).

and of thought. Ideas, he held, come from experience.[1] Observation "supplies our understanding with all the materials of thinking." But ideas have two sources. They come either from sensation or from reflection. Our minds are equipped not only with ideas directly derived from such sensory qualities as colour, temperature, and taste, but also from a variety of mental processes such as perception, thinking, reasoning, and willing. Our observation of our own mental operations gives rise to ideas which are not in themselves sensory.

Locke agreed with Hobbes that "simple ideas of sensation" are the properties of experience, and not of the objects outside us which excite these ideas in us. He proceeded, however, to distinguish between "primary" and "secondary" qualities.[2] Primary qualities, such as size and motion, produce in us ideas resembling the physical stimuli which excite them. On the other hand, secondary qualities are those aspects of external objects which produce in us ideas unlike anything really existing in the external world, e.g., such ideas as colour and taste. He supposed that some aspects of experience are genuine duplicates of patterns existing in external bodies, while others bear, in fact, no such resemblance to external bodies.

Ideas, however, may be either simple or complex. The mind creates complex ideas by combining simple ideas. Many of our ideas, designated by single words, can in fact be analysed in such a way as to show clearly that they are but combinations of simple sensory constituents. "Thus, if to substance be joined the simple idea of a certain dull, whitish colour, with certain degrees of weight, hardness, ductility, and fusibility, we have the idea of lead."[3] The principle was, as we shall see, far-leading. "Even the *most abstruse* ideas, how remote soever they may seem from sense, or from any operation of our own minds, are yet only such as the understanding frames to itself, by repeating and joining together ideas that it had either from objects of sense, or from its own operations about them."[4]

---

[1] The mind before all experience is "white paper." The Latin *tabula rasa* (wax tablet, smooth and ready for writing) is a familiar epitome of Locke's conception of a mind upon which experience has as yet written nothing.
[2] See footnote 1, p. 18.
[3] *Op. cit.*, Book II, Chapter XII, 6.
[4] *Op. cit.*, Book II, Chapter XII, 8.

Two things were needed to make a systematic psychology out of these principles. One was to lay stress upon and give content to the notions of " repeating " and " joining," which constituted the basis for integration of simple into complex experiences. The other necessary step was to postulate a physical basis for mental interconnections. Both steps were soon to be taken. In spite of Locke's study of perception, judgment, and other intellectual functions, perhaps his chief permanent contribution lay in making explicit the possibilities of an association psychology which should start with the data of experience and work out the laws governing the interconnections and sequences among experiences. The germ of associationism had, of course, been apparent in the work of Hobbes, which in turn went back to Aristotle. But Locke's lucid exposition of the implications of empiricism, and of the possibility, through analysis, of clearly understanding the origin and organization of ideas, gave empiricism an appealing quality which greatly contributed to its strength and influence.

Locke's distinction between primary and secondary qualities was systematically demolished by Berkeley.[1] He showed with an indomitable logic that there are no qualities in experience except those qualities which Locke had already described as subjective ; in other words, that there are no " primary " qualities. Berkeley asserted that these qualities are, as a matter of fact, not properties belonging to some external object, having mathematical character (location, size, shape, mass, and movement). We never know anything but experience ; the whole objective world is a pure hypothesis supported by no evidence whatever. In analysing our experience we notice that we have such qualities in ourselves as the colour of a rose, the prick of a pin, and so on. And when we talk of external *objects* we do not know what they are ; objects external to experience are nothing at all. He laid the corner-stone of that great edifice in modern philosophy, " subjective idealism," which portrays a world of experience-qualities, and denies, throughout, the existence of any other world whatever. This was the logical end of the train of thought which began with Hobbes's

[1] *A Treatise Concerning the Principles of Human Knowledge* (1710.)

teaching that experience is made up of sensory qualities alone.

But Berkeley was forced to find some kind of unity in mental life, something that should hold these mental states together. There is no intrinsic reason why pain should follow the thrusting of the hand into fire, or why the odour of a rose should accompany the visual and tactual experience of the rose. Why do two persons see the same object or sequence of events? And what is it that holds together one collection of experiences in a group designated " the mind," distinct from another group called " the mind of another " ? Why do not ideas from two separate minds become confused, if in fact there is no body which gives personal identity ? It is clear that breaking up the universe into bits of experience does not give personality. The soul must be assumed to exist. It is the invisible, unobservable, but logically necessary background of our experience. There must be a soul if there is to be experience. Furthermore, there must be an active cause for the succession of experiences, and this cause is to be found in God Himself.

Berkeley made a very important contribution to the theory of visual space perception.[1] He furthered the trend towards associationism. He got rid of the simple, atomistic mechanism of Hobbes, but he showed nevertheless how the principle of association must be used to explain some of the most complicated facts of perception. Locke had recognized that in the compounding of ideas elements might be drawn from two or more sense modalities. Berkeley went further with this analysis of the origin of compound ideas ; and theories of perception in general, and space perception in particular, were profoundly affected by his discussion.

In the consideration of visual experience, he knew that the retina is spread out as a surface. It happens to be curved, but as a surface it has an " up " and " down," and a " right " and " left." How can we by this surface perceive a third dimension ? Berkeley answered in terms of tactual experience. Through reaching and touching, the whole notion of distance is associated gradually with the elements given by the retina. The perception of the third dimension is not a unitary function. Touch qualities are not directly perceived when we analyse our visual perception of three dimensions ;

[1] *An Essay Towards a New Theory of Vision* (1709).

but somehow or other, when visual impressions are combined with tactual memories derived from reaching for objects, we find a three-dimensional quality in our objects. The retina " gives " us three instead of two dimensions. Since Berkeley used the notion of compounding sensory qualities, he became, unwittingly, one of the founders of association psychology. Although his fundamental motive was quite foreign to the mechanistic leanings of associationism, he contributed to it in spite of himself.

Now appeared one who questioned the premises and conclusions, the beginning and end of all these views which had been propounded with a confidence characteristic of the leaders of the Renaissance. The central psychological contribution of Hume[1] was the analysis of the stream of thought into one endlessly changing kaleidoscopic series of experiences. For Berkeley there had been the necessity of a soul to bring all these experiences together, to make a coherent sequence ; we must have some unity to tie together yesterday's experience with to-day's experience. Berkeley had separated the soul from its experiences. Hume declared that he had patiently examined his consciousness without succeeding in finding evidence for the soul. What one calls the " self " turns out to be a group of sensations from the body. For the description of personality all that was necessary was a series of experiences. The soul might be dispensed with. Each experience was sufficiently related to what followed.

Hume took the position toward which Hobbes had groped, that psychology deals with experience as it comes to us, and not with any logical postulate of the observer as a separate entity. Hobbes had not been able to see the real issue, because there had not been a Berkeley before him to make this sharp distinction between self and experience. Hume could do it because there *had* been a Berkeley. Hume, denying the validity of Berkeley's assumption of the soul, and of God as an active cause of experience, offered a psychology which was nothing but the study of a series of experiences combining and recombining, following one another in an endless chain. Here arose one of the central

[1] *A Treatise of Human Nature* (1739–40).

problems which association psychology had to face hence-
forward : what made these different bits hang together and
what made them follow in certain sequences ?   This was long
before the day of a detailed physiological psychology ; the
idea that there was an organism that holds things together
could scarcely be worked out.   The association psychology,
until its demise in the middle of the nineteenth century, made
a desperate effort to give continuity and unity to the various
experiences with which it dealt, by means of the continuity
of the physiological substrate.[1]

By the middle of the eighteenth century associationism
had begun to be the central point around which psychological
problems revolved.   But associationism as a psychological
system is usually traced to Hartley.[2]   He differed from his
predecessors not so much in his enunciated principles as in
the clearness with which he grasped the need of a thorough-
going physiological basis for association.   He undertook to
define the physical facts upon which memory images and their
sequences depend.   Greatly interested in Newton's study
of the pendulum, he held that if certain experiences follow
in a given order it means that nerve fibres must *vibrate* in a
given order.   When a stimulus arouses a sense-organ, and a
moment later a second stimulus arouses a second sense-organ,
the vibrations in the brain caused by the first are followed by
vibrations caused by the second.   The parts of the brain are
so connected that if now the first stimulus is again presented
and arouses the first brain region, the arousal of the second
region follows, with no need for the presentation of the second
stimulus.   A series of sensations *A, B, C, D*, forms such a
pattern in the brain that later the arousal of *A* will set going
b, c, d—that is to say, *memory images* of *B, C, D*.   These
images are produced by the vibration on a *small* scale of
nervous tissue previously stimulated more actively.

He realized that there was a resemblance between motor
habits—a series of acts in which, step by step, each act leads
to the next—and purely mental activities like memory,

---

[1] As is done by many schools of psychology to-day.
[2] *Observations on Man, his Frame, his Duty, and his Expectations*
(1749).   The preface to the work makes it clear that the core of his
system of thought was suggested by a " Rev. Mr. Gay," whose views
on association were stated nearly twenty years earlier.

where a series of experiences follows in a certain order because of past experience in a certain order. There was, moreover, a distinction between sensation and image only in so far as differences in *intensity* of nerve function were concerned ; the image had its seat in the *same region* which served as basis for the sensation.[1] He had therefore by physiological principles brought the whole realm of thought and of imagination into the same physiological terms as the perception of external objects, and had offered a clear theory to explain why ideas occurred in particular sequences.

Hartley accepted Locke's conception of compound ideas. A group of revived sensations might cohere so as to form a mental product. But this mental product was to be conceived as parallel to a physical product, a group of nerve-excitations. He delighted in reducing complex experiences to the elementary sensations which by association constituted them. Now Aristotle had laid down certain fundamental laws of association—those of contiguity, similarity, and contrast. Hartley reduced all these types of association to one simple physiological principle. First, as regards contiguity (in time or space). He reduced all *successive* association to sequence of one physical change upon another. Nor was any difficulty presented by the association of *simultaneous* events, because, if stimuli are presented together, there is simultaneous response in the brain. The nervous system furnishes, Hartley said, sufficient explanation of either type of association through contiguity in time. But things which are together *in space* are also frequently *observed* together, so that their perception involves contiguity *in time*. Contiguity either in space or time is another way of saying contiguity in experience, which is in turn stated in neurological terms.

Further, Hartley showed great originality in the treatment of association by similarity. He assumed that an idea (a complex experience or cluster of elements) may lead to another idea by virtue of a common element, an element which is a part of both experiences and therefore contiguous to the elements of each. Certain elements in any total situation are a little more active than others ; and of these bits, which we may designate A, B, C, D, one element, D, may have occurred together with E F G. To pass from one

---

[1] A refinement of Hobbes's statement as to the relation of image to sensation.

complex idea A B C D to another one similar to it, it is necessary only that D should have occurred sometimes in the context A B C D and sometimes in the context D E F G. This classical explanation of association by similarity is still to be found in current textbooks.

And association by contrast may be handled in the same way. Terms are not contrasted because they are really totally unlike ; contrasts have a great deal in common. " Good " and " bad " would never be contrasted were they not both terms of valuation having in common a constellation of similar ideas of value. We contrast things only when the elementary ideas which compose them are to a large extent identical. Thus Hartley reduced the Aristotelian laws to the one law of contiguity in experience.

For Hartley, as for Locke, the child begins life without associations. But rejecting the notion of ideas derived from reflection, Hartley held that the child has simply the capacity for *sensory* experience. In the course of time, sensory experience, by making endless connections and establishing trains of association, building up complex objects of thought, becomes more and more intricate ; and finally systems of thought, such as philosophy, religion, and morals, arise. Hartley had almost arrived at a complete psychical atomism. He and his followers had as their goal such a thorough understanding of association as would enable them to take a number of psychical elements and show how their combination in various ways, acting according to a few simple laws, could produce all known experiences. This fascinating game is one which had not yet been played with vigour and thoroughness.

There were many associationists in the half-century following Hartley's writings, but they added little of importance. Perhaps the chief contribution was Tucker's[1] elaboration of the notion of compound ideas. He emphasized cases in which the compounding of sensory elements produces a new synthesis wherein the sensory components can no longer be *separately* observed ; such compounds differ from those in which the elements are still introspectively observable.[2]

---

[1] *The Light of Nature Pursued* (1765–1774).
[2] The former are to-day sometimes called " blends," the latter " patterns." Hartley had himself noted the distinction, commenting on the fact that the flavour of a medicine is not the simple *sum* of the separate elements, but a fusion.

Though associationism continued to thrive in England, there was another direction open to post-Hartleyan thought. The whole tendency to simplify and mechanize mental processes led to a revolt, a revolt arising chiefly from religious and ethical sources. The reaction against Hobbes's mechanism, and, in particular, against Hume's indifference to the claims of the soul, was evident in the Scottish universities, where empiricism had made less headway than in England, and where intellectual circles were ready to support the claims of established religion against impending infidelity. The mind had been reduced, not only by Hobbes, to motion, but by Hume to a mere series of elements, and by Hartley to nerve-vibrations causing particular bits of experience to be fitted together in various ways—destroying not only the soul but the possibility of the soul.[1] This might be all very well as speculation, but it had moral implications. Religion and the State, which had been closely allied throughout the known history of western Europe, were alike threatened ; popular education (through the parochial schools) was taken in real earnest in Scotland as in few places in the world, and public opinion could not brook an attack upon the core of its ethical and religious structure. There was sure to be a reaction. Ever since the time of Knox and Presbyterianism there had been a cleavage between England and Scotland on religious grounds. Religious freedom was tolerated in some circles in England ; respectability did not necessarily involve orthodoxy in religious thought. But Scotch Presbyterianism of the mid-eighteenth century definitely and consciously undertook to create a philosophy that would combat a degrading mechanism. Universities looked about to find suitable champions.

The Scottish school began with Thomas Reid.[2] He undertook to show, in the first place, that the skepticism of Hume was absurd, that we know perfectly well that we have minds, the capacity to perceive real things, to think and to know. How could we be certain of all these things ? Reid appealed to the practical reliability of our senses, and

---

[1] Though Hartley was not himself a mechanist, but a parallelist, he was easily misinterpreted.

[2] *Essays on the Intellectual Powers of Man* (1785).

to common observation.[1] Do we not, for example, observe ourselves reasoning—that is, exercising a capacity which to the skeptics and associationists has become a useless term ? Can we not think mathematically and logically ? Have we not intellectual powers which actually work in solving all sorts of problems, making it possible to understand the external world, and to predict what will happen ? Does this not mean that the human mind is endowed by nature with the capacity to know the universe ? And how can we by a mechanistic philosophy explain the aspirations of humanity ? Not only the rational but the moral nature of man is unexplained by associationism. Moreover, no amount of pleasure or pain will give a child *concepts*. These come from powers of insight and analysis, which are inborn. The child is endowed likewise with the ability to classify things as good and evil. Do we not know, moreover, that we are free to choose between right and wrong ? Does not our moral nature defy the fundamental mechanism of associationism ? In all this Reid was not only trying to undermine the basis of association psychology, but to build up another system ; he appealed to common observation as against the subtlety—the sophistry, he maintained—of the empiricists.

This teaching was characteristic enough of the trend of the period. Such a revolution against prevalent philosophic thought would probably have taken in the thirteenth century, or in the sixteenth century, the form of an appeal to logical principles. Demonstration of the soul had then been effected by means of certain steps in deductive reasoning. But in the eighteenth century empiricism had taken such hold that rationalism was no longer trusted ; even the enemies of the empirical movement resorted to experience rather than to deductive logic as their defence. Reid says in substance : " there are the facts on which *you* rely, but look at *my* facts ; they are more conclusive than your facts." One of the last up-flarings of the dying embers had been Berkeley's demonstration of the existence of the soul. We shall not find any

---

[1] The Scottish school was called the school of " common sense," but the term is confusing. Aristotle had assumed a " common " sense through which the reports of the senses are apprehended. Dugald Stewart pointed out the confusion between the Aristotelian usage and the use of the term in the sense of " mother-wit." (See Hammond, *Aristotle's Psychology*, Introduction, li.)

thorough-going return to rationalistic principles in British thought.

Because of its insistence upon the unity and coherence of mental life, and because it pictured the individual as an active entity, not as a mere field in which capering ideas assembled and reassembled, the greatest contributions of the Scottish school were necessarily general, rather than specific.[1] It contributed but little to the solution of specific problems until the school became blended to some extent with the associationist movement. But Reid and his direct followers had great influence, not only in Scotland but later in England, France, and the United States, because they appeared to save the individual and society from intellectual and moral chaos. Something, also, was due indirectly to the intellectual activity apparent in Scotland at the beginning of the nineteenth century. Many business men (members of a class which had not heretofore thought such a process necessary) began to educate themselves. The Scottish school became genuinely popular.

There was another tendency at work which in part grafted itself upon the Scottish school, but also continued a separate existence in Germany, the " faculty psychology." This was never " founded " at any particular period ; we find it implicit or explicit in the psychology of some of the ancients and some of the Scholastics. As the soul carried out the activities, for example, of memory, reason, and will, it made use successively of the different faculties. It is ordinarily stated that the founder of modern faculty psychology was Wolff, whose *Rational Psychology* appeared in 1734. The central doctrine is simple and intelligible. There are definite and distinct faculties or capacities of the soul ; the soul enters for the time being into each activity, just as the whole body may at different times take part in widely different acts. But the soul remains a unity, never a mere sum of constituent parts. German thought remained for more than a century steadfast to this general principle.[2] For

---

[1] Reid did include the empirical findings of Newton and others on the senses.

[2] The profoundly significant teachings of Leibnitz concerning the mind-body relation and apperception bore but little fruit until they were transformed by the transcendentalists and the Herbartians. Kant gave new life to the doctrine of the faculties at the same time that he elaborated his own theory of apperception.

D

this school a *faculty* was the *capacity* of the soul to carry out a certain activity. This gives us a double enumeration of all mental processes ; there is not only the specific process of remembering, but the power of remembering. The distinction is convenient. But as a system, faculty psychology merely gives names to certain functions ; it cannot analyse these functions. Naturally, the Scottish school and the faculty psychology had something in common. Starting with the soul and the various ways in which it can act, the Scottish psychologists catalogued its capacities much as the Scholastics and the German school had done. If we say we have the power to reason, we use a term from faculty psychology.

Associationists denied the value of this approach. The individual's mind, they repeated, was blank at birth, and only by experience learned certain ways of functioning ; it had no innate capacities to do things. The associationists, therefore, and the faculty psychologists stood at opposite poles, with the Scottish school in general agreement with the faculty psychology.

We must next deal with some of the dominant tendencies in French psychology during the period just preceding and during the French Revolution, and the relation of these tendencies to British psychological and philosophical thought.

In the work of Condillac there arose a structure far more beautiful in its rigorous simplicity than anything of which Hartley dreamed. Condillac[1] held that no formulation of the principles of association, as entities added to our primitive sensory experience, is necessary. He asked his readers to imagine a *statue*, and to imagine what would follow if it were given sensation, and nothing more than sensation. The sum total of all possible human experiences, he held, would follow. We need presuppose no laws of thought. There was in his system such a dependence upon sensory factors that we are led to suppose that mere variations in the quality of sensation are capable of producing those judgments and comparisons which Locke thought required an inner sense. The fact of passing through experiences, one after another,

---

[1] *Treatise on Sensations* (1754).

is sufficient explanation of how judgments and comparisons arise. Operations and functions are not added to the elements ; the elements carry out their own functions. The mind is an assemblage of parts, and these parts, being what they are, give us, by definition, mental functions of all describable varieties. A point implicit rather than explicit in Condillac's system is the assumption that pleasantness and unpleasantness are inherent in the nature of the sensory process itself ; qualities of sense are by their very nature pleasant or unpleasant. He next assumes that pleasant experiences are inevitably (almost by definition) prolonged and repeated, while unpleasant experiences are as far as possible terminated. It is true that for Condillac's purposes we need consider only one of the senses ; the other senses would contribute other *qualities*, but the laws formulated from observing them would be identical.

His system of psychology is a logical creation as beautiful, probably, as is to be found outside of mathematics. We may, to be sure, smile and remain unconvinced as we read how the experience of one sensation followed by another gives us, *ipso facto*, a comparison of the two, or how an inherently unpleasant sensation constitutes directly, and without further assumptions, the will to terminate the experience ; but the logical construction comes to the modern reader as something exquisite in its simplicity and clarity.[1]

Condillac's teachings were influential during the French Revolution, especially in the educational system of the Republic. This attempt to picture mental life as an aggregate of sensory bits became the dominant philosophy for the remaining years of the century, until the idealistic movement came into vigorous life again. The success of Condillac's sensationism was due in large part to the intellectual soil of the " Enlightenment," to such influences as deism and the Encyclopædist movement. Though the system was of English origin, it was grafted, so to speak, upon French thought, with which it had a close affinity. The middle of

---

[1] A somewhat similar system, but with much more attention to physiology, was offered by Bonnet (*Essai analytique sur les facultés de l'âme*, 1760). Bonnet described memory in terms of alterations in nerve-fibres (in language similar to Hartley's). He performed a rough experiment on the " span of attention."

the eighteenth century had been a period of great mental activity throughout the cities of France, but concentrated above all in Paris. Here the influence of scientists and historians, especially of the anti-ecclesiastical group, had begun to simplify the picture of human life, as the English empiricists had done, by doing away with the super-natural and by making human experience the all-sufficient object of study. The great advances of physics, chemistry, and astronomy were making for the growth of the concept of natural law so important in the economic[1] and political policies of French statesmen both before and during the Revolution.

This scientific movement was destined to reach great heights in the work of two Frenchmen who are usually thought of as figures in the history of medicine, Cabanis[2] and Bichat. Living at the time of the French Revolution, they were the most brilliant exponents of the movement which aimed to unite the science of the non-living with the science of living things.

Cabanis first attracted attention as a student of a problem which arose from the facts of execution by guillotine. He was interested in the philanthropic question whether the guillotine hurt its victims or acted so swiftly as to be painless. By questions of this kind he was prompted to a study of reflex action and to the formulation of a concept which has become an important principle in physiological psychology to this day. We can summarize his conception in the term " series of levels." The spinal cord level was the simplest of a hierarchy ; it carried out reflex acts in response to stimuli. (The concept of the reflex had been put forth more than a century before by Descartes,[3] but it had now been enriched by many decades of research upon the central nervous system.) At a higher level, semi-conscious or semi-integrated activities were carried on ; and at the highest level were more complicated functions, thought, volition, and

---

[1] The beginnings of modern political economy are usually traced to the French Physiocrats in the generation preceding the Revolution. The doctrine of " laissez-faire " is an apt summary of their belief in the universality of natural law, as well as the general belief in the *beneficence* of natural law as contrasted with laws humanly enacted.

[2] *E.g., Rapports du physique et du moral de l'homme* (1799).

[3] See page 9.

the like.[1] Cabanis believed that unless the brain was involved there were no mental processes, but mere mechanical responses. On this assumption he concluded that the guillotine was not painful; movements in the body after execution were reflexes of the lowest level.

Having postulated these levels, Cabanis went on to suggest an explanation of cerebral activities on the analogy of more elementary functions. He showed evidence that the same mechanical principles which govern reflex activity govern cerebral activity; he made use of data indicating the relation of brain disease to mental disease. He ventured upon a systematic physiological psychology, replacing many of Condillac's assumptions by the postulation of neural functions which served as the basis for an active adjustment to environment. He made use of a genetic approach, making much of the fact of increase in mental complexity arising from increase in the complexity of the nervous system. Finally, he conceived of a social psychology, based on laws of individual behaviour and social stimulation, and was led to an empirical consideration of ethics. He was one of the first to realize that the biological observations of the eighteenth century had clear implications for social life. Starting from reflex action, he proceeded all the way to the most complicated problem with which psychologists have to deal, human conduct in its ethical aspects. He was a moralist, not in the sense of laying down dogmatic principles, but in suggesting modes of conduct which seemed workable and adapted to make the best of men as he pictured them—biological units interacting on one another in a material universe.

The writings of Cabanis were contemporaneous with the work of Bichat, whose medical researches led him also to the conception of a physiological psychology. From the time of Hippocrates, medicine had recognized the body as an assemblage of *organs;* in spite of the active prosecution of research with the aid of the microscope, the intimate knowledge of the composition of these organs had not been achieved. Bichat proceeded to carry the analysis into the

[1] This conception was greatly elaborated by Hughlings-Jackson nearly a century later. Jackson supposed that the levels most recently achieved through evolution were most easily deranged, and based a psychiatric classification upon this principle. (*The Factors of Insanities*, 1894).

realm of the structure of the *tissues*, and founded the science of histology. He showed that every part of the human body is composed of a few types of tissue which combine in various ways to form the vital organs, muscles, glands, etc. He came into contact, of course, with problems of neuropathology, and through these, with psychopathology. He thought of the forms of mental disease in terms of the abnormality of anatomical and histological structure. This type of psychology could not possibly have come into being had it not been for the development of physics and physiology in both Britain and France from the sixteenth to the end of the eighteenth century. Descartes and Hobbes had outlined a physiological approach to psychology ; Hartley had boldly attempted a detailed neurological system ; but a thorough-going physiological psychology could arise only on the basis of a fairly definite conception of the structure and functions of the nervous system.

Another French scientist seems to sum up all these tendencies, although his position as a humanitarian is perhaps even higher than his position in the history of science. Pinel was appointed in 1791 as director of an institution for the insane in Paris, the Bicêtre. Here he struck off the chains with which many of the insane were bound. He epitomized in this act a view which had been gaining prevalence steadily since the time of Sydenham, the conviction that the insane are diseased ; that instead of being simply queer, or immoral, or in league with Satan, these individuals suffer from sick brains. Pinel, therefore, epitomized on the one hand the great advances in neurology and pathology, holding that disorder in the brain meant disorder in the personality ; and on the other hand, the humanitarian movement, with its insistence on the mitigation of suffering. We break with the demonological conception of disease, which, although rejected by individuals in all ages, had held sway for centuries. Pinel was a practical psychiatrist of no mean ability. He won outstanding distinction in the classification of mental disorders, attempting wherever possible to correlate brain disorder with mental disease.

We have now to consider another movement which dominated British and French thought during the eighteenth century, and to which brief reference was just made in connection with "humanitarianism." The treatment of criminals had been carried on in much the same spirit as that of the insane. Among the factors responsible for the situation were the concept of original sin, and, on the other hand, the emphasis on the principle of the freedom of the will, which made each individual personally responsible for his wickedness. These factors added to the severity of the treatment accorded to the criminal, treatment which of course had been brutal even under the "pax Romana." Severe torture was in use in France until the Revolution. The most violent reaction now arose against such barbarous methods.[1]

Perhaps the humanitarian movement had its ultimate origin, as some economists have suggested, in the discovery of the New World and in the Commercial Revolution, the bringing in of new goods and the raising of the general standard of living. With the break-up of the feudal system and the rapid rise of democracy, traders began to compete with the nobility for economic and political power. In the Old World the guildsmen had raised themselves into a commercial class, and even those below them had risen to positions of genuine prosperity. And in the New World Europeans found a new opportunity to escape the oppression of a landed nobility ; they might claim land for themselves and take part in the establishment of a democracy. Their constant emigration contributed to a rise in wages in western Europe ; with the decrease of the number of available labourers, wages rose and the condition of the poor tended to improve.

Whether our emphasis on these factors be great or small, we find the humanitarian movement widespread by the middle of the eighteenth century. Pinel was expressing it in the field of medicine. It was even more strikingly apparent in the work of Beccaria,[2] the founder of modern criminological theory. He protested against the brutality and the futility of the heavy sentences imposed for all sorts of petty crimes ; capital punishment, for example, for petty larceny, seemed to him barbarous and absurd. He carried into

---

[1] Torture is, to be sure, still present in some American institutions Whatever the existing abuses, they can scarcely compare with eighteenth-century methods.
[2] *Crimes and Punishments* (1764).

criminology that system of thought known as psychological hedonism, which pictured each individual as motivated solely by desire for pleasure and aversion from pain. He outlined a theory of punishment which was designed to direct this human nature into conduct desired by the group. He argued that a man commits a crime only when he is impelled by a wish. A man steals bread because he is hungry; if he is terribly hungry, he steals more. If we institute a system of *graded* punishment, we may for each crime assign a punishment which will deter the individual from that act. This conception is an integral part of the humanitarian movement just considered. Had it not been for the violent repulsion against systems of torture and the use of capital punishment for dozens of crimes, such an application of hedonistic theory would not have been necessary.

Closely bound up with the humanitarian movement were the writings of the " utilitarians." Jeremy Bentham[1] was at the same time an incarnation of the humanitarian movement and the advocate of an ethical system widely influential in the newly risen " political economy " of the late eighteenth century. This was " ethical hedonism," the doctrine that the only individual or social good is happiness. The phrases " the greatest good of the greatest number " and the " sum total of human happiness " are characteristic of the system. At the same time he insisted upon " psychological hedonism," the doctrine that all human acts are self-interested.

It will be recalled that the physiocrats had maintained that wealth came solely from land ; in other words, from agriculture, and to some extent, from mining, forestry, etc. All other forms of human activity were parasitic. Soon Adam Smith in England began to see the inadequacy of such a simple formula. His *Wealth of Nations* treated of the principles involved in commerce ; why it is that men trade with one another, what satisfactions they obtain from exchange of goods. He grasped the need of a psychological background for economic processes, just as in his work on *The Theory of Moral Sentiments* he had already attempted a psychological explanation of morality. What had been a problem of mathematics with the French became a psychological problem with the English ; human motives were the key to social organization. Smith's psychology differed much

---

[1] *The Principles of Morals and Legislation* (1789).

from Bentham's, but Bentham and his school soon won the day. The *psychology* of the economists came to be based in the main on his principles ; to these we must give closer attention.

Bentham was the first to formulate systematically the universal principle of psychological hedonism, which many writers had assumed, but none had thoroughly worked out.[1] He sought to explain all social behaviour in terms of rational search for pleasure and avoidance of pain. He and his followers sought to show a way to use this self-interest motive of each individual in the interests of society as a whole ; in an ideal society, individual and social good would coincide. Just as Beccaria had explained that, if the punishment is just great enough, the individual will refrain from stealing bread, so Bentham built up the doctrine that men will work just so much for their bread ; that is, they will undergo labour and suffering only if their reward is sufficiently great. In his hands this became a method of explaining not only individual conduct, but the whole organization of society. The statesman's task is to find out the way in which these motives work, and to guide the social order so that each individual's conception of his own greatest good will be one with that of society's greatest good. Bentham's theory of motivation and his desire to use this motivation for the general welfare, accorded with the humanitarian movement ; and his doctrines were fused with those of Beccaria, of Pinel, and of the humanitarian wing of the deists and the French anti-ecclesiasts.

But there is one more link still to be fitted in. We have tried to make clear that the dominant influence in English psychology during the eighteenth century was associationism. What was the link between associationism and these other developments ? A very direct connection, a connection shown in the fact that Bentham himself was a great advocate of associationism. Bentham asserted that certain things, in themselves neutral, become sources of pleasure and pain, and come through association to influence us as though they were the pleasure and pain themselves. For instance, a piece of metal which has no use and which is not feared is neutral ; but if the piece of metal has become

---

[1] See p. 14. Ethical hedonism does not necessarily involve psychological hedonism, nor *vice versa*, but Bentham embraced both.

associated with value, it becomes as *money* a direct object of satisfaction. Every kind of conduct in which we may indulge may be pleasant or unpleasant, according to the association. Associationism and utilitarianism, therefore, become intermingled to a point where it is vain to try to disentangle them. Associationism is the intellectual background, humanitarianism the emotional and sentimental background, for the utilitarian movement.

A number of social and intellectual movements had now grown together. They constituted almost a systematic view of life. The Commercial and the Industrial Revolution ; the development of natural science ; the rise of political economy; associationism ; humanitarianism ; reform in the treatment of criminals and the insane ; deism and utilitarianism, as well as a number of other movements, had led to a new and " naturalistic " conception of human nature. A large number of contemporary historians of western culture would make the economic factors, especially those arising from the Commercial Revolution, the origin of most of the others ; for our purposes it suffices to note the existence of all these factors as they moulded British psychology.

Though all these movements were international, their influence on continental psychology was considerably less than on psychology in Britain. Before the Revolution every one of these movements was clearly active in France, but no psychological system such as those constructed by the associationists and the utilitarians existed. French psychology up to Cabanis and Bichat had merely continued the Cartesian tradition, and borrowed, through Condillac, part of Locke's system. During the Revolution and the Napoleonic era, French thought enjoyed no such freedom for development as that vouchsafed in Britain. Although there was some psychological work in the interests of education,[1] and although Pinel had led the way toward a new outlook on mental disorders, the necessity of waging war from 1793 until 1815, a constant war on many fronts, inevitably stifled to some extent the tendencies with which we are now concerned. This political situation had also some effect on Germany and Italy.

German psychology, as we shall see, was pursuing its independent career, and was but little affected by association-

---

[1] Headed by Condorcet.

ism and the kindred movements noted above. Association-ism had not been going on long enough to " catch," so to speak, in Germany. But beginning with the work of Herbart, it became in the nineteenth century one of the main currents in German psychological and educational thought.

We must next consider two phases of German thought parallel with the two British movements already discussed. It will be remembered that the " faculty psychology " of the seventeenth and eighteenth centuries, which had concerned itself with the various functions of the mind, maintained that a unitary soul was capable of acting in a variety of ways, but entered fully into each of its various activities at various times. This conception is closely related to a view which has been widely advocated in recent years, that each function is the function not of a part or element of the organism, but of the whole organism ; no experience or act can be viewed out of the context supplied by all other experiences and acts. The main purpose of faculty psychology was to describe the primary powers exercised by the soul ; memory, reason, the will, etc., were regarded as utterly distinct functions or activities. This approach was congenial to the rationalistic tendency pre-viously noted, because cognitive functions were accepted at their face value and freed from the humiliation of dissection into sensory bits in the manner favoured by the association-ists. Faculty psychology also emphasized the religious and moral functions of the soul. Growing in the soil of German religious intensity,[1] it became essentially and mainly " ideal-istic."[2]

Now in the course of time this faculty psychology, with its emphasis upon the " ultimate modes of psychical func-

[1] Much of the psychological work of Great Britain in the seventeenth and eighteenth centuries was done quite outside of the religious atmo-sphere ; and English empiricism, through Condillac, was amalgamated with French agnosticism. Germany was singularly free from these powerful agnostic trends. A strong empirical tendency flourished in Germany in the late eighteenth century, but it was unable to maintain itself.

[2] " Idealism " may be defined for our purposes as that type of philosophy which emphasizes the reality and value of mental processes which appear to be (at least relatively) remote from or independent of physical processes.

tioning," expressed itself more adequately in the writings of Immanuel Kant, one of the greatest figures in the history of thought. His celebrated doctrines received their initial impetus from the skeptical thought of Britain. Hume's skepticism was chiefly responsible for the injection of the critical spirit into the mind of Kant. "It was Hume," said Kant, "who awoke me from my dogmatic slumbers." Kant found it impossible by logical and deductive methods to demonstrate the reality of the soul. After centuries in which many men of great learning had undertaken to prove the reality of the soul, he was the first to show by deductive[1] methods the hopelessness of the attempt to define the ultimate properties of this invisible substance. We are forced, therefore, said Kant, to a new analysis, in order to discover the ultimate modes of experience. He found in the complexity of mental processes a variety of cognitive functions which he believed to be not further analysable. But psychologists are more concerned with the sanction he gave to the notion of the three great subdivisions of mental activity, knowing, feeling, and willing. Analysis of the process of knowing is set forth in his epoch-making *Critique of Pure Reason* (1781) ; the processes of feeling and willing, though less exhaustively treated, are handled in the *Critique of Practical Reason* and elsewhere. His influence upon psychology was not at all comparable to his influence on philosophy, and this just because he sought the ultimate, the transcendental, caring but little for the events of mental life as immediate data and entertaining no hope that they could become the subject matter of science. In our discussion of him we must omit important questions of purely philosophical significance, and be, as far as we may, simply psychologists.

Two phases of Kant's work have profoundly influenced psychology. In the first place, his insistence on the unity of an act of perception. This attacked the very heart of associationism ; many of the intellectual forces which in the nineteenth century contributed to the downfall of the associationist system are directly or indirectly traceable to Kant's emphasis upon the unity of experience.

When we cognize what we call objects, as in the case of

---

[1] Kant was much interested in *inductive* efforts to do so, as exemplified in Swedenborg.

touching a solid object with the fingers, we find certain mental states which are apparently composed of sensory qualities. We seem to find just that integration of bits of experience of which the associationists spoke. But we find these things coherent, meaningful; some operation has been performed by the mind, in organizing these bits into a unitary experience. This is more than mere association. Kant's term "transcendental unity of apperception" can be fully understood only after mastering his system of thought; but two definite contributions are evident at a glance, the notion of a self which organizes its experience, and the notion of space-perception and the perception of time-relations, as essential to that organization. We find in all "apperception" a number of constituent elements welded into a unity in experience. A man looks and sees a tree, he listens and hears a melody; but there must be some entity which carries on the act of experiencing or cognizing. In the nature of the case we cannot know what that something is.

In the second place, we have his clear exposition of the impossibility of treating the soul as the subject matter of psychology, and his appeal to experience as the only foundation for the formulation of psychological laws. Some of the associationists had taught that the "primary" qualities (size, shape, motion, etc.) are independent of the observer. But all primary and secondary qualities were equally secondary in the eyes of Kant. Nevertheless quantitative observations are relatively free from inconsistencies in the hands of various observers. Though they fail to measure the thing in itself, they give a systematic and orderly account of experience as qualitative observation cannot do. Kant sums up by saying that there is in any discipline as much of science as there is of mathematics. That is, science deals with quantities, but not with the quality or nature of the things measured; the rest is a study of experience subject to all the limitations of "knowledge."

Perhaps the most important of Kant's many epoch-making contributions was his demonstration of the relativity of knowledge. But although knowledge is relative, there seems to be some external agency at work, so that perception is fairly uniform for most observers; the congruity of testimony regarding experience suggests that there must be real things

acting upon us.   The subjectivism of Berkeley is replaced by
Kant's doctrine that there is a real world of "things in
themselves."   These things are presumed to arouse within
us sensory qualities built together into a unity by the process
of "apperception."   We see, for example, a watch.   The
only thing observable is our experience.   We do not know
the " real " object, but we find a certain unity in testimony
—white, black, certain shapes—these things distributed in
space and their motion distributed in time.   But outside of
experience, what that watch is in itself, beyond any quality
that may come into our consciousness, we cannot know.

A word may be added about Kant's treatment of willing
and feeling.   The process of willing, he held, is independent
of causality ; we are free in our activity.   This is part of our
moral nature.   Kant therefore leads us back to that religious
outlook and idealism which he had had to abandon in his
study of the process of knowledge.   He insists that the
ultimate moral and religious reality lies not in the field of
knowledge but in the process of the will.   His adoption of
the " faculty psychology " made feeling and willing each
quite separable from knowledge.

The transcendentalism with which Kant concerned himself
derives its name from the fact that its *ultimate* explanatory
principles lie outside of the content of any particular experience.   It was therefore in one important respect in violent
conflict with empiricism ; " experience," taken without reference to its transcendental laws, was for Kant simply a
meaningless chaos.   This is far more important for philosophy than it is for psychology.   But Kant showed psychologists that they must study experience rather than the soul,
and suggested that the data of true science must be stated
in terms of their quantitative relations—that it is only by a
quantitative study of events that a science can be built
up.

The transcendentalism of Kant shortly underwent profound modification in the hands of men who had much less
to offer in the analysis of cognitive functions, but who
reproduced more adequately the romanticism of their age.
Fichte begins his philosophy very much in the spirit of some
poets of the romantic period by positing that the soul's first

activity is the subdividing of the world of experience into the self and the not-self. The same tendency is evident in the writings of Goethe and the romanticists, who tired of endless rationalism. The two streams, transcendentalism and romanticism, which spring from very different sources,[1] come together in a strange kind of unity.

In many ways the influence of the Renaissance upon Germany had been delayed. It is true that as far as the fine arts are concerned there was a good deal of excellent work, particularly in the Rhineland, in the sixteenth and seventeenth centuries. It is true that some of the literary productions of the period had shown great depth and power. But Germany was on the whole under scholastic influences for a longer time than Italy France, or Britain. Experimental science, which had made rapid progress elsewhere, hardly brought an echo in Germany in these centuries, except among those educated in France. Germany was still locked in the mighty fortress of mediæval culture. Now there came at last not only the influence of British empiricism through the work of Kant, but a series of profound changes in the life and mood of the people, a rebellion against the didactic and the rationalistic.

One of the predisposing influences toward this " romantic " movement was the mystical attitude toward nature. The sixteenth century had shown a rapid development of interest in landscape painting and literary references to the beauty of nature ; these were but aspects of a vast movement. Something had happened in Italy, and then in France and England, and now with might began in Germany—a turning away from the study room into the bright day of nature. One of the greatest devotees of the cult of nature was Jacob Boehme (d. 1624) ; for him everything had a mystic significance ; every animal, every tree had a spiritual lesson for humanity. He was also interested in numbers in the manner of the Pythagoreans. The preoccupation with symbols seems to be characteristic of mysticism ; the mystic strives to grasp the meaning of something more than the perceptual aspect, attempts to regard things as symbols of something deeper.

In consequence of the mystical and romantic movements there rapidly developed within transcendentalism a specific form of philosophy the whole purport of which was to show

---

[1] Kant's transcendentalism sprang from intellectualist soil, and was critical and " cognitive " rather than poetic.

that nature is not merely a series of events but a system of interaction among spiritual entities.[1] From the contact of the post-Kantian transcendentalists[2] with the romantic movement there arose a philosophy which was transcendentalist in its approach, romantic in its motivation. It was called the "Philosophy of Nature." This became a prominent school in the early nineteenth century. It was by no means indifferent to the progress of the sciences ; its leader, Oken, did much to stimulate research, and it concerned itself constantly with newly discovered facts, especially with facts from the biological sciences. But it was not interested in the quantitative method except as that had spiritual meaning. It was dealing with the same subject matter as science, but according to a law of its own. It was ultimately incompatible with the science which it imitated. We shall see that this philosophy was one of the most potent factors in the early training of some of the greatest nineteenth-century physiologists. Its psychology was necessarily vitalistic rather than mechanistic, and its centre of interest lay in the fact of the richness of experience rather than in detailed analysis.

Let us briefly review these various schools with which we have been dealing so far, and see their mutual relations at the beginning of the nineteenth century. First, the Scottish school, with emphasis primarily on cognitive processes which were thought to be self-evident. It was glad, indeed, to borrow from the ethical doctrines of the new philosophy of the continent, but was in its ultimate make-up opposed to Kant's whole way of thought. For the Scottish school insisted still that we can by direct observation discover that we have souls and that our souls have certain ways of obtaining knowledge which are ultimately valid. In England the work of the empirical school went on, under Hartley's followers on the one hand, Bentham's and the utilitarians' on the other. French psychology was to a large extent modelled upon English, and in the opening decades

[1] Hegel went further than this, attempting to show that all human history is more than a record of external events ; there is a spiritual thread, a series of embodiments of the "Idea."
[2] Fichte, and notably Schelling.

of the century upon the Scottish school. The French had in the persons of Cabanis, Bichat, and many others, worked out with extraordinary vision a physiological psychology much in advance of that of Hartley. In Germany the rationalistic tendency prevailed, bearing fruit in the transcendentalism of Kant and others, which insisted on realities beyond experience ; and on the other hand, the romantic movement appealed directly to Nature, which under transcendentalist influence inspired the mystical Philosophy of Nature.

E

CHAPTER III

All our thoughts [the Stoics believe] are formed either by indirect perception, or by similarity, or analogy, or transposition, or combination, or opposition.—*Diogenes Laertius*.

WE must next take account of the influence of British associationism upon German thought. Transcendentalism had been gaining in momentum in Germany, but yielded to associationism in the doctrines laid down by Herbart[1], whose significance is equally great for the history of psychology and for that of education.

He began with those elementary bits of experience which we have heretofore called sensations. Just as Condillac and his followers had done before him, so Herbart now adopted the structuralism of the English school, reducing complex mental states to combinations of elementary sensory qualities ; these units by combining into groups make up our ideas. We have here a structuralism combined with a doctrine regarding the laws of association, all that is needed for a new school of association psychology. The passive linkages assumed by most of the English and French associationists were, however, replaced in Herbart's system by dynamic principles. The associationists had created a system very similar to a jig-saw puzzle ; it was never easy to see what power put the parts together. The parts or bits of sensory experience were there as units ; but even in Hartley's neurological theory associationism failed to face squarely the problem of finding the integrating mechanism.

Mental functions were regarded by Herbart as ways of manipulating elements, and were treated from a dynamic— and from a mathematical—point of view. Had he been more of a mathematician and less of a metaphysician he could perhaps have constructed his beautiful associationism without reference to *forces*, the notion of which had come down

---

[1] *A Text Book in Psychology* (1816).

from the physicists of the seventeenth century and especially from Newton[1]. But Herbart not only constructed a mathematical system to explain how bits of experience become associated ; he not only showed the formulæ by which we can create a calculus of the mind ; he gave us the principles according to which something, as yet unknown, actively puts these parts together. He closely interwove these distinct conceptions, a mathematical system and the doctrine of an activating principle. The bits of experience coming through the senses combine with each other, not by virtue of mathematical principles alone, but through the operation of certain forces in the mind as in the physical world.

Now there are two ways in which elementary bits of experience may interact. First, they may combine harmoniously into wholes ; the resulting composite ideas are closely similar to those described by Locke and Hartley. But secondly, there are, Herbart taught, ways in which ideas may come into relation with each other through conflict or struggle. That is to say, ideas which are incapable of combining compete with one another in consciousness. A systematic theory of the conscious and unconscious becomes necessary. In following out the dynamic implications of the system, a system in which ideas were active forces, Herbart had to show not only what happens when ideas combine, but also what happens when they compete and exclude one another from consciousness.

For Herbart there were three different relations which the bits of elementary experience may bear to consciousness. They may be plainly conscious ; these include the things to which we are attending. There are also ideas in the very margin of consciousness which may easily lapse from it in a moment. There are, thirdly, some which may be forced out of consciousness altogether. Herbart proceeded to discuss the phenomenon of " opposition " between ideas.[2] He needed a category into which to put the ideas which had been repressed from consciousness. For when an

---

[1] Burtt, *Metaphysical Foundations of Modern Physical Science* (1925).
[2] Recent authors point out that objects of thought do not conflict with each other because they are in logical opposition, but because they lead to divergent lines of conduct. Ideas are in conflict if they lead us to do opposite things. This is one reason for serious doubt as to the indebtedness of psychoanalysis to Herbart.

idea is repressed it is not *lost:* it may reappear later in consciousness. How does it come back? Either by the weakening of the idea which repressed it, or by its combination with an ally, a co-operating idea which may join with it, and through joining forces, enable it to regain supremacy in consciousness. This means that there is a multitude of tendencies which later lead to the recurrence of ideas which have once been banished. Herbart felt that no purpose was served by trying to describe the *nature* of such ideas as were not in consciousness, but might later come back. He was interested in such ideas in terms of their functions, not in terms of their structure or being. When ideas leave consciousness they simply have a tendency to return. There is a vast company of " ideas " which have once gone and may return. This is a clear recognition of the fact that psychology must deal not only with what is present in consciousness, but with psychological factors beyond the reach of introspection; and it also involves a theory so free from ambiguities that it can be applied to the phenomena of memory and to all phases of mental conflict. As the ideas in the field of consciousness pass from it they cross a " threshold "; the same threshold is crossed in the reverse direction when the idea reappears. Or the idea may be exactly at the threshold. It was over fifty years before a more adequate description of the unconscious in terms of empirical findings was attempted.[1]

This conception of a sharp and definite line between conscious processes and other somehow similar processes occurring outside of consciousness, has been a storm-centre in psychology for a century. Some regard it as a very unfortunate and superfluous assumption, one that is entirely unnecessary for empirical psychology, one which clutters up psychology with confusion almost as devastating as the doctrine of conflict is enlightening. Others have found in the sharp separation of " conscious " and " unconscious " the only salvation from bad metaphysics and worse logic.

How does this theory of association relate to the Hartleyan system? Herbart rejected categorically the neurological

[1] By Janet, James, Freud, F. W. H. Myers, and Höffding. The theoretical studies by Schopenhauer and von Hartmann seem to have been less important forerunners than the clinical work of Charcot.

formulæ which had been current from Hartley onwards, a period of about seventy-five years. He wanted a purely psychological statement without assumptions regarding echoes and re-echoes of the nerve substance. Further, he wished to be able to describe all mental phenomena in terms of the time-relations of the processes. He sought to do so by means of mathematics applied directly to mental processes themselves, using force and time as two of the variables which preside over the uprisings and down-sittings of all the different bits of sensory experience in their different combinations. If we have learned a certain order or series of experiences, we establish certain dynamic relations, depending on the speed of learning, the amount of repetition, and so on, and our mathematical formulæ enable us, if we know the factors operating at a given moment, to predict future experience. In place of Hartley's statement of associative sequence through patterns once established in the brain, we have in Herbart a series following in order because certain dynamic relations inherent in the ideas themselves have been set up.

The constant tendency of some ideas to come into consciousness pushes others out of consciousness. Of course, there are two kinds of factors which make for this predominance of some ideas over others, internal factors in the ideas as such, and the initiation of ideas from without, that is, from new stimulation. Many of our sensory experiences are not attributable solely to a new stimulus, but are rather due to a stimulus augmenting an unconscious deposit of experience. This is equivalent in some cases to the statement that although we had not noticed a stimulus before we now have the background to notice it as soon as it is presented. We may take as an example the case of a professional tea-taster looking for a particular flavour or quality. Most of us might seek in vain for a certain quality present, but the tea-taster has so frequently given attention to a certain sensory quality that now, when the stimulus is presented, he is able to detect it because of his accumulated past experience ; it rises into his consciousness.

This brings us to Herbart's most famous conception, the *apperception mass*. This is a name for all those past experiences which we use when we perceive something new. In the illustration used, the perception of a certain quality in the tea is dependent upon the fact that there is a myriad of past tea-flavours in the man's accumulated experience, and the elements of flavour immediately find a place and are assimilated in consciousness.

Herbart applied his theory extensively in education. The child is learning, for example, the meaning of numbers. If he has observed his fingers often enough and has learned a group of words which apply to one, two, and three fingers, and so on with other objects, and if we now attempt to teach him the general idea that one plus two equals three, he can assimilate this idea because he has observed it in specific cases. Similarly, in the process of learning geography, he can understand a map of Europe if he knows how land, water, and mountains are represented on the map of a region he already knows. His teacher builds in his mind a certain structure (say, a series of geographical symbols) and now gives him a map of Europe. Immediately all these new sensory stimuli combine with the ideas which lie already assimilated in his mind. This background of ideas constitutes apperception mass. Instead of merely gazing at the map, he apperceives it. The term " apperception " has for Herbart much the same meaning that it had for Leibnitz, with whom it began ; it borrows also from Kant. The process of apperception is a combination of a number of sensory bits into a unity. But instead of emphasizing an innate unifying power, as did Kant, Herbart presupposed that a background already in our mind makes possible the assimilation of a new idea which could never otherwise be learned.[1] This seemingly obvious common-sense doctrine has enjoyed the most extraordinary influence in education.

A revolution in educational theory and practice was taking place in the closing years of the eighteenth and the opening years of the nineteenth centuries. It came mainly in the form of a protest against the mechanical implanting of information. It emphasized the new idea of developing the child's inherent capacities. Rousseau, in his time, had done much to disseminate this doctrine in speaking of the natural as opposed to the artificial. The aim of education should be

[1] Herbart did indeed regard the soul as necessary to the coherent function and organization of mind. But this is little more than lip service to it, as the apperception mass sets the limit on what the soul can do, and is throughout Herbart's treatment the central agency in the process of learning and knowing.

to bring out the natural responses of the child.   But no one knew just what was " natural." It remained for Pestalozzi (at the end of the eighteenth century) and Froebel (a little later) to clarify the idea.   Pestalozzi, a Swiss, developed an experimental school in which he departed radically from the educational system of his day and undertook to bring out the native powers of observation in the child.   He was interested in the systematic interrelation of all parts of self-development. He was far from being a mere student of the sense-organs for their own sake ; he believed one must start by developing the child's ability to observe.   He did not confine this doctrine to class-room instruction, but applied it to work on the farm, in the garden, and in the home.   The implanting of information in the child's mind was reduced to a very subordinate position.   Froebel, a German, borrowed much from Pestalozzi and carried the idea further.   He emphasized the use of vivid stimuli, bright colours, toys, etc., as means of attracting and holding attention, and exercising the child's capacities for dealing with things ; he made much of the educational value of play and founded the *Kindergarten* as a means of making use of the easy or " natural " in the child's development.

Herbart made good use of these contributions.   He realized in the first place the great importance of this emphasis upon observation.   He saw that there were all kinds of ways of reacting to stimuli, depending upon how much background we have.   He saw that Pestalozzi was right in emphasizing objects of observation in which the child is interested and relating them to his activities.   He felt that education could make use of this principle throughout the whole course of life, starting with physical stimuli, gradually reaching more and more complicated forms of experience. He believed that systematic use could be made of his doctrine of apperception.   Just as counting the fingers may lead to a general knowledge of numbers, so each contact with the world gives a background for the handling of more and more complex situations.   But we must make sure that each idea is put to the child's observation only after the child has so co-ordinated his *past* observation as to be ready to assimilate the new.   This led to the idea of a curriculum so devised that the child constantly passes from familiar to closely related unfamiliar subject matter.   The entire curriculum should be presented systematically in accordance with the child's ability to assimilate it.

These ideas were epoch-making. Educational method became an empirical study. Herbart established an experimental school ; he conducted classes for teacher-training, and made comparison of different methods of presenting school material. And although the mathematical aspirations of Herbart's work were destined to receive no great fulfilment,[1] being rejected as though by common consent, his general conception of mental organization was the basis for educational theory and experimentation for many decades, and remains widely influential to-day. He hoped to make psychology an *exact* and an *empirical* science ; he failed in the former, but did much to advance the latter purpose.

Except in the case of his theory of apperception, it is difficult to appraise to-day the historical significance of his system. The theory of the threshold and the doctrine of conflict keep reappearing in nineteenth-century psychology ; but the threshold in Herbart's sense is obscured and frequently forgotten through the different use of the concept in the writings of Weber and Fechner,[2] while modern emphasis on conflict and struggle seems to owe more to Darwinism[3] and to psychiatric experience.

Herbart's relation to the history of associationism is unique. He was the only associationist for whom the elements of experience were measurable entities ; on the other hand, his interest in the soul (and his whole metaphysical interest) constitutes a direct rejection of the method of most of the English empiricists. He had but little influence on subsequent associationism, which continued its course in Great Britain ; his influence consists rather in helping to overthrow the faculty psychology, in the emphasis upon psychological factors outside of clear consciousness, and in the advancement of educational theory and method.

---

[1] His mathematical methods did, as we shall see (p. 195), influence Ebbinghaus. He contributed also to the quantitative conception of mental abnormality, regarding mental deficiency, for example, as a matter of *degree*, levels of intelligence departing to a greater or lesser extent from the normal.

[2] See pp. 81 and 89f.

[3] Not, of course, to Darwin's conception of the conflict of organisms, but to that of dynamic patterns or " instincts " within the organism.

The German psychological literature in the age of Herbart was of considerable quantity, but most of what was written was ephemeral. Our selection of authors and tendencies must be based, as usual, upon the sole criterion of their significance in relation to our contemporary psychology.

One heterogeneous group of thinkers comprised the " anthropologists."[1] They occupied themselves with the dream of a science of man which would correlate data from physiology, psychology, ethics, and epistemology. Kant may in some respects be classified with them. This group was eager to make use of the accounts of primitive cultures in relation to those more complex ; the raw material of travellers' records and memoirs was woven into a system of conceptions about man in his " natural state "[2] and as a social being. There appears to have been a considerable increase during the eighteenth century of the practice of travelling for its own sake. The improvement of roads in France and later in England was important in knitting together more closely the nations of western Europe,[3] while longer journeys ceased to be ventures of discovery and became almost a part of a liberal education. The services of the traveller von Humboldt in unifying the intellectual life of western Europe were typical. The growing knowledge of many civilizations, primitive and advanced, gave therefore an inductive basis for the work of these " anthropologists." But they needed a theory as to how the mind works ; they were forced to build some kind of bridge between the mind of the individual and the life of the group. The first vague intimation of " folk-psychology " is found in this period, particularly in the writings of Kant.

One of the most significant of the anthropologists was Fries.[4] He felt forced to admit the fundamental accuracy of

---

[1] Not, of course, to be confused with the more critical and methodologically uniform work commencing with Bastian and Ratzel in the middle of the nineteenth century, now generally known as " cultural anthropology."

[2] The reader will recall that Hobbes and Rousseau, among many, had pictured a non-social human existence ; such fervid and uncritical descriptions of primitive societies as had been offered by Montaigne served as material for Rousseau's " noble savage."

[3] Sterne, *A Sentimental Journey:* " they order . . . this matter better in France." Goldsmith's *Traveller* is an equally celebrated expression of the tendency noted.

[4] *Handbuch der psychischen Anthropologie* (1820–21).

Kant's analysis and the futility of hoping to know anything ultimate about reality.   All we have is experience, and that is relative.   But the process of cognition, instead of being attributed to a soul or a self which lies beyond experience, was for Fries a function of the constitution of the organism. That is, a person born with a nervous system and sense organs is forced by his biological make-up to see things in a certain way.   Let us, he said, grant Kant's principles, that we cannot know anything in the absolute and that all is mere experience, and that our only methods of dealing with reality are through certain categories or forms which give patterns to our experience.   Our minds cannot get out of the ruts in which they must run.   But instead of introducing a transcendental principle, we should attribute human perception and reasoning to laws inherent in organic make-up.   In other words, the Kantian categories, instead of being transcendental, are empirical.   Anthropology proceeds to construct on the basis of man's observation the ways in which he adjusts himself both to his physical and to his social environment.

In the work of such men as Fries anthropology was trying to join the natural sciences.   It was as an empirical student of man, making use of general biological principles, that Fries took his stand, insisting on the necessity of empirical methods, applying these even to the study of the methods themselves.   He was of importance to mid-nineteenth-century thought in other sciences than psychology; he served to bring Kant's doctrine of the relativity of knowledge into general use.   Fries was significant also in keeping alive the idea of *degrees* of consciousness which had come down from Leibnitz—that there is at any moment a margin as well as a central field of greatest clearness.

At the same time that these rather academic modes of thinking were going on, an extremely wide-spread movement was taking place which enormously exceeded in its popular influence any of the writings just discussed.   With the possible exception of Rousseau, none of the authorities that we have had to consider had enjoyed what we might call a genuinely popular standing.   But with the founding of phrenology by Gall[1] early in the nineteenth century a tendency began which was destined to attract wide attention. Gall started with a series of hypotheses in which the doctrine of the faculties was worked out in relation to cerebral anatomy.

His first hypothesis was that the mind or personality or self has a number of entirely distinct functions which overlap only in the sense that two may combine in a given process. They are independent in the same way that the movement of the right hand and of the left may be independent, although both hands may be used at once. There are in human beings a certain number of specific and definite functions whose activities are located in various parts of the brain. The last vestige of doubt that the brain was the seat of mental life had disappeared as a result of clinical investigations. Nor was the subdivision of the brain into regions possessing certain independent functions original in itself. But Gall enumerated these functions with a vastly greater care than any one had before given to them. Of this kind of thing the phrenological models are illustrations, with their location of such traits as imitation, the poetic gift, destructiveness, and so on. Gall made a list of more than thirty faculties, and the list was expanded by his followers. This scheme was diametrically opposed to the association psychology of the period. When we speak of atomism breaking up mental life into pieces, we are referring to quite another thing. Gall did not teach that mental life is an integration of bits of experience. He thought in terms of a total individual whose *activities* could be classified and labelled.

Another of Gall's assumptions was that the exercise of a definite mental function depends chiefly upon the development of its own part of the brain, a development which may be ascribed to heredity. Such development of the brain tends to exert local pressure on the skull and to press it outwards in the form of a " bump." The final assumption was that feeling the skull with the finger may detect those regions in which there is rich endowment, and thus make possible an analysis of the individual's chief traits.

This not only had a certain fascination as a game, but, like

---

[1] *Introduction au cours de physiologie du cerveau* (1808).

telling fortunes and casting horoscopes, it immediately dragged down what might have been a serious contribution to a mere charlatanism. The hypotheses, with the exception of the one relating to the pressing out of the skull, seemed plausible enough at the time. Unfortunately the results of Gall's measurements of heads appeared to him to confirm his assumptions. Instead of seeking clinical evidence, men went on the road to lecture and to study character on the basis of " bumps." The practice came very rapidly into vogue in France, England, and America, and, indeed, still survives. It is impossible to deny the hold it has had on western European and American thought. In a series of lectures on " Domestic Duties " for young housewives, popular in the 'thirties, the well-informed young woman is warned against the hasty acceptance of the generally discussed tenets of phrenology. The continuance in popular speech of such phrases as " the bump of locality " shows, to be sure, no adoption of phrenological dogmas. But it does show the continuance of the doctrines of faculty psychology through the vehicle of phrenological terms ; the phrenological scheme has reinforced faculty psychology by keeping alive the notion of independent mental functions.

Gall borrowed from Cabanis and others the concept of definite innate reaction tendencies of the organism which enable it to adjust itself. Many of the instincts, he thought, have their accompanying emotional quality.[1] This was fifty years before the publication of the *Origin of Species*, and the resulting emphasis in psychology upon instincts. Both in relation to the idea of specialized cortical areas, and in relation to the necessity for dynamic units in the study of behaviour, Gall was a person of no mean significance. He had a theory of motivation which was decidedly more fruitful than that of associationism, or the idealistic reaction of the Scottish school.

Nevertheless, he fared but ill in academic circles. His unverifiable assumptions and the popular degradation of his system led to the general neglect of his work among psychologists and physiologists.

---

[1] Compare McDougall's analysis of instinct in his *Introduction to Social Psychology* (1908).

As we turn to the development of psychology in France, we must remember that there had been in French psychological work only one really long-lived movement. This had started with the introduction of the association psychology into France in the middle of the eighteenth century, and had attained a beautiful elaboration in the writings of Condillac. Cabanis had filed a formal protest against some features of this system. Where Condillac had taught that we learn through experience that certain things bring us pain or discomfort, that we love things because we learn from experience that they bring us pleasure, Cabanis insisted on inherited reaction-patterns. We ought not to start with sensations, he asserted, but with reactions. Instead of analysing experience, we should begin with the study of the physiology of reflexes of various levels. He protested that ideas as such have no energy, no tendency to connect with each other; dynamic principles must be introduced to show how experience becomes organized as life goes on. All these assertions arose from the acceptance of a physiological starting-point. However, the brilliant contributions of Cabanis as a physiologist, important as they were for psychology, enjoyed but a short life. His system suffered from the growing unpopularity of the mechanistic tendency. When the school of Cabanis was beginning to take hold of the French intellectual world, two adverse movements interfered. The Napoleonic wars created new political and economic problems; and for this and other reasons the attack on the Church and on accepted religion lost ground. On the other hand, partly through the dissemination of Scottish influences,[1] an idealistic movement was rapidly coming into its own.

The spirit of the revolt was largely empirical. Thomas Reid, in founding the Scottish school, had tried as we have seen to base his psychology not on dogma but on confidence in the trustworthiness of the senses. Even those who attacked the empirical findings of mechanism used empiricism as a method. The same thing is true, to some extent, of the new French idealism.

Biran began with an attempt at empiricism : the analysis of the genesis of habit, will, and self-consciousness in the

[1] And, of course, partly through a number of other social and intellectual forces too complex to be briefly appraised.

child. His chief concern was the development of the self, of a personality which is capable of truly integrated activity. He represented, moreover, a reaction against the mechanistic method, believing that the self is, after all, an experiencing *agent*, and something more than a series of experiences; it is a unified spiritual principle. Now the self is not at first aware of itself. It is, to begin with, not directly experienced. But, by the process of adjusting itself, it becomes conscious of the distinction between the self and the not-self. There are two steps in this process. Such activities as crying and movement of the limbs are first called out mechanically. They take place by virtue of those principles which Cabanis had emphasized. But when the same stimulus is repeated later there is in the field of experience a division into two parts, the object or thing upon which we react, and the self that reacts. In other words, the exercise of will is the first and dominant principle which causes the development of self-consciousness. It is because of our reactions, especially when resistance is offered to them, that we become aware of ourselves as individuals. This is definitely a dynamic psychology. As activity becomes more complex, self-consciousness develops greater richness.

This contribution was more important as giving a certain turn to French thought than as a specific, constant endowment for later generations. As a matter of fact, the details of Biran's system of psychology had little influence even in France a generation after his death, and extremely little outside of France. He remained a sort of guardian spirit constantly present with French psychology, not indeed as a stimulus to the use of the genetic method, but as an embodiment of voluntarism. It was not for his most original contribution that he was remembered.

The Scottish school had a simpler and more popular approach, which the French school adopted in preference to Biran's genetic method. For the writings of Royer-Collard, who became professor at the Sorbonne in the year 1811, were simply continuations of the work of Reid. But in giving psychology a " spiritual "[1] interpretation, the school of Royer-Collard naturally made use of many of the doctrines

---

[1] The term *spiritualisme*, which is still in general use in French psychology, corresponds, roughly, to our " idealism."

of Biran. In the first place, he had postulated a soul, in place of the raw " experience " of the mechanists. In the second place, he had emphasized the fact of *activity*, which the associationists had almost without exception disregarded. His voluntarism had opened the way for a psychology which could meet their requirements. It was to some extent the influence of Biran which made the will dominant in French psychology for the next forty or fifty years (idealism almost necessarily clings to the will as an independent function). But no clear facts about the will were available. With Biran as their presiding genius and Royer-Collard as their recognized head, French psychologists now settled down into an extraordinarily unimaginative and unproductive eclecticism. In the second quarter of the century the greatest figure was Cousin, whose contribution lay more in wide scholarship than in original observation.[1] Eclecticism was so general that during the entire half-century which followed Biran French psychology may be characterized as the influenced rather than the influencing psychology of western Europe. But, as we shall see, France did more than her share in the development of psychiatry and in the task of bringing psychiatry and psychology together.

Thomas Brown[2] was a representative of three schools of thought, Scottish, English, and French. He was Scottish in his background, his education and his academic position, ideally fitted for his post as Professor of Moral Philosophy at Edinburgh. He dominated the psychology of the day ; for he had a gift of exposition, the capacity to illustrate clearly, copiously, and in detail, which drew people of intelligence and influence.

He never abandoned that claim to prestige which the Scottish school had maintained through its emphasis upon the dignity of man and man's religious nature. He therefore maintained, both with scholars and with the public, the high position which the Scottish psychology had held before him. And he derived from the Scottish school one cardinal doctrine, the conception of unitary substance or principle ;

[1] The survival of voluntarism is indicated in his doctrine of the " spontaneity of the will."
[2] *Lectures on the Philosophy of the Human Mind* (1820).

in other words, the soul, whose affections and functions are the phenomena of psychology. This was the central Scottish teaching, in opposition to the notion of bits of experience fitted together by association. The mind was not a mosaic of pieces, but a unity of substance with varying manifestations. But he borrowed copiously from the associationists. Antipathy to physiological explanations was skilfully reconciled with a cordial assimilation of many associationist principles and constant recourse to their methods of observation. Beginning with the work of Brown, the Scottish school came definitely under the influence of English tradition. We must, therefore, consider Brown's work first of all in relation to the theory of association which had been so prominent for a half-century.

While accepting the principle of association as a key to psychology, Brown objected to the word " association." He used in its place the term " suggestion." " Association," through its derivation, implies that two things have become one. Association involves unification. Brown held that we find nothing in our mental life which shows that one piece of experience has been unified with another. Suppose that " four " makes us think of " five." This does not mean that these figures enjoy some kind of absorption in one another. Brown's term " suggestion " meant merely the process by which one idea *arouses* another. But this is no mere verbal manipulation ; Brown felt the need for an empirical treatment of the problem of mental connections.

It will be recalled that the Aristotelian principles of association by contiguity, similarity, and contrast had been reduced by Hartley to one fundamental pattern. Brown accepted Hartley's reduction of mental connections to one basic principle, which he called " co-existence " ; but this basic principle manifested itself in three forms, dependent on *resemblance, contrast*, and *nearness in time and space*. But now we come to this vital problem : when one thing is somehow connected with *two* or more other things, what is it that determines each particular course of association ? When, for example, *tiger* resembles both *leopard* and *lion*, why does *tiger* in some cases make us think of *leopard* and in other cases of *lion* ? Hobbes, in the middle of the seventeenth century, had vaguely seen the problem (see p. 19) but had given no satisfactory solution. Over one hundred and fifty years passed before anyone undertook a more detailed analysis of the principles determining particular associations. Hartley had gone into great detail with regard to the nature of association. He had considered, for example, such specific problems as the influence of emotion upon association, and had concerned himself with the analysis of complex life situations. But he had never undertaken to show how his laws worked in the determination of particular sequences to the exclusion of others ; he was not prepared to explain, for example, why one person when thinking of a bear thinks next of a lion, whereas another person is reminded of the practice of teaching bears to dance. We think of a great variety of things about bears, depending not only upon our past experience, but upon such things as the mood we are in, our constitutional make-up, and the like. Brown, grasping the significance of the problem, undertook an analysis of the many factors determining the course of association, the celebrated " secondary laws of association." These have a peculiarly modern ring. Much of the weakness of nineteenth century associationism could have been avoided if their importance had been recognized ; it was not until the last decades of the century that German and American experimentalists[1] discovered the necessity of taking such an analysis into account.

The first four of Brown's secondary laws have perhaps the most vital significance, but all are important as modifications of the associationist tendency to oversimplify. Brown's laws are thus summarized by Warren.[2]

(1) The relative *duration* of the original sensations : " The longer we dwell on objects, the more fully do we rely on our future remembrance of them."

(2) Their relative *liveliness :* " The parts of a train appear to be more closely and firmly associated as the original feelings have been more lively."

(3) Relative *frequency :* " The parts of any train are more readily suggested in proportion as they have been more frequently renewed."

(4) Relative *recency :* " Events which happened a few hours before are remembered when there is a total forgetfulness of what happened a few days before."

[1] Notably Külpe and Calkins.
[2] *A History of the Association Psychology* (1921), p. 73.

F

(5) Their coexistence in the past with *fewer alternative associates :* " The song which we have never heard but from one person can scarcely be heard again by us without recalling that person to our memory."

(6) *Constitutional differences* between individuals modify the primary laws : They give " greater proportional vigour to one set of tendencies of suggestion than to another."

(7) Variations in the *same individual,* " according to the varying emotion of the hour."

(8) " Temporary *diversities of state,*" as in intoxication, delirium, or ill-health.

(9) Prior *habits of life* and thought—the influence of inground tendencies upon any given situation, however new or irrelevant the experience may be.

The general laws of " suggestion " were now seen to operate in terms, for example, of the relative *recency, frequency,* and *liveliness* of particular experiences. The emphasis on emotional and constitutional factors was also significant and quite in contrast with the associationists' usual neglect of individual differences. It was a contribution of great moment, both to see the need of working out specific laws and also to think in terms of the individual as a whole in the determination of each specific sequence of thought.

Brown borrowed another important point from the English school, this time not from Hartley but from Locke. He returned to Locke's position as to the presence in our minds of certain capacities of a reflective nature as well as those of a merely sensory nature. Locke had taught that in addition to ideas derived directly from the senses, we have ideas derived from *reflection* upon the data given by the senses. Hartley had abandoned this position, believing that he could reduce all experience to the association of sensory elements. Now Brown, being unwilling to use the nervous system as an explanatory principle, could not regard images or ideas as mere reverberations of sensations. He could not reduce the idea to a faint copy of the original. Admitting no neurological explanations, he had to regard memory as a function independent of perception. The memory elements were not for him identical with the sensory elements ; they were independent entities. But if two objects are observed at the same time, and if we immediately become aware of the relation between the two, this is not a sensory function ;

it is a function definitely performed by the mind, as a mind. To perceive, for example, that one book is of a darker shade of red than another is to grasp a *relation* present in experience. If we see a large piece of chalk and a small one at the same time, we perceive instantly that one is larger than the other, and the perception of " larger than " comes into our minds not as a sensory element, but as a *relation*. This was another blow at associationism. Mental life was not a mere concatenation of sense-data, but was characterized by capacities to grasp relations. This was called by Brown " relative suggestion," as opposed to the " simple suggestion " by which one idea follows another by virtue of sensory experience. Strangely enough, " relative suggestion " was not treated as a part of perception, but was emphasized only as it appeared in such processes as comparison and judgment. These relational elements have been successively forgotten and re-discovered. Bain, for example, recognized them ; German psychologists re-discovered them in various guises late in the century. They have again come into their own in connection with the *Gestalt* school in recent years.

In addition to these obvious influences of the Scottish and the English schools, we have to take into account the fact that Brown had immersed himself in the writings of those French philosophers who were gently but effectively reinstating idealism in opposition to the mechanistic trend of the late eighteenth century. It was noted above that both Condillac and Cabanis had been popular because their mechanistic systems were in harmony with a widespread revolt against religious and spiritual interpretations. Similarly, the return of the pendulum to religion after the Revolution gave strength to the hands of those who sought to overthrow the mechanistic schools. The followers of Condillac[1] were amending his system by attributing some degree of *activity* to the individual ; and Cabanis, though himself a mechanist, had helped to point out the significance of activity in personality. An idealistic and religious turn of mind found therefore close at hand the materials for the construction of a new system. This group of " ideologists " took hold upon that polite part of society which was interested

---

[1] Among their greatest names were Laromiguière and De Tracy ; the former, greatly influenced by Biran's activism, influenced in turn the work of Brown.

in philosophy.   They were gentlemen of a sedate yet genial temperament.   They would not call ideas by unpleasant names, such as " mere sensation.''   But they were not so direct and flamboyant as Thomas Reid.   Their protest was orderly and courteous.   They represented a mild revolt against mechanism, but in terms compatible with good manners.   Their central principle was that mind is not a passive instrument for receiving impressions.   In specific revolt against Condillac they held that mind is essentially a thing which reacts, which has spontaneous activities of its own.   But theirs was scarcely a constructive move-ment.   It was an attempt to restore the broken handle rather than to mould a new vessel.

This philosophy had all the necessary elements to become popular in Scotland.   It was not only in harmony with the spiritual views of the Scottish school ; it had, in fact, much that had been absorbed indirectly or borrowed directly from Scotland.   Its specific alterations of associationist doctrine were useful and welcome to the Scottish school.   Brown mastered both Scottish and French systems ; his introduction of the French viewpoint and the French critique was, in fact, an enriching influence in his own system, and responsible in part for his popularity.   It was through French conceptions rather than Scottish ones that he saw how he could safely use the methods of the associationists while still rejecting their viewpoint.   Regarding the soul as a living and acting entity, he could without compromise accept most of the empirical analysis of Hartley and his followers.

One point in which French influence was especially clear was his emphasis on the " muscular sensations," the sen-sations which give awareness of the position of the limbs, and of opposition which they may meet in contact with out-side objects.   Some attention had been given to the muscle sense by physiologists ; its introduction into psychology was, however, chiefly the work of Brown.[1]   The muscle sense, said Brown, gives us our notion of resistance.   This was an elaboration of the ideologists' position ; it was similar also to the point which Biran was making, the idea that the " self " is in fact engendered by the resistance offered to the blind

---

[1] An addition to the traditional five senses naturally had to meet some opposition ; cumulative evidence from physiology led to its general acceptance by the middle of the century.

movements of early infancy. But Brown's treatment of the concept differs materially from Biran's. Instead of Biran's poetic and mystic treatment of the " will," leading to self-consciousness in the child, Brown's was a downright simple statement of the part played by muscular sensation in giving us awareness of the solidity of material things.

Brown's chief significance lay perhaps in the fact that he served to make the Scottish school more empirical. He made the school so closely acquainted with empirical and analytical methods that it could never quite go back to the firmly implanted dogmatism of its founder. The Scottish school began to become amalgamated with empiricism and associationism, and to lose its identity. But in Brown's hands associationism had for the first time undertaken a specific narrative of why we think and act in the particular ways forced upon us by particular occasions, while the interaction of " ideas " was replaced by acting individuals. Psychic atomism remained, to be sure, for a while ; as we shall see, it was incorporated in the thorough-going associationism of James Mill, with whom it reached its logical perfection and systematization. But Brown's work was the beginning of the end both of associationism and of the Scottish school. He had seen the necessity of empiricism, and had given new life to many of the bold endeavours of those who wished to analyse and systematize the furious complexity of experience. He had put an end for ever to the naïve formalism and pompous barrenness of the Scottish school. At the same time his conception of personality as a unity did much to give associationism that maturity and caution through which it attained its greatest achievements in the work of Spencer and Bain.

CHAPTER IV

THE origins of experimental psychology in Germany are to be sought in the intellectual development of western Europe in the late eighteenth and early nineteenth centuries; and most of all in the progress of other experimental sciences in France and Germany. We must turn first to the progress of the exact sciences, particularly mathematics, chemistry, and physics; next, to that of the biological sciences.[1] For experimental psychology grew out of the soil of an experimental physiology which was dependent upon all of these for its existence.

Experimental methods had yielded many and cumulative results in the natural sciences since the days of Gilbert and Galileo. The Newtonian mathematics had been eagerly adopted and developed in France, and became the central feature of French science. Whereas the experimental approach was more characteristic of English science, the most characteristic feature of French science was rather the development of mathematical methods. By the middle of the eighteenth century French mathematicians had won pre-eminence in the world.

In the middle of the seventeenth century the French Academy of Sciences found favour with Louis XIV; and from that time on it served as a central repository of scientific methods and results, as well as a centre for the mutual stimulation and encouragement of scientific men, a centre not merely for France but for the world. This was utterly unlike anything to be found in Britain or Germany. It is true that Newton took a leading part in the activities of the " Royal Society " in England, but it was never favoured by much royal support. A great British astronomer of the

---

[1] For a fuller treatment of the history of science in the eighteenth and early nineteenth centuries see Merz, *History of European Thought in the Nineteenth Century*, upon which I have chiefly relied.

period was forced to give part of his time to tutoring in order to get the wherewithal for his researches. The French, on the other hand, offered much encouragement to astronomical work. This matter of patronage was a prominent factor in causing the leadership of Newton in mathematics, great as it was, to give place to the leadership of the French school. There sprang up departmental centres for scientific study and research all over France, so that French science attained some degree of integration. French students everywhere co-operated ; local groups had opportunities to exchange ideas with one another, and many individuals went to Paris for study. Such close affiliation for scientific work was not dreamed of in England, nor in Germany.[1] Another instance of French leadership lay in the establishment of journals of mathematics in the decades just preceding the Revolution.

But the departmental centres and the journals were dependent on an all-important element, without which French intellectual leadership would have been frustrated, namely, national solidarity and a unity both political and cultural. Among the many economic factors which contributed to this national unity was the excellence of the French roads. The improvement of English roads through the introduction of French methods in the late eighteenth century seems to have done much to knit together groups whose intellectual co-operation had previously been hampered.

Whichever of these advantages we see fit to emphasize, the pre-eminence of the French in the exact sciences was apparent. The French had borrowed to such an extent the mechanical view of the universe, founded upon Newton's work, that we begin to find literary expression of it in the mid-eighteenth century, e.g., in Voltaire and Fontenelle. This gave to the reading public the unified view of the mechanical universe which had been discovered outside of France by Kepler, Galileo, and Newton. Voltaire was almost a popularizer of Newton ; he occupied himself with the task of turning over to the public that conception of the world which mathematics and physics had outlined.

[1] The German States which were parts of the Empire were held together in the loosest fashion ; while Prussia, though powerful, had a negligible influence as yet in the intellectual integration of the German-speaking States.

This task of popularization did not, of course, in Voltaire's time, really reach the masses ; it spread rapidly among the élite, but it was scarcely adapted for the labourer and the peasant. The Revolution brought about an immediate change. Educators sought to dispense with traditional subjects, and to found the whole system of public instruction upon natural science. Condorcet made the point that the mathematical sciences were of immediate importance to the public ; they strengthened the powers of observation, and the capacity for clear thinking. Moreover, they were of practical value in the problems of industry and war. Engaged, as France was, in war with most of the powers of western Europe, the use of mathematics for artillery, and of chemistry for explosives, was sure to be emphasized. Biological science had its place because of its relation to the training of military surgeons. Condorcet undertook then the task of educating the whole Republic in the exact sciences.

The Revolution inevitably interfered at first with research work, but it is surprising to note how much scientific investigation, even in fields not immediately practical, was carried on during this period of French isolation. Some individuals suffered, but most of the scientific work in progress was publicly recognized. And Napoleon acknowledged the importance of science and mathematics, for this added to his own personal prestige as well as to the value of his engineering and artillery officers.

Some of the specific contributions of French science may serve to show its spirit. By means of the differential and integral calculus it had been possible to work out the laws of the movements of heavenly bodies more adequately than seventeenth-century mathematicians had dared to dream. A little more than a century after Newton's *Principia* (1687), Laplace published his great books on celestial mechanics. He undertook to describe the evolution of the solar system from nebular substances (the view known as the " nebular hypothesis "). Laplace won wide recognition also through his " theory of probability." Tables showing the annual number of births, marriages, and deaths within a given group had been in use for more than a century ; but a sound mathematical understanding of the means of prediction from such tables (and the likelihood of variations of different magnitudes) was much needed. Laplace supplied the mathematical theory necessary for the first steps, so that, although his interest lay chiefly in pure rather than in applied mathematics, it was but natural that he should become statistician to Napoleon. The relatively simple conception of *quantities*, offered by Newton, was also subjected by French mathematicians to a critical analysis.

The discovery of oxygen by Priestley is another instance in which British work led rapidly to French elaboration both in theory and in practice. Almost all the chemists of first magnitude in the late eighteenth century were Frenchmen. It was Lavoisier who, just before the Revolution, succeeded first in laying down those general principles which made a unified experimental chemistry possible. Chemistry had been full of alchemy and a host of occult ideas ; there were no unifying laws which could be quantitatively stated. It was chiefly through the work of Lavoisier that a quantitative chemistry came into being. He also made many specific contributions ; he discovered, for example, the nature of respiration (the union of carbon with oxygen), one of the most important discoveries in physiological chemistry. The scope of chemical experimentation is indicated by the founding of journals for the publication of chemical research. This advance of chemistry in France was slow in reaching other nations, as the military situation tended to isolate France in respect to both pure science and its applications. Furthermore, the tradition of the isolation of individual investigators from one another still held sway in Great Britain, in sharp contrast to the co-operation and centralization which characterized French research.

On the other hand, it happened through a fortunate concatenation of circumstances that Germany began, early in the nineteenth century, to occupy herself with chemistry and physics. Chemistry in the German universities had been very dependent on French sources.[1] Practically all textbooks in the exact sciences in use in German (as in British) universities were in French, or were translations from the French. But within the university system of

[1] The dissemination of French science into Germany had, of course, been possible to some extent even during the Revolution and the Napoleonic era. A prominent figure in this task was von Humboldt, whose wide travels and international spirit had done much to acquaint Germany with French problems and methods.

Germany there began to arise shortly after the close of the Napoleonic era a group of men (some of them trained in France) who were prepared to introduce French ideas. The first decade of their work was essentially a continuation of the French tradition, but German chemistry soon acquired a distinct individuality.

Liebig founded in 1826 a university laboratory for the systematic study of chemistry. He became, indeed, the founder of a new division of chemistry; he devised suitable methods for the chemical study of some of the functions of living creatures, and for these the term " organic chemistry "[1] came into use. Borrowing, indeed, freely from contemporary French work, he probably did more than any other man to give German chemistry its enviable position in the three generations which have followed. Wöhler, his pupil, succeeded as early as 1828 in actually creating synthetically an organic compound, urea, and thus in throwing a bridge across the gulf which separated the inorganic from the organic.

At the same time other investigations which served to establish connection between the physical and the biological sciences were going on in many other countries. Galvani discovered (1791) the electrical current generated by stimulation of the frog's sciatic nerve. This was conceived by many to have tremendous philosophical significance. Some hastened to conclude that the intimate nature of life processes had been found, and that these processes were fundamentally different from the mechanical processes supposed to dominate the non-living. On the other hand, mechanists derived an equal consolation from it. It proved for them that physical principles were sufficient for the explanation of life. The same comment holds for Humboldt's discovery of the electrical discharge from the torpedo-fish. Men dreamed of bringing together on a scientific level those disciplines which we call physical on the one hand and biological on the other. The dream had been dreamt by many before; but these strange electrical phenomena which were actually under investigation gave new ground for the hope of unifying the physical with the biological sciences.

---

[1] The term gradually acquired its present meaning, the study of the compounds of carbon.

Contributions in the same direction were made by a series of discoveries in acoustics and optics. Chladni's work in acoustics was followed by Sir Thomas Young's celebrated statement of the wave-theory of light.[1] There followed throughout the first two decades of the nineteenth century an active controversy between the adherents of the Newtonian or corpuscular theory and those of the wave-theory. Optical phenomena necessitated physiological and psychological assumptions ; and Young himself formulated a three-colour theory (later supported by Helmholtz), according to which the retina is equipped with three kinds of colour-receptors, whose co-operative function gives the entire range of colours experienced. The Bohemian physiologist, Purkinje, made important observations on the brightness of colour in relation to the intensity of light. From such developments followed that experimental physiology of audition and vision which was later on to play so great a rôle in the establishment of an experimental psychology.

We may now turn our attention to the development of biological science. The first great step, perhaps, in the organization of modern biological research was the classification of species. As Cuvier very aptly remarked, to name well one must know well. Ray's seventeenth-century classification of species was extended by Linnaeus. Not only did Linnaeus know and classify thousands of plants (and animals), but, more significantly, he devised a *system* of classification, grouping individuals into species and species into genera, and indicating both by Latin (hence international) names. The conception of a " species " has undergone notable changes ; but the Linnean system has been of inestimable value.

The work of classification was carried forward and greatly enriched by Cuvier. His many contributions extend through the Revolutionary and Napoleonic eras. They give him rank with Bichat and Cabanis as a representative of French biological work as brilliant, though not as abundant, as the work in the physical sciences. His contribution consists

[1] *E.g., Course of Lectures on Natural Philosophy* (1807). The general conception goes back to the pioneer work of Huygens, in the Netherlands.

first of all in carrying out Linnaeus's idea of systematically grouping organisms, and noting the elements of similarity and difference observed in members of various species and genera.   He sought to make possible a classification which would not only give names to organisms, but would show their true resemblances and differences by noting which similarities were significant and fundamental, and which were superficial or without significance.   In spite of the lead taken by Lamarck, Erasmus Darwin, and others, Cuvier definitely opposed the evolutionary theory,[1] which would have been most useful as a genetic method of classification. But he was an anatomist of such insight that he was able to lay down fundamental principles of wide general validity ; he is generally recognized as the father of modern comparative anatomy.   It is interesting to note that Cuvier relied chiefly not on the structure of bones, muscles, or sense-organs, but on the central nervous system, as the most reliable single criterion of classification.

Another feature of importance in Cuvier's career is the fact that he was the first person to make a systematic survey of all the scientific work done each year.   These surveys were in the form of reports to Napoleon.   Together with *Éloges* delivered upon the deaths of great scientists, these mark a further advance in the establishment of central storehouses of scientific information.   The group of physiologists and anatomists to which Cuvier belonged gave France—in fact we may say specifically the city of Paris—almost as definite a position of leadership in biological science as it enjoyed in physical science.

But in the early nineteenth century a variety of forces became apparent, by which a new place in the study of the biological sciences was won by Germany.   To understand these, attention must be turned to the German university system, in which, during the eighteenth century, a series of important developments had been taking place.   We must take account of some of the intellectual trends of the period, in order to see how Germany was able to make contributions in physiology which it had been denied France to accomplish.

The German university during the Middle Ages typically included three faculties : a faculty of theology, a faculty of

[1] See p. 118,

law, and a faculty of medicine. These three faculties were virtually professional schools. No general or liberal arts course was provided. If a student went to the university he usually prepared himself for one of these three professions (or he might become a doctor of the civil and canon law at the same time, taking the degree of *Doctor of Laws*, the origin of the honorary LL.D.). There was a general neglect of scientific courses, except as they forced themselves into the medical curriculum. In the eighteenth century (in the year 1734, to be exact) a faculty of philosophy was founded at Göttingen, the aim of which was to give instruction not for the specific purpose of training for a professional career but for the purpose of providing what we should now call a "liberal education." This involved the establishment of chairs for some subjects which had traditionally been a part of the three older faculties, and some chairs for subjects newly introduced. The faculty of philosophy included such subjects as mathematics and physics ; history ; history of literature ; oriental languages; as well as two chairs for various subdivisions of philosophy, and a professorship of philosophy "without special definition." Carlyle's Teufels-dröckh, professor of "things in general," was perhaps a reminiscence of such chairs without portfolio. This new faculty was rapidly copied all through the German-speaking world.

During the eighteenth century science became an important part of the German university curriculum ; but "science" (*Wissenschaft*) took on a distinctive meaning. In France, science had come to mean mathematics or "exact science." German scholars attacked the problem of phonetics and of language ; they developed philological technique. At the same time they were applying critical methods to the study of literature, developing in particular the technique of Biblical criticism, and working out general principles by which it was possible to ascertain, for example, the date and authorship of ancient manuscripts. They improved the methods of history and archæology. They devoted themselves to the problem of evaluating historical source material. Baumgarten's attempt to found a science of æsthetics, Kant's critical approach to the process of cognition, and Hegel's revision of logic under the term "dialectic," are parts of an extensive movement already well under way ; they were works of *Wissenschaft*,[1] just as truly as were experiments in physics. The application of critical methods to such a variety of subjects, and the interdependence of all these, brought it about that the German university teacher and student had but little of the departmental turn of thought which inevitably influenced the French student. The German faculty of philosophy served as a means of attaining a broad view of civilization as a whole. The German university was an engine with which to create a unified knowledge of the world.

Together with this ideal of the unity of all human knowledge—the idea that a scholar should be equally versed in history and mathematics, in oriental languages and in contemporary political issues—there was also the feeling that the phenomena of life, as represented by the biological sciences, were to be viewed not merely in the perspective of chemistry and physics, but in their relation to these other disciplines. No single approach could suffice in the study of so complex a thing as life ; there must be in life some kind of unity or connection, at least in treatment if not in subject-matter. There had been in both Britain and France a considerable skepticism about the possibility of building up a scientific technique for the study of living things. But in the German university the phenomena of life were subjected to the same critical treatment and seen in the same perspective as was required in any other specialty. The study of life must be undertaken from a unified philosophical world-view.

It is natural to ask how there could be uniformity of treatment in spite of the fact that there were over twenty universities in Germany, politically separated, each man teaching from his own point of view. Such a possibility resulted from the exchange of professors between universities and the students' habit of moving about from one institution to another, customs still prevalent and vitally important in the unification of German thought. It never occurred to the German student that there ought to be any local continuity in his course towards a degree. This exposure to many influences augmented the tendency to seek for a unified view of the world and the desire to see life as a whole. The

---

[1] Such " cultural sciences " (*Geisteswissenschaften*) are distinguished from the " natural sciences " (*Naturwissenschaften*).

secondary schools received to some extent the benefit of such interchange. Teachers in the secondary schools were promoted to higher teaching, and teachers in the universities went back at times to the secondary schools.

One who did a great deal to point out the unity between the sciences was Haller, the physiologist of Göttingen, who flourished in the middle of the eighteenth century. Profoundly influenced by his teacher, the Dutch physiologist Boerhaave, he sought to treat human and animal life, chemistry and physics, as a unity. He gave to German students the conception that the empirical approach—in particular, the experimental method—which the British and French were using in the physical sciences, could be applied to life processes ; in other words, the notion of physiology as an experimental science was established. The importance of this conception can only be realized when we consider the extraordinary degree to which biological science had been occupied with the astrological and the occult. Even the great teacher, Paracelsus, who did so much to establish a chemical view of life processes, made extensive use of astrological principles ; even the intrinsically helpful notion of humours in the blood was confused with much that was incapable of any sort of verification. Haller has been called the father of modern physiology.[1] He published a textbook which remained for three-quarters of a century the standard text on physiology for the world.[2]

The university system, and the leadership of Haller and his pupils, are thought to have been mainly responsible for the fact that the biological sciences came into a certain vogue in Germany towards the end of the eighteenth century ; the science of living things absorbed more attention than was given to the physical sciences. We may say, to put it negatively, that the reason why the French and British had given biology a secondary place was their preference for quantitative analysis. They could approach physics and chemistry with mathematical methods. They could not understand that the biological sciences could be experimentally or mathematically approached. While the

---

[1] Harvey had, of course, shown the way, and many clinicians had contributed important empirical studies of physiological functions, side by side with the rapid progress of anatomy.

[2] Until the publication of Johannes Müller's text book. See p. 99.

British and French thought the biological sciences incapable of being genuinely scientific, the Germans thought every field of knowledge could be equally scientific. Even the analysis of the knowing process itself (as Kant undertook to show) could become an exact and systematic discipline.

But we have to consider another factor which this statement disregards. We may recall the extraordinary development of the interest which Germany of the "romantic" period showed in living things, as something distinct from the world of matter and motion. Something in the German temperament of the time reached out toward the comprehension of life.[1] There is, of course, no need to designate this as a permanent national trait ; the same general tendency was apparent in Italy during the Renaissance. One might be tempted, and not entirely without justice, to say that this is the arrival of the Renaissance in Germany. One might be tempted to say that Germany, isolated from the rest of western Europe through a series of wars and through such influences as the surviving feudalism of the Holy Roman Empire, had its awakening in the eighteenth century, so that problems of the nature of life won a prominent place outside of as well as within the university system. All this development of the biological sciences in Germany might be regarded as part of a general cultural movement. It would be too dogmatic to say that the German university was the sole explanation for the popularity of biology.

A familiar illustration of the German spirit of the time is the personality and career of Goethe, who was so great as a poet that few people thought of him as a scientist. But he was, in fact, responsible for two important biological contributions. He was one of the first of the moderns to put forward a theory of organic evolution ; and he elaborated a significant theory of colour vision.[2] In opposition to Young's three-colour theory, he undertook to show that one cannot account for the facts of colour-blindness, colour contrast, and negative after-images without postulating at least four primary colours. Goethe made also a number

---

[1] Eighteenth-century France and Britain witnessed, of course, striking romantic movements. But the tendency to speak of the "romantic movement" as essentially German is perhaps evidence for the view suggested. But we are dealing with a question of degree and definitive demonstration of the point is, of course, impossible.

[2] *Farbenlehre* (1810).

of contributions to botany, which would have sufficed to render him illustrious, were they not overshadowed by his position in literature and philosophy. It was not only in the universities that the growing study of life processes was manifest.

On the other hand, the main current of this development undoubtedly did flow in the universities. It reached its greatest height after the Napoleonic period in the brilliant physiological researches of Weber and Johannes Müller and their pupils. (To these men we shall later devote special attention; for the present it is important only to show their relation to the general movement indicated.) We saw above how Liebig and Wöhler worked together to found the science of organic chemistry, and how a link had been forged between the inorganic chemistry of Lavoisier and the study of life. While this was going on, botanists and zoologists sought with the aid of the microscope to discover a connection between physical principles and the principles of form which underlie the structure of living things. They were trying to do in the field of morphology what Liebig had done in the field of chemistry. A great step had already been taken in France in the closing years of the eighteenth century by Bichat's demonstration of the relation between organs and the fundamental structures (the tissues) which composed them. In Germany a new step was now taken by Schleiden, who demonstrated in 1838 that all plant tissues were made up of cells, each cell being in some respects an independent unit. Two years later Schwann succeeded in showing that the same principles held for animal tissues. The study of life processes was enormously furthered by these two epoch-making discoveries; the knowledge of the cellular constitution of living matter made possible the analysis and classification of microscopic structures. The discovery of such structural units was of far-reaching consequence, not only for anatomy but for physiology. The science of embryology was also established in Germany[1] in the period under discussion.

Germany held, by the middle of the century, a position of leadership in biological science, which, as we have seen, was due very largely to a certain background of intellectual history that differentiated its specific problems from those

[1] By von Baer.

of France and Britain. While this widespread movement was going on in Germany there were many brilliant biological researches under way in England, in the hands of individuals who enjoyed no such co-operation and no such profound intellectual stimulus as were vouchsafed to the German scientist. The most notable of these was Sir Charles Bell's discovery of the principle of differentiation of sensory and motor nerves. Galen, to be sure, had known of sensory and motor nerve-functions. But it was supposed that nerves possessed in general *both* sensory and motor functions, and it remained for Bell to show that some structures are sensory, others motor—that immediately before entering the spinal cord the sensory fibres group themselves into the dorsal, and the motor fibres into the ventral, root of each nerve.[1] He laid the foundation for a detailed study of nervous physiology in terms of the incoming and out-going pathways. He suggested also that the division of labour might be still more detailed ; that in spite of mor-phologic similarity the *variety* of mental functions might be based on a variety of specialized tasks carried out by many functionally distinct nervous elements.[2] The lack of inter-national co-operation in this period is well shown in the fact that many years passed before Johannes Müller[3] undertook the elaboration of these two doctrines of Bell, experimentally verifying the former and stating the latter in the famous formula of " specific energies." Bell's epoch-making dis-covery regarding sensory and motor roots seems in fact to have attracted but little attention until Müller's time.[4]

[1] His *New Idea of the Anatomy of the Brain* (1811) was followed by a number of papers read before the Royal Society. See Carmichael, " Sir Charles Bell : A Contribution to the History of Physiological Psychology," *Psychol. Rev.*, XXXIII, 1926.

[2] In essence, the idea is really a very old one, and the eighteenth century had revived it. Bonnet had grasped it quite clearly : " . . . there are in each sense certain fibres which are appropriate to each kind of sensation. . . . There are consequently still among the fibres of vision certain differences corresponding to those which exist among the rays."—*Analyse abrégée de l'essai analytique* (1779–83), VI, X.

[3] See p. 96.

[4] Though Magendie, in France, did experimental work on the problem in the 'twenties.

PART II

From Weber's Experiments to the Age of Wundt

CHAPTER V

THE BEGINNINGS OF EXPERIMENTAL PSYCHOLOGY

The art of measurement would do away with the effect of
appearance. . . . They err not only from defect of knowledge in
general, but of that particular knowledge which is called measuring.—
Plato.

THE rise of the biological sciences in Germany led quickly
to a brilliant personification of the movement in E. H.
Weber. He was one of three brothers illustrious in the
natural sciences. Whereas the others devoted themselves to
physical science, his own work was centred in the physiology
of the sense-organs. Research upon the sense-organs and
their functions in Germany, as well as in France and England
had been confined almost entirely to the higher senses,
seeing and hearing. His work consisted largely in opening
up new experimental fields, notably research upon the
cutaneous and muscular sensations.

He began shortly before 1820 to teach anatomy and
physiology at the University of Leipzig, where he remained
throughout his career. His life was characterized by the
constant publication of new work and the stimulation of a
large number of students ; medical students for the most
part, for medicine held the supremacy among the biological
sciences, and physiology as an independent science did not
yet exist. He was more or less under the influence of the
" philosophy of Nature," with its belief in spirit expressing
itself through physical symbols, and in the realization of
values not found in the mechanical world. Weber was,
nevertheless, a physiologist who separated his philosophy
from his experiments. His results stand solid, and
independent of his attachment to the more or less
speculative viewpoint of the period.

He conducted classical investigations on the temperature-sense and on the sense of smell. He offered a theory to the effect that the experience of warmth and cold is not dependent directly on the temperature of the stimulating object, but on the *increase* and *decrease* of the temperature of the skin. If the hand is placed in warm water, the rising temperature of the skin leads to the experience which we call warmth. The skin temperature may rise or fall without occasioning the experience of warmth or cold if the change is very gradual. This theory accounts well for the adaptation or habituation which makes warmth or cold less noticeable after the skin has been exposed to it for some time. Another of his minor experiments aimed to determine whether liquids or gases are the true stimuli for the sense of smell. He put a ten per cent. solution of *eau de cologne* into his nose, and tilted his head so as to bring the liquid into contact with the nasal mucous membrane. Finding that no sensation of smell was received, he concluded that liquids are not direct olfactory stimuli.

He experimented also upon vision and hearing. As an example of the experiments in vision, we may name one in which he undertook to determine the smallest arc that would permit discrimination of two lines. When the lines are exceedingly close together we get the impression of one line, while if they are not so close we see two distinct lines ; he measured the arc necessary for such distinction. Instances of his work on audition are the discovery that if he held a ticking watch at each ear he was less proficient in judging whether the ticks were simultaneous than if the two watches were held at the same ear.

To one experiment of Weber we must give much more attention.[1] It had to do with the distance that must separate two stimuli applied to the skin, in order to bring about the perception of doubleness. This was, of course, the same experiment within the field of *cutaneous* sensation which we noted above in the field of vision. Precautions being taken to exclude the use of vision, the subject's skin was stimulated, sometimes with one compass-point, sometimes with two, the distances between the two points being

[1] Wagner's *Handwörterbuch d. Physiol.*, III, ii, 529 f., (1846) ; separately published as *Der Tastsinn und das Gemeingefühl* (1849).

constantly varied. As the distance increased, with two-point stimulation, the subject passed from the impression of one clear-cut stimulus to an impression of blurring, or uncertainty as to whether there was one or two, and thence on to a state where he was quite definitely aware that there were two points of stimulation. There was, in other words, a threshold (*limen*) to be crossed before the impression of doubleness could be evoked. He established a " two-point threshold." The concept of the *threshold*, so widely used in the measurement of stimuli and the relations between them, was first systematically used by Weber. Now Weber found that the two-point threshold, the distance necessary to make possible the discrimination of doubleness, varied in different parts of the body, in fact, varied enormously. It was smallest on the tips of the fingers and the tip of the tongue. It was somewhat greater on the lips, greater still on the palm and wrists, and increased toward the shoulder. Further, the threshold for a given region varied with different individuals.

Weber concerned himself with the theoretical interpretation of these results ; and for about fifty years his interpretation, although distinctly secondary in importance to his results, attracted considerable attention. He put forward the hypothesis that the " sensation circles " (areas within which doubleness is not perceived) must contain a number of nerve-fibres, and that unstimulated fibres must lie between the two stimulated, if doubleness is to be perceived. Weber himself refused to resort to the simple assumption that there is *one* nerve fibre for each circle. Serious difficulty was encountered in the fact that subjects showed marked effects of training ; the circles became smaller with practice. Other difficulties have arisen, and the theory has lost ground.[1] Weber's experimental method was, however, of much more permanent significance than his explanation of the results.

Even more important, perhaps in Weber's own mind the most important of his contributions, was his examination of the muscle sense.[2] It was while exploring the muscle

[1] The work of Blix and Goldscheider (see p. 179) showed that there are many " touch-spots " in each sensation-circle.

[2] Published in instalments (1829-34), reprinted under the title *De Tactu* (1851).

sense that he made the discovery with which his name is chiefly identified. Physiologists had come to recognize that sensory impulses arise not only from the outside but from the interior of the limbs. Thomas Brown had emphasized the important part which these muscular sensations play in detecting resistance offered to our movements. Weber undertook an experiment to find out to what extent muscular sensations function in the discrimination of weights of different magnitude. He found that if the subject lifted weights with his hand in such a way as to experience not only tactual sensations, but also muscular sensations from the hands and arms, he discriminated very much more accurately than when weights were laid upon the resting hand. He made use of four subjects whose results were quite consistent in showing the great superiority of those judgments in which the muscle sense was used. Weber worked with two sets of weights, the standard weight being 32 ounces in the one set and 4 ounces (32 drachmæ) in the other. He later undertook another series of experiments with a standard weight of $7\frac{1}{2}$ ounces. In the latter experiment the conditions were systematically varied ; the weights were, for example, applied both simultaneously and successively. In all these experiments, the fact emerged that discrimination depended not upon the absolute magnitude of the difference between two weights, but upon the ratio of this magnitude to the magnitude of the standard. Under the most favourable circumstances, the difference between the weights was correctly perceived when they bore roughly the ratio 29 : 30. Using touch alone, the necessary difference was roughly one-fourth of the standard weight, but again proved to be not an absolute quantity, but a fraction depending on the relative magnitude of the stimuli. From these facts of muscular and cutaneous sensation he reached the conclusion that the ability to discriminate between two stimuli depends not on the absolute magnitude of the difference, but upon a relative difference statable in terms of their ratio to one another.

He saw that the " just noticeable difference " could be stated as a fraction, which, though constant within a given sense-modality, varied with the sense tested. This led him to inquire whether there was not evidence from other sense-modalities to support the general principle that discrimination depends not on the absolute difference of stimulus magnitudes but on their relation to one another. Accordingly, he undertook experiments in vision which bore on the same problem. He presented pairs of straight lines, requesting the subject to state which of the lines was longer, if either was judged longer than the other. The results of this experiment confirmed the principle of " relativity " which he had already found. Here the fraction was even smaller than in the case of the muscle sense experiments ; visual discrimination between two lines was possible if one was from a hundredth to a fiftieth longer than the other, that is, one or two per cent.[1] The fraction for a given subject at a given time was roughly constant, and independent of the length of the " standard " line. This led Weber to the bold hypothesis that we can lay down for *each* of the senses a *constant fraction* for " just noticeable differences." He was misled, however, by his experiments with visual stimuli ; these really involved to some extent sensations from the external eye-muscles, and did not directly settle the question of the discrimination of visual intensities.

Just before the period of these experiments Delezenne,[2] who was working in the field of acoustics, had hit upon the fact that if a wire of a certain length and tension was struck, and its pitch compared with that of a similar but slightly longer wire, a constant difference in the length of the wires was necessary to make possible a correct pitch-discrimination. He worked with 240 vibrations per second as a standard, and found how much higher the pitch of the second tone had to be in order to enable the subject to distinguish it from the standard. Weber seized upon this observation as another instance of his law. But, as Delezenne had used only one standard, Weber was mistaken in utilizing this conclusion in support of his own. From the results of all the experiments noted, Weber believed that his general principle was founded on facts from the skin, muscle, eye, and ear.

---

[1] This holds for simultaneous presentation. With successive presentation a five per cent. difference was needed.
[2] *Recueil des travaux de la société des sciences de Lille* (1826).

It would be hard to over-emphasize Weber's importance in the genesis of an experimental psychology. His interest in physiological experimentation served to turn the attention of physiologists to the legitimacy and importance of approaching in the laboratory certain genuinely psychological problems which had throughout history been neglected. Not only did he set problems which occupied men of the ability of Helmholtz, Fechner, and Lotze, but he himself attacked a great many of these problems, and pointed the way to their systematic study.

An illustration will show the extent to which he could transform the problems of the physicist and the physiologist. An experiment had been carried out in France (by Bouguer) a generation before Weber's time, in which the sensitiveness of the eye to light was measured by varying the relative positions of candles and pinholes through which light reached a screen beyond. In order to make a faint shadow distinguishable from a shadowed area adjacent to it, it was found that the illumination of the two must differ by one sixty-fourth. The problem led to no principle of any particular consequence. Yet it was in embryo the problem of " just noticeable differences." It was just such a problem as in the hands of a Weber might have become a corner-stone of epoch-making research.

It is no accident that work like Weber's came when and where it did. German intellectual history for a century had paved the way ; the influence of Haller still lived, enriched by the brilliant French discoveries of the late eighteenth century, which had been adopted with new energy by the German universities in the early years of the nineteenth century. Important as it may be to plant wisely the seed of an experimental project, the soil is no less important. When Hamilton, a few years later, undertook to study experimentally some problems in attention, nothing of significance resulted in British psychology ; associationism and the Scottish school were alike uninterested. The crucial point was that in Germany experimental physiology was solidly established with quantitative methods and with a wide outlook. These many investigations conducted by Weber, such as the problem of the " just noticeable differences ", were throughout envisaged in quantitative terms ; and the last of these was experimental in the more restricted modern sense, several different factors being varied in order to isolate the significance of each. Weber ventured, moreover, to bring together an array of results under a common law, a universal principle. Important as this law was to become as a hypothesis for voluminous research, Weber's greatest significance lies rather in his conception of an experimental approach to psychological questions, and in the stimulation of research through which ultimately a vast variety of problems other than his have been inductively studied.

Nothing could be more misleading than to study Fechner as a follower of Weber, as if he were simply an echo or a reflected light from the great physiologist. A moment's glance at Fechner's early life shows how soon his characteristic genius displayed itself.

He started his career as a student of medicine, and of physics and chemistry, at Leipzig, where he began to give instruction a few years later. He interested himself especially in contemporary discoveries in mechanics and electricity. His earliest writings, consisting of scientific treatises and translations from French experimental contributions, show how, as a young man, he mastered the physical sciences of his day. But he began before long a series of brief articles of purely literary design. Among these, one of the purest gems is the *Little Book of Life After Death* (1836). In this he strove to show how we are, as it were, all parts of one another, living in each other so fully that, as long as human life continues, no individual can die. He was studying the philosophy of Fichte and Schelling also, and beginning to give literary expression to the feelings it kindled within him. And he was very deeply stirred by the "philosophy of Nature," which was dominated by the desire to find a spiritual meaning in all the events of the natural order.

The source of this many-sided distribution of interests was the problem : " How can quantitative science teach us to study the human spirit in its relation to the universe ? How can those exact methods which have been applied so successfully in the natural sciences be turned to advantage in the study of the inner world ? How can we ever see the

soul under conditions of direct and reportable observation ? "
As we are told by J. T. Merz :

> " He became acquainted with the philosophy of Schelling,
> Oken, and Steffens, which dazzled him, touched the poetical
> and mystical side of his nature, and, though he hardly understood
> it, had a lasting influence on him.   The simultaneous occupation
> with the best scientific literature of the day (he translated French
> text-books such as those of Biot and Thénard, and verified Ohm's
> law èxperimentally), however, forced upon him the sceptical
> reflection whether, ' of all the beautiful orderly connection of
> optical phenomena, so clearly expounded by Biot, anything could
> have been found out by Oken-Schelling's method ? '   This mixture
> or alternation of exact science and speculation, of faithfulness and
> loyalty to facts as well as to theory, runs through all Fechner's
> life, work, and writings."[1]

It is easy to see why he was both a follower of the
" philosophy of Nature " and one of its most ardent
opponents.   He did not come to this attitude hastily ; he
felt about for a way.   He knew vaguely what it was that
he sought, but there was no movement which undertook
the thing he wanted, no school with which he could affiliate.
Reaching in one direction and another, he was bewildered
by the complexity of the spiritual heritage, and the futility
of stating and cataloguing it in the terms of those sciences
in which he was at home.   He began then, in a series of
satirical writings under the name of Dr. Mises, to assert
a negative expression of what he felt ; he began to satirize
mechanistic science.   The attempt to bring the biological
sciences into terms similar to those of mathematics and
physics seemed to him to involve the repudiation of biology
and psychology, because this attempt seemed to repudiate
life and mind at the outset.   The attempt to transfer the
methods of physics and chemistry into biology and
psychology meant for him a retreat from the self-evident
world of life of which we are a part ; it meant also the denial
of the living reality of the whole universe, every fibre and
atom of which was for him equally alive and meaningful.

From these satires it is apparent that he had not achieved
in his own mind the first statement of his problem.   He
could not begin to solve his problem because he could not
quite state it.   He felt, on the one hand, the need of an
exact method in order to make headway in biological and

psychological science ; but, at the same time, the existing methods could never interpret the events which they recorded. While he groped about, satirizing quantitative science under a pseudonym, he was at the same time carrying on exact research in the field of physics—was identified, for example, with investigations into the atomic theory. While teaching in the class-room the physics of the day, he was constantly trying to see a way in which satire could be replaced by a new understanding of the subject-matter of science, an understanding which would make both the human soul and the objects which it knows equally accessible to methods by which real knowledge can be amassed.

During this period Fechner suffered from a progressively severe illness ; perhaps it was the sort of illness that is now vaguely called a " nervous breakdown." He persisted in increasing his difficulties by undertaking the study of positive after-images from bright stimuli, particularly the sun. Violent pain in his eyes and partial blindness resulted, from which he did not recover for several years. The earlier disorder, complicated by the inability to read, and apparently even the inability to think clearly without great difficulty, caused something verging upon a collapse. His wife, however, brought him through this difficult time and he gradually recovered.

As the vigorous use of his mind returned to him, he began to ponder again on the relation of mental to physical pro-cesses, and the possibility of discovering a definite relation between them. One day the discovery burst upon him that there is one sort of quantitative relation observable in daily life, namely, that the intensity of sensation does not increase in a one-to-one correspondence with an increasing stimulus, but rather in an arithmetical series which may be contrasted with the geometrical series which characterizes the stimulus. If one bell is ringing, the addition of a second bell makes much more impression upon us than the addition of one bell to ten bells already ringing ; if four or five candles are burning, the addition of another makes a scarcely dis-tinguishable difference, while if it appeared with only two its psychic effect would be considerable. The effects of stimuli are not absolute, but relative ; relative, that is, to the amount of sensation already existing. It occurred to him that for each sense-modality there might be a certain relative increase in the stimulus which would always produce a certain intensification of the sensation ; and this ratio would hold for the entire range through which the stimuli might be made to increase. We might say, for example, that sensations increase arithmetically, according to a formula in which we need only to know the constants which determine the rate of geometrical progression for the different sense-modalities. This he stated as :

$$S = C \log R$$

where S is sensation, C is a constant for each of the different fields of sense, and R is the stimulus.

In this same period (1851) he published a sort of philosophy of Nature of his own, entitled the *Zend-Avesta*, its title reflecting the incursion of the philosophy of Asia during the middle of the century. The Persian system, with its fundamental dualism, in which good and evil centre in personal beings, laid hold upon Fechner's imagination ; through it the world could be seen to be really personal, really alive. It absorbed Fechner partly because it made possible the personal interpretation of the natural world, a world not seen, however, as an antithesis between natural and supernatural, but natural and spiritual at once. This gave him the desired antithesis to the science of his day ; it gave the universe a soul, or rather a plurality of souls. In the *Zend-Avesta* Fechner mentioned that he had recently discovered a simple mathematical relation between the spiritual and the physical world.

He now undertook a series of experiments on brightness and lifted weights, visual and tactual distances, to test his hypothesis regarding the relation of sensation-intensities to stimulus-intensities. Immediately after beginning these he happened upon the work of Weber, which had commenced a quarter-century before. Weber had shown that there appeared to be a definite law governing the relation between the intensities of stimulation and the ability to distinguish which of two stimuli was the greater. The " just noticeable difference " is a constant fraction of the standard stimulus. This principle, laid down by Weber, seemed to Fechner to be a mathematical generalization of great importance. Fechner saw its relation to his own hypothesis. He seized upon it, made much of it, and proceeded to extend enormously the experimental work to confirm it. But the difference between Fechner's hypothesis and Weber's is immense. Weber had concerned himself with " just noticeable differences," but Fechner could only be satisfied with a mathematical statement of the relation of the physical to the spiritual world.

Fechner's formula had to be put to the test of long and arduous experimentation. He had, of course, to use two supplementary hypotheses : first, that sensations can be measured (for example, three units of loudness), and second, that there is a zero point for all sensation (leading to mathematical difficulties in handling the sensation when the stimulus decreases below the zero-point of the sensation). Both points became the subject of endless controversy, but both, as Fechner realized from the beginning, were essential to the very core of his purpose. For in this measurement of sensation, as he explicitly stated over and over again, his one purpose was to find the quantitative relation of the objective to the subjective world. The longing to grasp the meaning of the world in terms which would articulate with the scientific methods of his day, that is, to find the relation between the qualities of experience and the quantities of science—this was the thing which forced the treatment of qualities into the quantitative mould. If he laid a foundation for one great subdivision of experimental psychology, seeking to confirm his law in as many fields and through as many methods as possible, it was in the service of a struggle to find confirmation for his mystical conviction. The magnitude of the man is shown not only by the elaborateness and ingenuity of the experimental approach, but by the patience and honesty with which errors and discrepancies, pitfalls and disappointments, were recognized.

A closer examination of the most important of Fechner's psychophysical methods is necessary. Weber's law remained his guiding principle. He carried on his experiments, stimulated by this discovery, for seven or eight years before he gave any account of his methods or his findings to the public. The first presentation of his work (1858) was a paper on mental measurement, a forerunner of the *Elemente der Psychophysik*, which appeared in 1860. In the *Elemente*,

psychophysics was defined as an exact science of the functional relations or relations of dependence between body and
mind.   Its sphere included sensation, perception, feeling,
action, attention, etc.   He selected sensation as most susceptible of measurement at that stage of the science, and
developed his methods on the basis of the fundamental
principle that sensation is a measurable magnitude.   That is,
any sensation is the sum of a number of *sensation-units*, and
these units can be standardized by the aid of the correlated
stimuli.[1]

Weber had, it will be remembered, used the method of
" just noticeable differences."   This method Fechner
developed during the course of his work on vision and
temperature sensations.[2]   He used Weber's method of
presenting two like stimuli and increasing or diminishing
one of them until a difference became noticeable.   Fechner,
however, recommended approaching the just noticeable
difference from both directions, and averaging the just
noticeable differences obtained from the ascending and
descending approach.[3]

---

[1] Of course, the ideal of psychophysics is to measure the relation
of subjective intensities to the bodily intensities which accompany
them, *e.g.*, to compare sensations with brain changes.   This realm
of " inner psychophysics " was regarded by Fechner as free from
those inconsistencies and errors which attend " outer psychophysics "
(in which the stimulus rather than the bodily response is compared
with subjective intensities).   Outer psychophysics was accepted only
because it was more immediately practicable.

[2] Fechner's insistence on the psychophysical value of the method
of just noticeable differences is not justified by the results of
experimentation since his time, although the *psychological* value of
the method remains almost undisputed.   See Titchener, *Experimental
Psychology* (1905), II, Part 2, cxiii.

[3] He did not sufficiently appreciate the value of making a carefully
graded approach from a difference greater or less than the just noticeable difference.   This modification was made by G. E. Müller (*Zur
Grundlegung der Psychophysik*, 1878), who did not, however, make
large use of the method.   Wundt worked out the method with this
modification of small gradations, and extended its use under the name
of the method of " minimal changes."   Wundt insisted that judgments
of just noticeable difference were determined under the cumulative
influence of previous judgments, and that their significance was,
therefore, psychological rather than psychophysical. (*Principles of
Physiological Psychology*, 1873-4, pp. 295 and 326 f.)   Wundt emphasized
also the method of " mean gradations," in which the subject adjusts a
stimulus so that it seems midway between two others.

The method of "right and wrong cases," although originated by Vierordt,[1] was developed and established as a tool for psychophysics by Fechner. It was the method which Fechner used in his elaborate work with lifted weights, involving over 67,000 comparisons. In contrast to the method just described, in which the stimuli vary and a constant judgment is sought (the judgment of the just noticeable difference), the method of right and wrong cases depends on constant stimuli and varying judgments. The aim of the method, according to Fechner, was to measure the difference between stimuli which was required to produce a given proportion of right judgments. Fechner found it possible, by the use of an intricate mathematical formula, to simplify the procedure of measuring sensitivity by this method. Thus, instead of arriving at the desired difference after experimentation with a number of differences, one small difference was decided upon with which the series of judgments was to be made. This difference was large enough so that it would be recognized most of the time, but not large enough to be recognized invariably. The right, wrong, and doubtful judgments were computed to give the measure of the perceptibility of this chosen difference. The formula, based upon the theory of probability, then made possible the computation of the difference required to give the percentage of right cases desired.[2]

In co-operation with Volkmann, Fechner developed the method of "average error" (already in use in astronomy) for use in visual and tactual measurement. The procedure is based upon the recognition that errors of observation and judgment depend not only on variable factors in the situation or within the observer himself, but, most significantly, upon the magnitude and variability of the observer's sensitivity, or the amount and variability of the difference between stimuli required to be noticeable. This method involves

---

[1] Hegelmayer, *Vierordt's Arch. f. physiol. Heilkunde*, XI, 1852.
[2] G. E. Müller (*op. cit.*) objected that Fechner did not distinguish between the measure of precision of the observer and the true difference required for correct judgments ; he also objected to Fechner's method of disposition of the doubtful judgments by dividing them between the right and wrong judgments. He worked out formulæ for the right, wrong, and doubtful cases, and measured both precision and sensitivity.

the adjustment of a variable stimulus to subjective equality with a given constant stimulus. Under controlled test conditions the mean value of the differences between the given stimulus and the " error " stimulus (adjusted by the observer) will represent the subject's error of observation. When applied to lifted weights the method is simply as follows : the subject takes an accurately measured weight as the norm, and attempts to make a second (or " error " weight) equal to it. When he is satisfied of the equality of the two weights, he determines his error by weighing the second weight. The errors through many experiments are averaged to give the " average error."

Although Fechner's confidence in the psychophysical significance of his methods was not shared by his successors, and although his methods have suffered devastating criticism and provoked endless controversy,[1] his contribution, as the real creator of psychophysics, was of immense importance. It was largely through these investigations that Wundt was stimulated to conceive of an exact science which should study the relations of physical stimuli to mental events. Indeed, Fechner's long and careful research did much to give Wundt and his contemporaries the plan of an experimental psychology.[2]

When at last his *Elemente der Psychophysik* was published, Fechner was beginning to turn to other fields of investigation in a way that would tempt one to think that he pretended to finality. As a matter of fact, however, the work went on and on. Through his contact with Wundt and the latter's laboratory investigations and publications, Fechner was constantly occupying himself with the writing of new articles and with answering objections.

In this period he began to concern himself with a further

---

[1] " Those who desire this dreadful literature," said James, " can find it ; it has a ' disciplinary value ' ; but I will not even enumerate it in a footnote." (*Principles of Psychology*, I, p. 549.) The historian cannot escape so easily. The principal criticisms by Müller and Wundt are contained in the works already cited, but the following are also important : Müller, *Die Gesichtspunkte und die Tatsachen der psychophysischen Methodik* (1904) ; Fechner, *In Sachen der Psychophysik* (1877) and *Revision der Hauptpunkte der Psychophysik* (1882). Additional references are to be found in Titchener, *op cit.*, II, Part 2, xlvii. More recent material is given in Fröbes, *Lehrbuch der experimentellen Psychologie*, I, 3rd ed. (1923), p. 463 f.

[2] Titchener, *op. cit.*, II, Part 2, xx.

statement of his philosophical position, and as time went on gave it more adequate expression. This statement he called " the day view opposed to the night view."[1] In it we find a magnificent insistence upon the meaning and value of all the known universe, expressed with a lyrical beauty which moved William James many decades later to an outburst of enthusiastic welcome to a most kindred spirit. The universe, said Fechner, is an organism with articulate parts, living and rejoicing in living. Each of the stars and planets, each stone, each clod of earth, has its organization, and organization means life, and life means soul. Everything is imbued with a consciousness of itself and a response to the things about it. This view Fechner carried into the foundations of a system of philosophy which is as utterly and absolutely monistic as was the materialism of the nineteenth century, but as pantheistic as Hinduism. It is a far cry from this, to that parallelism which says that mental processes and brain processes go on without relation like two trains moving on tracks side by side. Fechner was assumed to be a parallelist ; few took the trouble to understand him, and he has contributed, strangely enough, to the spread of parallelistic ideas in modern psychology. But for him the world had become one ; the experience which men have as persons is of the very substance of the universe, all of which is throbbing with life and experience. This life we may, if we choose, study quantitatively ; we may study it in the physical laboratory or in measuring the intensity of sensations.

Both experimentally and logically, therefore, Fechner's purpose seemed fulfilled. But he was not content, and, pushing forward to new worlds to conquer, he laid the foundations of the science of experimental æsthetics.[2] Just as he had protested against the vague symbolism of the " philosophy of Nature," so he protested against the æsthetics " from above " which undertook to lay down the principles of beauty from which the beauty of the individual object might be deduced. He began to measure books, cards, windows, and many such objects of daily use, to find what quantitative relations of line are judged to be beautiful. He carried this into the study of the master-

---

[1] *Die Tagesansicht gegenüber der Nachtansicht* (1879).
[2] *Vorschule der Aesthetik* (1876).

H

pieces of pictorial art, undertaking to find those linear relations which the artist has unconsciously used. This æsthetics " from beneath " was to offer the same humble but endlessly careful approach to the problem of beauty which the psychophysics had offered toward the mind-body problem.

As little as in the psychophysics were his hopes destined to be fulfilled. Time has gratefully taken his methods and his data and gone on with them, to be sure, to a rich harvest. The problem, however, for which he sought a solution was not so easily met. Fechner's mystical grasp upon the unity of life and of the world lives and seems to grow apace, not as an adjunct to an experimental problem, but as the fulfilment of both an intellectual and a spiritual need. It is to-day as if, in the white heat of his glowing personality, quantitative science and mystical intuition had become one ; outside the flame of that personality the fusion will not take place, and the two stand starkly opposed to one another. Perhaps his was a synthesis more artificial than real ; perhaps it was a synthesis which only the rarest metal can attain. The struggle which goes on to-day to find the relation of the mystical to the natural world is at any rate less agonized, more insightful, than it could have been without Fechner.

In 1833 Johannes Müller became Professor of Physiology at Berlin, the first man to hold a position under that title at any university. As an experimentalist, especially in the physiology of the senses, he ranks among the greatest of the nineteenth century ; but his enduring influence is due much more to his success as a teacher, as a systematizer of knowledge, and as a writer. Before his time physiological experimentation was carried on by physicians and teachers of medicine, partly in connection with clinical practice and partly as an adjunct to anatomy ; Müller's career marked the emancipation of physiology from the practical demands of medicine.

He was interested in a number of specific problems in sense physiology, most of all in optics. The best known of his investigations are those which dealt with the external muscles of the eye and with the problem of space-perception. His researches were inspired in part by Kant's doctrine of the innate character of space-perception, and the qualifications apparently needed in the theory as a result of Herbart's analysis from a radically different viewpoint. Kant had laid down the principle that space-perception is given to us by virtue of an innate capacity. Space was for Kant a mode of experience beyond which we can never hope to go with our finite minds. But Berkeley had prepared the way for an " empirical " theory by asserting that the third dimension, as we know it, is built up through experience; it is necessary only that the different elements of the retina and skin should be stimulated simultaneously. Herbart had gone farther, maintaining that the world of space is organized through the integration of a vast number of particular experiences. The debate over "nativism" and "empiricism" which was to occupy much attention throughout the century was already in full swing when Müller approached the problem. No one had made possible any kind of compromise between the two views. They stood flatly opposed to one another. They were stated in such arbitrary terms that no genetic analysis of the facts was possible. Müller put the problem in such a way as to make use of the arguments of both schools, and in a form to some extent experimentally verifiable. This opened a field for research. His position was as follows : We are endowed with a general ability to perceive space as such, but not with the specific capacities to judge distances, size, and position. We learn by experience whether a given object is within reach or not. But we could never learn such specific relations, were we not endowed with a general capacity to perceive in spatial terms. Müller borrowed from Berkeley and Herbart the idea that we build up a spatial order through experience. Important in this connection was his study of binocular vision and of the nerve pathways in the chiasma.[1] We shall see later that the problem of the empirical derivation of the spatial order (learning to judge distances, learning to recognize at what point we are stimulated, and so on) was carried further by Lotze (p. 157).

Another striking contribution was the experimental study

---

[1] Wheatstone's discovery of the stereoscope in 1833 gave a technique for the further investigation (notably by Helmholtz) of this problem. Müller had made at least one phase of the problem amenable to experimental attack.

of reflex action. This was inspired partly by the teaching of Descartes, and, more immediately, by Bell's study of the functions of the spinal roots. The theory demanded experimental verification to support anatomical analysis. It was Müller who supplied the necessary data, from experimentation with frogs. He showed that reflex activity comprises three steps : (1) impulse from sense organ to nerve centre *via* the dorsal root, (2) connection in the cord, and (3) impulse going out *via* the ventral root to the muscle.

The most important theoretical contribution which he offered was the doctrine of " specific energies."[1] The great physiologist Bell had suggested that each sensory nerve conveys one kind of quality or experience ; visual nerves carry only visual impressions, auditory only auditory impressions, and so on. Müller realized the importance of such a view. He realized that, if it were true, the whole nervous system could be regarded as a company of specialists, each performing its own task, but unable to take over the functions of another. Might it not be true, he asked, that the various qualities in experience can come to us only through the specific qualities or energies of particular nerves ? Some nerves, for example, are specialized to give us vision ; that is their function. Just as the eye is specialized to receive light, so the optic nerve is specialized to give visual qualities. No other nerve could ever take over these functions ; these mental qualities come from physical qualities intrinsic in the nerve tissue.[2]

It occurred to Müller that there is perhaps another way of defining specialization in the nervous system. Not the nerves, but the terminals in the brain, may give specific qualities. Perhaps the nerves are nothing but " wires " which connect the sense organs with the brain tissue, and perhaps the different parts of the brain are themselves specialized. Müller's problem was this : do visual qualities result directly from the stimulation of the optic nerve or, on the contrary, do they arise from the excitement of a specialized visual area in the brain, the optic nerve serving merely to transmit the various stimuli impressed on the retina ? He believed both alternatives defensible, the

[1] *Elements of Physiology* (1834–40), Book V.
[2] Thus the doctrine reasserted the principle that the qualities of experience are not the qualities of an external world (see p. 18).

evidence being inconclusive in favour of either. He decided, however, in favour of the theory of specific energies in the nerves themselves. This view clinical work has now discredited, but it seemed not unreasonable in Müller's time.

His conclusion was of the greatest significance for the generation which followed. It implied that the qualities of experience are given us not by the sense organs alone but by the very constitution of specialized parts of the nervous system. The reason why we have visual experience is that we have brains containing within them specialized tissue which causes the particular kind of experience to appear. This view led to a physiological psychology in which mind and body were even more intimately related than in the systems of Hobbes, Hartley, and Cabanis. It helped to drive from the field the doctrines of Cartesian dualism and its congeners, which were indeed already dying of inanition. Whereas earlier physiological psychologists had contented themselves for the most part with showing a correspondence between brain *connections* and mental associations or *connections*, Müller's reasoning sought to find in the brain the physiological basis for difference in the elementary *modes* or *structures* of experience. Whichever of Müller's alternatives be emphasized, our variety of experiences must be due to the functioning of a variety of tissues in the central nervous system. Not, of course, that such a conception put an end to dualism in psychology. Müller's own views tended, indeed, as we have seen, to differentiate mental from physical events. But the dualisms which have taken account of Müller's principle have necessarily narrowed the scope of the " mental " to a central governing principle, the particular varieties of experience being stated more and more in terms of physiological events.

Few physiologists clearly grasped the fact that the problem of specific energies was very similar to that of local specialization within the nervous system, as it had been stated by Gall and the phrenologists. Müller had seriously entertained the possibility that the different parts of the brain might have their specific qualities. We have seen that phrenology, in defending a rather similar position, fell on evil days. Flourens'[1] experiments on the brains of pigeons,

---

[1] *Recherches expérimentales sur les propriétés et les fonctions du système nerveux dans les animaux vertébrés* (1824).

leading to the conclusion that the brain acts *as a whole*, and that no local specialization exists, were generally accepted to the discredit of phrenology ; yet without in any sense dislodging either of Müller's versions of the principle of specific energies.   Flourens' work put an end for the time being to what little reputation the doctrine of cortical localization enjoyed.   But it did not affect Müller's position at all.   He had in fact given preference to the alternative of specialization in the peripheral as against the central elements.   His theory of specific energies remained as orthodox as did Flourens' view that the brain functioned as a whole.   In the latter part of the century clinical studies[1] led to a revival of the concept of cerebral localization, while studies of nerve anastomosis served to discredit the doctrine of specific energies in the form preferred by Müller.   Nevertheless the plasticity of the theory gave it long life, while its attempt at definiteness made it useful as a hypothesis in experimental psychology.[2]

The next contribution to the problem of localization came not from experiment but from the collection of clinical material.   Suggestions during the 'twenties and 'thirties as to the definite localization of speech functions led in 1861 to the declaration by Broca[3] that injuries to the third frontal convolution of the left hemisphere were the cause of motor aphasia, the loss of voluntary speech.   This statement of Broca attracted attention, and soon came into wide acceptance.   This was the first case of definitely accepted cortical localization for a specific function, antedating by twenty years the definite location of any of the sensory centres, and antedating by ten years the *experimental* demonstration of the location of the motor functions.[4]   In general, from the time of Müller and Flourens until the work of Broca there was a widespread belief that nerves had within them the capacities to produce various qualities of experience, but that the *brain's* response was general and integral, without definite local specialization.   But the clinical and experimental study of cortical localization became after

---

[1] See p. 200.
[2] Helmholtz's colour theory and Blix's studies of cutaneous nerves are two familiar examples. See pp. 149 and 179.
[3] *Bulletins de la Société Anatomique.*
[4] First in the dog, subsequently in other mammals. See p. 200.

Broca so rich a field that we shall have to postpone its consideration.

While Johannes Müller was devoting himself to special problems of this kind, he was also concerned with the relation of physiology to other sciences. It is interesting to see on the one hand the eagerness of his research and on the other hand the perfectly clear allegiance which he felt to Kant and to the philosophy of Nature. He tried to reach a philosophical understanding of physiology. One of the clearest illustrations of this was his long and detailed discussion of the difference between the " mental principle " and the " vital principle." It is evident, he said, that the vital principle which distinguishes living from non-living processes must exist not only in certain parts of the body but in all the body. That which distinguishes living from non-living is diffused ; it is not confined to any particular part of the body. But the *mental* principle is not so widely diffused. Johannes Müller was inclined to accept the mental principle as distinct from the vital principle, and as residing in the nervous system and not in the other tissues. The brain was the chief seat of the mental principle. His concern with this question is important simply for the light it throws upon the nature of some of the problems with which physiologists were still occupying themselves one hundred years ago. Müller was also drawn into the maelstrom of the controversy concerning the nature of living matter and the whole problem of vitalism, for the excitement engendered by the discovery of electrical phenomena in the living body had gained rather than lost in intensity in the opening decades of the century. The prevalent vitalism, and the bold romanticism of the philosophy of Nature left their mark upon him.

Perhaps more important than any of these things was his production of the first great textbook of physiology since the time of Haller. Müller's *Elements of Physiology* (1834-40) quickly became not only the national, but the international standard. Since it brought together all the notable results of European research in the whole realm of physiology, it was quite naturally accepted by physiologists and served literally as an international storehouse and authority. But from a modern viewpoint the book treats not only physiology but anatomy. In fact, it is interesting to see the list of tissues and organs whose gross anatomy and histology Müller knew without knowing anything about their physiology. The description, for example, of the structure of the sympathetic nervous system and the glands of internal secretion reads much like that available in contemporary handbooks ; but on many pages Müller contents himself, after describing the structure, with the brief statement that the functions are unknown. In spite of, or perhaps because of, the breadth of outlook and the eclectic spirit in which the book was compiled, it is quite futile to search in it for a consistent point of view. Indeed, the very fact that Müller had an impartial avidity for all sorts of physiological data did as much as any other factor in the first half of the nineteenth century to turn German physiology from its abject position under the philosophy of Nature to its independent magnificence in the hands of Helmholtz. It was indeed this quality which led men like Helmholtz and Du Bois Reymond to study with him ; it was this that made his work the point from which discussion began and from which research followed, and marked him as the great master by whom all others were to be measured.

Contemporary with Müller were several psychologists who, though not experimentalists, marked an equally definite rebellion against the prevailing transcendentalism. Greatest among them was Beneke, the caption of whose work, *A Textbook of Psychology as a Natural Science* (1832), indicated the adoption of that spirit which had guided the English associationists. He borrowed, indeed, more of their spirit than had Herbart, though with less of their content. His central problem was that of the origin of personality ; how it is that the chaos of the newborn child's experience becomes organized into a coherent unity. There had been two traditional answers to this question. One was in terms of experience, the other in terms of the unfolding of " original nature." There had been the associationists' answer, most clearly stated by Hartley, maintaining that all experience comes through the senses, and that separate experiences are associated to make more complicated forms of experience. On the other hand, Descartes, Cabanis, and others, had maintained that we are born with reflexes, instincts and

" passions," which must function in a particular way. (From the standpoint of the Scottish school and the transcendentalists, innate tendencies were equally important, but emphasis was to be placed rather upon innate capacities to remember, reason, will, etc.) While associationism had assumed that the child begins with nothing but sensation, other schools, despite their enormous differences, had agreed in endowing him with the miniature patterns of his later adult activities. They had taught that when a sense-organ is stimulated a certain reaction follows by virtue of original nature ; the mind is not at birth Locke's " white paper," but a bundle of *tendencies* ready to be aroused. Beneke felt that neither of these systems was at all satisfactory. A child begins life with a capacity for a great number of single activities, but not with the complex capacities of the adult ; he manifests neither perception nor judgment, neither reason nor will. We are born with a number of specific *elementary* capacities of mind and body. For example, we are not born with the ability to perceive space ; we are born with many part functions (" fundamental processes ") which are integrated in the total process through which space-perception is achieved. Space-perception is learned, if we wish to use the term, but learned not through the agglutination of sensations but through the aid of various processes. The same method of approach characterizes Beneke's treatment of such traditional faculties as memory, reason, and will. Beneke may be reckoned as one of the most important of the nineteenth-century contributors to the dissection and hence to the disappearance of the " faculties " which still throve in German psychology.

Perhaps the chief *specific* contribution of Beneke was the doctrine of " traces." His view closely resembled that of Herbart (he devoted, in fact, much attention to the refutation of the Herbartians' charge of simple plagiarism from their master). Herbart had taught that the ideas lying outside of the field of consciousness have a *tendency* to reappear in consciousness. Similarly Beneke postulated traces by which each idea is linked to another. He refused to state this in physiological terms and insisted on the right of psychology to treat of its laws without recourse to the data of another science. Beneke made use of these traces to explain how an experience may be brought back into consciousness, that is, remembered. The disappearance of an idea from consciousness simply leaves a trace which serves as basis for the later revival of the idea. A present impression is capable of bringing back a previous experience. The substance of this teaching obviously differs but little from that of Herbart ; but the viewpoint and the terminology are significant in their attempt to set for psychology an empirical task. For Beneke it was all-important that memory as a faculty should be dethroned ; the traces were for him a simple and empirical explanation of all memory phenomena. The value of his analysis is of less interest to us than his influence in undermining the complacency of the transcendentalists.

But Beneke's task was not an easy one. So solidly entrenched was the habit of recourse to the transcendental that Beneke's book, on the " Foundations of a Physics of Morality," caused the loss of his right to teach at the University of Berlin. The Prussian Minister of Instruction explained " that it was not single passages which had given offence, but the whole scheme, and that a philosophy which did not deduce everything from the Absolute could not be considered to be philosophy at all."[1]

[1] Merz, *History of European Thought in the Nineteenth Century*, III p. 208n.

CHAPTER VI

OUR next task is to note the beginnings in Britain of the decline of that tradition which had held sway from the time of Reid, and its amalgamation with the empirical or associationist school.

We shall find some interesting parallels between Britain and Germany in this period. Germany had been dominated during the interval from the time of Kant until the middle of the nineteenth century by two philosophical schools. One was transcendentalism, its characteristic appeal being to reality beyond experience, and the second the philosophy of Nature, its key-note being an attempt to interpret nature symbolically and spiritually. Here and there a man made his protest; but in psychology proper (apart, of course, from physiology) only two figures of note, Herbart and Beneke, had seriously shaken these systems. And physiology, too, as represented by Weber and Johannes Müller, was considerably influenced by the philosophy of Nature and the accompanying vitalism. But it did succeed in making headway on empirical lines, because physiology was an independent discipline; another half-century was to pass before psychology was to have its independent position as an experimental science. Psychology, as the German intellectual of 1830 knew it, was a mixture of transcendentalism and the philosophy of Nature. It was this psychology against which Beneke had, not very successfully, rebelled.

This same attempt at an empirical psychology, to supplant the current philosophy of mind, was going on in Scotland. Religious and ethical dogmatism was beginning to yield to associationism. The tendency, inaugurated by Thomas Brown, to borrow from the associationists, was destined within a generation to bring an end to the independent existence of the Scottish school. Some steps in the process are suggested by the work of Sir William Hamilton and James Mill.

Hamilton began as a young man to be drawn towards contemporary German philosophy. He travelled through Germany to acquaint himself in detail with the transcendentalist movement. This transcendentalist approach he succeeded in unifying with the spiritual and ethical tradition which had been a part of his heritage as one educated in the Scottish universities. In 1836 he became the most influential teacher of psychology in Scotland. His work was distinguished equally by his mastery of the history of philosophy and by his ability to grapple with the psychological problems of his contemporaries, especially those raised by the associationists. In learning he stood head and shoulders above all in the Scottish school, even Thomas Brown. His methods of debate were much less inclined to be of a merely popular type ; they were aimed rather at scholars, and dealt with crucial problems which the Scottish school had in general neglected. Through his fusion of German and Scottish thought, and the critical spirit which he imparted to the latter, he became an organic part of the idealistic tradition of the nineteenth century.

Accepting the faculty psychology in the form advanced by Kant, Hamilton's first principle was the unity and activity of personality.[1] He refused to admit the usefulness of either the analytic or the physiological assumptions of the associationists. For him the main problem was not to explain how integrated experience is formed from past experiences, but how the underlying unitary substance manifests itself in a variety of different situations. This position gradually fused with the tradition then taking shape, which we may characterize by the general title of " British idealism," later represented by T. H. Green and Bradley. The Scottish school definitely ended with Sir William Hamilton, not because his ideas died, but because they became assimilated with another movement, the idealistic movement, which was interested primarily in the conservation of the same spiritual values which we have seen in the Scottish school.

His greatest psychological contribution lay in a theory

---

[1] *Lectures on Metaphysics* (published posthumously, 1859–60).

as to the nature of memory and association, a theory which showed in clear form the difference between Scottish and English traditions as they then existed. This conception, known as " redintegration," was to the effect that each impression tends to bring back into consciousness the whole situation of which it has at one time been a part. It will be recalled that orthodox associationists, from Hartley on, had maintained that when A, B, C, D are actual sensations following in a given order, the sensation A will, when later presented alone, be followed by the memory images b, c, and d. This meant that the only part of consciousness with which the psychologist was concerned was that which lay in the centre of attention. Psychology, in its whole history from the Greeks onwards, had been primarily a study of focal or attentive consciousness[1] ; and those who had presumed to study seriously the marginal aspects of consciousness were few indeed. Hamilton held that the difficulty with Hartley's formula was in the first place that it presupposed the exis- tence of individual *parts* of the mind, each of which sets going another part of the mind without any unifying principle to make the parts hold together. (Brown had vaguely realized this difficulty when he objected to the term " asso- ciation " because it implied that mere sequence could give organic unity.) Going further, Hamilton showed that the associationists, in their statement of the sequence of mental events, had written as if the remembering mind contained (or rather, were) one *single* idea at a time. Hamilton taught that the process of perception is such that *any one* of the elements simultaneously experienced is capable, when presented later, of bringing back the *total* experience. If a person hears another pronounce a series of numbers he may, indeed, recall them in order ; but he actually recalls many other details besides. Hours later, a whole constellation of memories comes back at once, as soon as the experiment with the numbers is mentioned. The subject redintegrates in memory the original situation ; he recalls not a series but a pattern. Hamilton, like Leibnitz and Herbart before him, was trying to call psychologists away from their over- simplified schematizations. He realized that any given mental process is only part of a much larger whole.

---

[1] Since Aristotle, the most important exceptions had been Leibnitz and Herbart.

Hamilton overworked his hypothesis, omitting, as Brett[1] remarks, to explain the process of *forgetting*. Memory items not only often fail to bring back their whole context, but even fail to bring back anything recognizable. Associationism could not, of course, be dislodged with a single blow ; and Hamilton had clearly gone too far in neglecting both the facts of serial association and the frequent ineffectiveness or absence of the redintegrating principle. Neither Hartley's nor Hamilton's position stated the whole truth. But we still know very little about either forgetting or remembering, and such insight as we have is partly traceable to Hamilton's doctrine that the mechanism of association operates not simply as in a chain of elements, but, so to speak, as a net-work, an interconnection of parts. Bain, James, and many others have insisted on the importance of Hamilton's contribution. Even aside from the theory of memory, the emphasis upon the whole of experience rather than upon the centre of attention was of great importance.

The Scottish school ceases to occupy us from this moment onwards. After Hamilton's death the school survived only in admixture with idealism, associationism, or both. For James Mill,[2] though a true Scot, and brought up under Scottish influences, identified himself with the English school, and attained the most complete and most rigorous expression of associationism.

His unity of thought, and the severity and rigour of his ethics and his logic, mark him as a very unusual personality.[3] He studied theology, but quickly found himself out of sympathy with the doctrines of the Church, and became an agnostic.[4] But though he abandoned the Church, the fierce severity of Calvinism glowed in his devotion to a philosophy of self-renunciation.

---

[1] *Op. cit.*, III, 27.

[2] *Analysis of the Phenomena of the Human Mind* (1829).

[3] The opening chapters of John Stuart Mill's *Autobiography* give a most vivid picture of his father.

[4] He arrived at a complete agnosticism of a kind which was rare even among " free-thinkers "—neither affirming nor denying the existence of Deity, and convinced that " concerning the origin of things nothing whatever can be known."

He concerned himself with the problems of history, political economy, and science ; he is better known to-day as an economist and historian than as a psychologist. He was employed in the British India Office, having written a *History of British India* (1817) which gave him a nation-wide reputation.[1] His system of political economy was closely allied to that of Bentham, with whom he enjoyed the closest friendship. He borrowed Bentham's pleasure-pain philosophy, the doctrine that human actions are motivated solely through self-interest. He borrowed also the ethical conceptions of Bentham's school, the view that the wise organization of society is that which brings about "the greatest happiness of the greatest number."[2] In seeking to outline a comprehensive political economy, Mill had to include a treatment of ethical and psychological questions. In general, Mill and the utilitarians favoured the principle of free exchange without government interference ; they believed that individual self-interest would bring about social welfare, if economic (that is, from Mill's viewpoint, psychological) laws were left to themselves.

His psychology was definitely related to these other aspects of his life. In the first place, the agnosticism which had taken hold of him made him go further in his tendency to mechanistic theory than his discipleship to Hartley required. He reduced mental life to elementary sensory particles, conceding nothing to the claims of the soul. He went the whole way in making perception a process by which a number of bits are put together to make a single perceptual whole. *How* the parts are held together he did not explain. At the same time, the process of association was regarded as passive. Sensations were presented in a certain order, and later, when one of these was presented, the others followed mechanically. Elements in

---

[1] His position as an authority is indicated by the fact that, though he gave attention in the frankest terms to the abuses in the Indian government, all was done so fairly and temperately that he suffered no personal reverses.

[2] The widespread suffering of the factory workers in the newly-established industrial order served to make the ethical aspects of political economy particularly acute. Partly because of the migration of agricultural labourers into the cities, there was a disturbance in the food supply. An increase in the population augmented the difficulty. Practical political problems such as the " repeal of the Corn Laws " were considerably influenced by the agitation of the utilitarians.

experience were, so to speak, movable, or interchangeable with one another.

One feature of his treatment which differed from the work of any previous associationist was a *tour de force* in getting rid of all the laws of association except for simple contiguity in experience. Hartley had attempted to do this, but had really left association by similarity as an entity quite distinct from ordinary contiguity association. Mill taught that there was no such thing as association by similarity or contrast. The reason why one tree makes us think of another similar tree is simply the fact that " we are accustomed to see like things together." His explanation of association by contrast was equally simple. " Dwarf " does not make us think of " giant " by virtue of logical contrast, but simply because both depart from a common standard. We need, thought Mill, no associative laws but "contiguity"; similarity and contrast have no influence on the course of thought.

Another aspect of Mill's psychology, destined to be of importance because of its influence on Bain, was his concern with the task of reducing complex emotional states to simple sensory terms. Following the suggestions of Hartley, he undertook a genetic and analytic study of such complex phenomena as conscience, religious attitudes, and the like. In him associationism and hedonism were thoroughly fused, and the dream of eighteenth-century psychologists of reducing every experience to sensory components under the guidance of the pleasure-pain principle was realized.

Associationism came to maturity. The uncompromising rigidity and consistency of Mill's system gave much to Bain and Spencer, and much of it still lives in modern psychology. But its consistency showed where its weaknesses lay, and in the generation which followed, the inevitable reaction set in. Mill, its most thorough-going advocate, was willing to face the most complicated aspects of life in terms of sensation and association ; no one after him dared to venture so far.

The reaction against extreme associationism was evident in John Stuart Mill's notes[1] upon his father's work. Much of the economic teaching of his father he did, indeed, accept ; in particular, he elaborated and popularized the ethical

[1] He collaborated in the editing and republication of the *Analysis* in 1869.

aspects of utilitarianism. His prestige also helped to strengthen and further the popular belief in the adequacy of the pleasure-pain philosophy to explain human conduct. Nevertheless he had at times serious misgivings about the adequacy of the pleasure-pain principle (psychological hedonism) as well as about the mechanical conception of association. In James Mill's complicated and rigid system there was no active principle, nothing but the constant addition of new experiences. This was in direct lineal descent from the views of Hartley, which denied all independence of mind as an entity. For John Stuart Mill the mind was an active, not a passive thing. Furthermore, in its activity the mind made new syntheses. Just as seventeenth and eighteenth-century psychologists delighted in drawing analogies from the rapidly growing science of mechanics (as in Hartley's concern with vibrations), so John Stuart Mill in the middle of the nineteenth century borrowed an analogy from the increasingly popular science of chemistry. " Mental chemistry " is the most celebrated of his doctrines. By this he meant the process by which sensory elements become so fused in a new compound that the psychologist must recognize an essentially new entity, which is more than the *sum* of the constituent parts.[1]

A man of far greater significance for psychology than either of the Mills was Alexander Bain. He devoted much energy to grammar, rhetoric, and education. He spent much of his long life in administrative activities of one type or another ; and his chief university position was a chair not of psychology but of logic. But in spite of this scattering of his energies he mastered the Scottish and English, as well as much of the German psychology, and brought together a vast quantity of material, ably organized and with great originality of treatment. His two greatest works were *The Senses and the Intellect* (1855) and *The Emotions and the Will* (1859).

Bain's approach was through physiology, particularly the work of the German physiologists ; he incorporated in his

[1] The doctrine was, of course, not new ; *e.g.*, it differs only in name from Tucker's conception of fusion (see p. 26). But it is significant in that it shows how short a life was granted to James Mill's purely *mechanical* conceptions.

I

works a great quantity of empirical material. We find, for instance, Weber's experiments on the two-point threshold and on the temperature-sense. Although the titles of his two celebrated works suggest the continuation of the old subdivisions of *knowing, feeling,* and *willing,* these titles are but cloaks for associationism. It was, however, an associationism based upon physiological findings far more detailed than had been available for any previous scholar. In Bain we have for the first time physiological explanations sufficiently elaborate to be taken quite seriously. The psychologist began to think of experimental physiology as fundamental to his science. The sense-organs, the sensory and motor nerves, the brain and the muscles were considered in detail. The reflex-arc and the instincts were regarded as elements of behaviour, and human acts were presented as wholes whose parts had been studied by the laboratory method. Specific contributions of physiology to psychology took the place of the general ones which had been popular among the associationists.

His view of psychology was relatively comprehensive. Its most serious gap lay in the neglect of material (then being collected by neurologists) which showed the relations of abnormal mental processes to abnormal brain processes. But he furnished a rich and vivid picture of an immense variety of mental states and processes, many of which lay within the field now vaguely defined as social psychology. He concerned himself, as James Mill had done, with the origin of those complex attitudes and sentiments which we call æsthetic, moral, and religious ; these he related to his physiological principles.

Perhaps we may best illustrate the kind of associationism that Bain formulated by citing an extreme case, his famous explanation of the behaviour of a mother fondling her child.[1] It is clear, said Bain, that things which are warm are pleasant ; so also are things which are soft ; hence maternal joy.[2] (William James suggested that lonely parents might

[1] *The Emotions and the Will,* pp. 126–40.

[2] There is nothing new under the sun. Many psychological schools to-day reduce maternal behaviour to elements dependent on quite simple sensory gratifications. See Allport, *Social Psychology* (1924), p. 68 : " The caressing which children commonly receive and solicit is associated with sensitive zone stimulation. Their cuddling of dolls and toys, and expressions of love toward these objects, have their root in the same source " ; and the rest of the paragraph.

be supplied with pillows heated to the necessary temperature.[1]) The same kind of thing had of course been
done before by Hartley. Bain was concerned simply with
carrying out to its logical implications the doctrine of association wherever it could work.

Bain was not a denier of original nature. He was, in
fact, much more concerned with " instincts," innate dispositions to action, than any previous associationist. He
was much interested in the mechanics of their function.
But his chief contributions were written shortly before the
publication of Darwin's *Origin of Species*, and although
he lived to see the spread of Darwinism, he never remodelled
his psychological conceptions upon Darwinian lines. Nevertheless he was, throughout, thinking in terms of inborn
reaction-tendencies, tendencies which underwent modifications
through experience.

But the best known of Bain's specific contributions is his
treatment of learning and habit. Elaborating some suggestions of Spencer, he stated learning in terms of (1) random
movements, (2) retention of acts which bring pleasant
results, with elimination of those bringing unpleasant results,
(3) fixation through repetition. His maxims on habit were
quoted and elaborated by James ; they constitute, together
with some of Carpenter's observations, much of the pith of
what is so frequently referred to as " James's wonderful
chapter on Habit."[2]   This is but one example of the position
of authority which Bain enjoyed throughout the second
half of the century, and the way in which his writings have
been incorporated into the writings of others.

No one else had ever attempted, as he did, to cover the
entire range of normal human experience in a system of
psychology.   Of course, among all associationists there were
efforts to get universal principles, and with Brown an important list of secondary principles had been included.   But
no one before Bain had tried to analyse such a wealth of
particular situations.   Everything psychological, from the
experience of a man jumping a ditch to the mental operations
of a creative artist, was the perfectly legitimate concern of
the psychologist.   No other man had been so prolific in
descriptions of human experiences, so serious in trying to

[1] *Principles of Psychology*, II, 552.
[2] In the *Principles of Psychology* (1890).

give a colourful and exhaustive picture of mental life. It was as if previous authors had said, " Take these key-principles, and you may enter any room within the house of psychology." Bain said, " Here is the key to room 113, you will find there a table and three chairs ; here is the key to room 114, which contains two desks and a book-case." He was interested in providing not merely an entry into every mode of experience, but an analysis of its contents. This was the chief reason why he was so readable. Never had a psychologist been so widely read in his own day. He exerted as great a personal influence in psychology as did John Stuart Mill in political economy. Associationism became through him almost " popular." But he borrowed much from the works and from the spirit of the Scottish school, and he did not irritate his readers, as most of the associationists had done, by the apparent crassness of a mechanistic system. He made use of physiological principles for their practical usefulness, not for philosophical purposes. He was genuinely and consistently a psychologist ; he might fairly be described as the first to write a comprehensive treatise having psychology as its sole purpose.

This work of Bain in the field of physiological psychology, if we may call it such, summed up and crowned the achievements of physiological as well as of introspective work up to the middle of the nineteenth century. Another great contribution of Bain was the founding in 1876 of a journal for the publication of psychological articles. Psychological writings before this time had for the most part appeared as independent books or pamphlets, or as contributions to philosophical or physiological journals. The journal *Mind*, although of a philosophical cast, was from the first concerned chiefly with psychological material.

Another psychologist with a physiological approach was Carpenter. His *Mental Physiology* (1874), and the writings of Maudsley, served to popularize the idea that physiological conceptions were the groundwork of psychology. This idea was also becoming popular in France, especially through the writings of Ribot.

But with Bain the classical outlines of associationism were already beginning to fade. Immediately after his chief volumes there came the publication of Darwin's *Origin of Species* (1859). The evolutionary theory substituted for associationism two definite working concepts which changed the whole background of psychology. The concept of heredity was all-important, both for the understanding of uniformities of mental structure and for the interpretation of permanent and stable differences from one individual to another ; and the idea of the adaptation of the individual to environment was immensely significant. The biological outlook, emphasizing such concepts as the *functions* of an *organism*, had indeed been apparent in some quarters ; but after Darwin the term " biological " became a symbol for a new way of thinking, in which every organ and function was understood in terms of its history and its relation to the life of the creature which displayed it. Such an approach could not have been made before Darwinian evolutionism, and could not be avoided after it. These fundamental changes destroyed associationism.

The growing strength of the movement which we have called British " idealism," with its emphasis on the unity and activity of mind, was indeed pressing associationism hard from its side. Just as a " Radical " and a " Conservative " coalition may throw out a " Liberal " ministry, so associationism was attacked with equal vigour by those who thought it too biological and by those for whom it was not biological enough. Not that the central doctrines of the associationists have disappeared ; and not that the wealth of their specific contributions has been forgotten. On the contrary, the attention given to memory and learning in the late nineteenth century inevitably involved much use of associationist contributions. Students of the conditioned reflex in modern times have freely drawn upon associationist doctrines, while substituting for them a description in terms of overt responses rather than of " ideas." But, however much associationism left behind it in these as in more subtle ways, the movement itself may definitely be said to have died with Bain.

Herbert Spencer[1] is sometimes regarded as sharing with Bain in the last defence of associationism ; it is more nearly true to say that he was the first of the evolutionists. He

[1] *The Principles of Psychology* (1855).

does, indeed, seem less important as a psychologist than he did in his own day. But he had the enormous advantage over Bain that he was an evolutionist before Darwin ; as early as 1850 he had begun to write on evolution. His system attracted wide notice, so that when Darwin's *Origin of Species* was published his own more speculative evolutionism drew strength from it, a fact which made possible the preservation of many of his ideas that would otherwise have been lost.

Spencer undertook to create a synthetic philosophy, in which everything in the universe should be related to everything else, a scheme in which all parts should be organically connected. The most significant part of his system was his evolutionism. The world, he believed, began as something very simple, quite inchoate, yet homogeneous, which as time went on began to be subdivided into parts, each one of which became specialized. These parts began to integrate or make combinations with other parts. So, in place of a formless unity, a diversity of specific parts developed, integrated with other parts in such a way as to make articulated wholes. Fifty years ago people loved to quote Spencer's definition of organic evolution as "a change from incoherent, indefinite homogeneity, to coherent, definite heterogeneity." Increasing integration is the key-note of Spencer's system. We can find this process going on everywhere, Spencer held, in the physical sciences, in biology, in psychology, in sociology. For psychology this meant that the increasing complexity of the nervous system was paralleled by an increasing richness and variety in the forms of experience and in the types of association. Together with increase in complexity of structure come higher and higher integrations of function. There is also in the *individual* life, from birth to death, the constant integration of experiences. Association was regarded as an integrating mechanism, by which a more and more complex type of experience becomes possible. The psychological and biological viewpoints were worked out harmoniously.

Spencer was the first to elaborate the conception that the mind is what it is because it has had to cope with particular kinds of environment.[1] He laid great emphasis on

[1] Though suggestions in this direction had been given by several, *e.g.*, Lucretius among the ancients, Schopenhauer among the moderns.

the adaptive nature of nervous and mental processes, and on the notion that increasing complexity of experiences and of behaviour is a part of the process of adaptation. This doctrine, though part of a speculative system, was singularly similar, as we shall see to the conclusions which followed upon all the inductive work of Darwin. A more adequate and detailed application of evolutionary principles had to wait upon the accumulation of data by Darwin and his followers. Whereas Spencer's psychology never attained the popularity enjoyed by Bain's, his evolutionary teaching contributed indirectly to the widespread adoption by psychologists of biological conceptions, especially those relating to the principle of the adaptation of an organism to its environment.

One specific psychological doctrine of Spencer attracted attention and is still well-known, his theory of the relation between mind and body. We may regard the mind, said Spencer, as a series of events, and the physical processes in the brain as a series of parallel events; but both of these arise from a deeper underlying reality which is the basis for both.[1] This basic entity Spencer regarded as unknowable. He was, for practical purposes, a parallelist, like those we have already had to consider. But, unlike Leibnitz and the strict parallelists, Spencer believed that mental and physical events were intimately and organically connected; not that either was the cause of the other, but that both sprang from the same soil. Carrying the point further, he supposed that a single stimulation of a nerve causes a single nervous impulse, or, as he called it, "nervous shock." The *rate* of these shocks determines the *quality* of consciousness, different rates producing variations of this quality. "A single primordial element of consciousness, and the countless kinds of consciousness may be produced by the compounding of this element with itself and the recompounding of its compounds."[2] Some modern descendants of this "double-aspect" theory will be considered in Chapter XXII.

---

[1] This is of course reminiscent of Spinoza's monism.
[2] *Op. cit.*, I, p. 150.

CHAPTER VII

THE THEORY OF EVOLUTION

The majority naturally perished, having too weak a constitution.—
Hippocrates.
Our present ways of living have, I think, been discovered and
elaborated during a long period of time.—*Hippocrates.*

THOUGH it is natural to think of evolutionism and Darwinism
as synonymous, evolutionism had been one of the outstanding features of the thought of the last half of the
eighteenth century and of the first half of the nineteenth.
Quite aside from contributions made in the field of biology,
men were thinking in evolutionary terms.

The world was changing very rapidly in social organization,
as shown not only in political revolutions but in the Industrial
Revolution, with profound upheaval in the life of individuals
and institutions. The romantic movement had itself done
much in the eighteenth century to disseminate the idea of
diversification and progress. Thus Goethe, one of the most
illustrious of the romanticists, found evolutionary conceptions
useful in his studies of botany, and in fact worked out a
theory of organic evolution. Such thinking, in terms of
struggle and change, also displayed itself in some of the
philosophical writings of the time. These began to express
the idea of progress, a series of changes through which
humanity must pass. Among the French, Fourier constructed a theory of human destiny in terms of many
thousands of years that must be spent in each stage of
growth. The same tendency was expressed in Hegel's
conviction that civilization must be worked out step by
step according to a universal plan.

In the scientific thought of the period we may distinguish
two types of evolutionary doctrine : first, the theory of the
evolution of the inanimate physical universe, the study of
inorganic evolution ; second, the study of biological or
organic evolution. There had been in antiquity many

attempts[1] to explain the origin of the world without recourse to the idea of special creation. Laplace developed in connection with his mechanics the theory commonly known as the *nebular hypothesis*. This sought to explain the origin of the planets through the interaction of gravitational and centrifugal forces in a rotating nebula.[2] In geology, Lyell was making investigations from 1830 to 1860 to show how rock strata were formed by a series of changes in the earth. The late seventeenth and the early eighteenth centuries had marked the beginnings of this type of research; by the early nineteenth century the data permitted a systematic and coherent demonstration that the different strata had been built one upon another in a certain sequence, occupying definite periods of time. The various organisms whose fossils were found in these strata must necessarily have lived at different times, in periods corresponding to the strata where the fossils were found. Lyell enunciated the theory that the earth itself had gone through an orderly series of changes in which a chaos of elements had gradually been superseded by differentiation and separation. Thus different kinds of rock had been formed and had become relatively fixed and immutable. This form of thought was as foreign to the idea of special creation as was the Darwinian theory itself; and Lyell, though a deeply religious man, had to face serious religious opposition. He had undertaken to show that the earth itself reveals stages requiring vastly greater time than the six days allowed in the book of Genesis. As a matter of fact, Lyell was not the first nor the last, but in terms of scientific as well as popular influence he was by far the greatest of the geological evolutionists. He prepared the way in a definite sense for the habit of thinking of growth in terms of changes in living organisms. Lyell's evolutionism was, indeed, a direct stimulus to the work of Charles Darwin.

We may now turn to theories of organic evolution. Buffon, in the third quarter of the eighteenth century, outlined an evolutionary theory. Erasmus Darwin (the grandfather of Charles Darwin) at the close of the century stated such evolution in terms of heredity and adaptation to environment. Lamarck (*Philosophie zoologique*, 1809) elaborated

---

[1] *E.g.*, that of Lucretius.
[2] Kant had suggested a similar view as early as 1754.

Erasmus Darwin's conceptions in a system which became widely popular. His work has the very great merit of combining an enormous amount of biological knowledge (Lamarck was already a zoologist of some standing) with a theory which for the first time faced in detail the problem of why particular changes in organisms take place from generation to generation. The fact that he mastered both zoology and botany, and the fact that he had made elaborate studies and published dozens of volumes on different phases of the biology of his time, gave weight to his theory and demanded for it serious consideration. Lamarck's theory involved three steps. In the first place, in confronting the physical environment, the organism has needs, it meets situations to which it must adapt itself. Secondly, these situations demanding adjustment cause the animal to exercise certain parts of its body. Thirdly, the exercise of a given part of the body makes that particular member develop to a point sufficiently advanced to cause the change to appear in the offspring as an acquired characteristic. We may illustrate these three steps from the famous passage which explains why the snake has no legs. The snake is derived from the salamander or lizard. Some of these salamanders left the water and came to marsh-ground, where there was grass. Here they had to keep out of sight. So, in meeting this situation, they crouched down, and finding their legs useless (as a matter of fact, a hindrance) they must get rid of them. In the course of time, as their legs dwindled and disappeared, each generation was born with shorter and shorter legs, until the legs disappeared altogether.

Shortly after Lamarck put forth this theory, which was destined to be the greatest of the evolutionary theories before Darwin, a debate began (1830) between St. Hilaire and Cuvier. St. Hilaire championed Lamarck's doctrine of the transmutation of species (though differing from him as to its mechanism). Cuvier refused to entertain an evolutionary doctrine, simply because of the inadequacy of the evidence. And this debate was bound to be decided in scientific circles of the day in favour of Cuvier, because, in the first place, he was right—there was not enough evidence—and in the second place, because of his immense prestige. This very question of the inadequacy of the evidence during the first half of the century leads us, therefore, to a consideration of the task of gathering data bearing directly on the reality of evolution, as well as on the mechanism by which it was effected, a task chiefly associated with the name of Charles Darwin. Darwin's importance lay not in his thinking in terms of evolution and the struggle for existence, but in the fact that he, like Cuvier, recognized that the problem could be solved only by the accumulation of enormous masses of evidence.

His trip on the *Beagle* through the South Seas (1831–6) gave Darwin a magnificent opportunity to observe and collect plants and animals. Returning to England, he gave himself over to the intensive study of a few particular forms, not undertaking to master the essential economy of all forms of life (as he did later). This detailed study began to lead him to inquire why it was that forms of life were so perfectly adapted to the environment in which they lived. In his notebook of 1837, he tells of his concern with the problem of selection. He had noted that out of every generation some individuals were eliminated, although apparently constructed much like their brothers and sisters. What made some die and others live ? What was the mechanism of selection ; how did nature choose from the many ?

In 1838 he read Malthus's *Essay on Population*, a treatise written forty years before. This essay discussed the problem of the relation of the death-rate to the birth-rate in human societies. Malthus had been impressed by the industrial and political changes of his day. He thought that the improvement which might be made in the methods of getting food would tend to follow an arithmetical progression. But increase in population would inevitably conform to a *geometrical* progression. If, for example, each family has four children, and if three of them live and have offspring, the number given by the geometrical ratio must, in time, surpass the number that can be fed. So long as one ratio is arithmetical and the other geometrical there must follow an *excess* of population. Some individuals must be eliminated in one way or another. Malthus thought that there were two possible ways of elimination ; one through the natural struggle due to starvation and disease, which would take place as a part of what we call normal life, and the other through war. There was no escape from these hard alternatives. It was a rather loosely worked out hypothesis, but it had the advantage of envisaging human society in biological terms. The hypothesis that the number of offspring is usually greater than the number that can subsist implied that there must be a struggle for existence, the elimination of some and the saving of others.

The reading of Malthus's essay, interpreted in the light of Darwin's own observations, suggested an answer to his problem. He began to outline the theory of evolution which he later published. The theory was based, in the first place, upon the fact that in most species the total number is stationary ; yet there are more offspring than parents. In fishes there may be a hundred thousand eggs for each two parents ; there must be an elimination of all but two individuals. This leads directly to the idea of the " survival of the fittest." An organism is " fit " if in a given environment it is well adapted to the task of getting food and warding off its enemies. It has to maintain its own bodily structure, and get food until it is able to reproduce its kind. But if there is survival of the fittest, and at the same time adaptation to the environment (which is the necessary condition of the survival itself), this adaptation to environment must mean survival of those who are fittest *in the particular environment*. If those which are fittest for the particular environment survive, and if now there is a change in the environment, it inevitably follows that there must be a change in the organisms themselves. Selection is effected from among variations which are regularly observable among individuals of the same parentage.

What causes these variations ? Darwin did not profess to know, and the problem, though much studied, cannot as yet be answered in terms of any valid generalization. But that they do occur is evident, and when we find them we know that those individuals or species which survive could not do so if they were conspicuously lacking in adaptation to the environment. Darwin noticed in the South Sea Islands that certain species showed differentiation even on the same island ; the struggle for existence had selected one type of individuals for the shore, another for the interior, etc. One species, by migrating into two environments, might become in time two species. Now if there is some cataclysmic change, some tidal wave or volcanic eruption, all sorts of changes in environment are manifest through a wide area. The offspring which tend to survive are slightly different from those which have tended to survive before the cataclysm.

After his first rough formulation of the theory, he set for himself the task of collecting data on a scale large enough to permit the verification or refutation[1] of the hypothesis. By 1858 he had a large amount of material and had achieved, through a variety of publications, general recognition as a naturalist. He was nearly ready to publish the book which was to advance his theory and the supporting evidence. In that year he received a letter and manuscript from a young Englishman in the East Indies, Alfred Russel Wallace. Through an extraordinary coincidence, Wallace, while pondering on Malthus's *Essay on Population*[2] had formulated a doctrine much like Darwin's. During an illness he had worked out in a few hours the main outlines of a very similar evolutionary theory. In sending his manuscript to Darwin he asked for his opinion as to its merit, and whether he would help him to get it published. Darwin was in a difficult position. He must be fair to the man who had prepared a statement of the theory before his own had appeared. Yet Wallace's manuscript contained no such mass of data as Darwin had collected. So he submitted Wallace's work and an abstract of his own theory to Lyell. The latter decided that both must be submitted to the Linnean Society. Some portions of Darwin's forthcoming book were read, together with Wallace's manuscript.[3] In 1859 Darwin's *Origin of Species* was published.

Evolutionary theories were not, we must remind ourselves, new ; and even the hypothesis as to the mechanism of evolution had been in some respects anticipated. The chief significance of the book lay not in the newness of the theory, but in the mass of relevant data presented, and the compelling force with which they commanded serious attention. Darwin's work led before long to the acceptance by biologists of the central fact of the transmutation of species. A

[1] Keeping, in fact, a careful record of cases which seemed to count against his own view.

[2] Which he had read a few years earlier.

[3] The joint essay was read on the first of July, 1858, and appears in the Linnean Society Journal for that year.

general storm, however, was precipitated—partly on scientific, though chiefly on religious grounds—and some of the most violent battles in intellectual history took place. Spencer had prepared the intelligentsia for such doctrines ; Huxley was one of the greatest of those who took Darwin's side[1]; Haeckel saw the whole world-view inevitably involved in the theory. But during the 'sixties there was much acrimony even among scientists. Many were not ready to capitulate at once. Agassiz, probably the most eminent biologist in the United States, died without accepting the evidence. By the decade of the 'eighties, however, the last actual opposition to the theory of evolution as such disappeared among biologists.

The influence of Darwinism upon psychology during the last quarter of the nineteenth century probably did as much as any single factor to shape the science as it exists to-day. Psychology was certain to become consistently more biological ; mental processes tended more and more to be stated in terms of the functions served in the task of adjusting to the world. Darwin himself in the *Descent of Man* (1871) emphasized similarity between human reasoning and similar processes in the higher animals, and in *The Expression of the Emotions in Man and Animals* (1872) suggested an evolutionary interpretation of the characteristic facial and postural changes during strong emotion. The *comparative* viewpoint, although present here and there in the eighteenth and nineteenth centuries, could come into its own only when evolutionism had become the groundwork of psychological thinking. As a natural consequence, interest in animal psychology rapidly increased. Many books[2] appeared which concerned themselves with the nature of instinct and with the phylogenetic study of intelligence. Experimental studies of animal behaviour, though few, were accepted by psychological journals. The great gulf established by Descartes between human and animal behaviour had been bridged. The life of the organism was seen as a whole. Human psychology was to be seen in relation to all the phenomena of life.

[1] Huxley is also known for his championing of the still popular doctrine of " epiphenomenalism," which asserts that consciousness is a mere by-product of life-processes, playing no active or causal rôle in behaviour.

[2] *E.g.*, those of Romanes, Lloyd Morgan, Hobhouse, G. H. Schneider.

Francis Galton was the greatest of Darwin's immediate followers in the field of psychology. In fact, he was the first who attempted in a thorough-going way to apply the principles of variation, selection, and adaptation, to the study of human individuals and races.

He published in 1869, a decade after the publication of the *Origin of Species*, a book entitled *Hereditary Genius*, the aim of which was to show that individual greatness follows certain family lines with a frequency and a certainty that may oppose any explanation in terms of environment. These studies were, for the most part, investigations into family-trees of eminent jurists, scientists, authors, and so on. He collected data to show that in each case these men not only inherited genius, as shown by a long line of persons before them, but that they inherited *specific* forms of greatness. A great jurist or barrister comes from a family which has attained not only *eminence*, but eminence in the *law*. It was Galton's belief that there are specific legal gifts, medical gifts, and the like, transmitted by heredity. The theory presupposed that there have been, at some time in the past, variations within the human stock, and that these variations have been able to survive. Galton believed that the Darwinian principle of accidental variation about the average or norm of the group applied as much to the general and specific gifts of man as to the length of a bird's wings or the length of a polar bear's hair ; and that these variations tended to persist.

Such *individual differences* had not been seriously treated as part of the subject matter of psychology before the days of Galton. Perhaps their neglect had been the most extraordinary blind-spot in previous psychology. It was Darwinism, rather than the previous history of psychology, which brought about an interest in the problem. A few of the fragmentary studies of the subject in the nineteenth century, before Galton, may be noted. Thomas Brown had included, in his secondary laws of association, the factor of constitutional differences in persons. Herbart, about the same time, had written of differences in association accompanying various degrees of intelligence. Among experimentalists, Weber, Fechner, and Helmholtz had found individual differences, but had not systematically studied them ; Donders, as we shall see later (p. 148), met the problem in the 'sixties, but did singularly little with it. Galton was the first important figure in the exploration of the field.

Galton undertook also[1] to compare the various human races in respect to their hereditary make-up, and to show that the different races have been evolved because of their adaptation to their particular environment. Darwin[2] had pointed out instances in which the skin, the proportions of the limbs, and the like, are adapted to the mode of life of given races in a particular climate. Galton held not only that variations occur from one individual to another, but that there may be widespread variation and selection so that new races are evolved. He even suggested that the culture of the Greeks had been due to a favourable variation in the Hellenic stock.

Galton's faith in the all-importance of heredity could scarcely be better indicated than in the following two passages. After reference to anthropometric studies on the " criminal type," he proceeds to these generalizations :

> " The deficiency of conscience in criminals, as shown by the absence of genuine remorse for their guilt, astonishes all who first become familiar with the details of prison life. Scenes of heart-rending despair are hardly ever witnessed among prisoners ; their sleep is broken by no uneasy dreams."[3]

Galton assumed that all this was biologically conditioned ; individuals are born not only to peculiarities of skull or feature, not only to genius or imbecility, but to intrinsic criminalism. This is perhaps the most extreme case of neglect of the *environmental* factors which we have to consider in all our studies so far, just as associationism in general represents the most extreme neglect of the hereditary factors. The second passage indicates an even more picturesque application (or abuse) of Darwinian principles.

> " I may take this opportunity of remarking on the well-known hereditary character of colour blindness in connection with the fact, that it is nearly twice as prevalent among the Quakers as among the rest of the community, the proportions being as 5.9 to 3.5 per cent. We might have expected an even larger ratio. Nearly every Quaker is descended on both sides solely from members of a group of men and women who segregated themselves from the rest of the world five or six generations ago ; one of their strongest

---

[1] *Inquiries into Human Faculty* (1883).
[2] *Descent of Man* (1871).
[3] *Op. cit.*, Section on " Criminals and the Insane."

opinions being that the fine arts were worldly snares, and their most conspicuous practice being to dress in drabs. A born artist could never have consented to separate himself from his fellows on such grounds ; he would have felt the profession of those opinions and their accompanying practices to be a treason to his æsthetic nature. Consequently few of the original stock of Quakers are likely to have had the temperament that is associated with a love for colour, and it is in consequence most reasonable to believe that a larger proportion of colour-blind men would have been found among them than among the rest of the population."[1]

After establishing in *Hereditary Genius* the pedigree method of studying mental endowment (a method quickly turned to account in the study of mental deficiency, beginning with Dugdale's *The Jukes*, 1877), Galton turned to the construction of more refined quantitative methods in prosecution of the same problem. In his *Inquiries into Human Faculty and its Development* (1883) he outlined the procedure and results of two epoch-making studies. The first was his experiment on free association, the essentials of which he had already outlined.[2] Associationism had lived its whole life without any recourse to experimental procedure. Galton undertook to study quantitatively the appearance of various types of association. He prepared a list of seventy-five words, each word on a slip of paper which he placed underneath a book. He looked at them one at a time, using a spring chronometer to measure the time it took to form two associations with the word thus drawn. The associations might come spontaneously and immediately, or only after a pause. Many of the associations were themselves single words, but there were many cases in which there came to mind not a word but a mental picture, an image ; and this image had to be described. Either a word or an image satisfied Galton's definition of an " association," but all were reduced to verbal form. These associations were analysed with reference to their probable origin in his experience, in particular with reference to the time when the given association seemed to have been first established. One of the most definite of his discoveries related to the great frequency of associations from early boyhood and adolescence.[3] He classified associations according to decades,

[1] *Op. cit.*, Section on " Unconsciousness of Peculiarities."
[2] " Psychometric Experiments," *Brain*, II, 1879–80.
[3] An example of a boyhood association was the appearance of images recalling the scene of a laboratory where he had been allowed to dabble in chemistry.

K

finding the more recent associations relatively few. This was one of the earliest attempts to show the significance of very early life, particularly childhood, on adult personality, and to demonstrate the amount of childish material that remains. But the conception of an experimental study of association was vastly more important than the results. Galton's association experiment was quickly adopted with greatly improved technique by Wundt, who had just founded his laboratory in Leipzig.

A second and equally significant contribution was the publication (also in the *Inquiries into Human Faculty*) of an extensive study of " mental imagery."[1] It was carried on by " questionnaire " rather than by experiment ; it was, in fact, the first extensive psychological use of the questionnaire. Galton put before his subjects the task : " Before addressing yourself to any of the questions on the opposite page, think of some definite object—suppose it is your breakfast-table as you sat down to it this morning—and consider carefully the picture that rises before your mind's eye. (1) *Illumination.*—Is the image dim or fairly clear ? Is its brightness comparable to that of the actual scene ? (2) *Definition.*—Are all the objects pretty well defined at the same time, or is the place of sharpest definition at any one moment more contracted than it is in a real scene ? (3) *Colouring.*—Are the colours of the china, of the toast, bread-crust, mustard, meat, parsley, or whatever may have been on the table, quite distinct and natural ? " One of the most noteworthy things about this experiment was its use of quantitative method. Images were arranged in serial order from 0 to 100, according to their intensity or likeness to sensation. Galton found evidence that some individuals have no imagery whatever within certain fields. Even some well-known painters reported little or no visual imagery. There were, however, some individuals for whom it was a common experience to have images nearly as intense as full-fledged hallucinations.[2] The study of imagery lent itself, as the association experiment had done, to refinement as an experimental problem ; before the close of the century

---

[1] The imagery of several individuals had been reported by Fechner, *Elemente der Psychophysik*, II, p. 469 f.

[2] The *Society for Psychical Research* published in 1894 an elaborate *Census of Hallucinations* (Proceedings, *S.P.R.*, X).

the investigation of imagery became a standard problem in German and American laboratories. Imagery proved to be one of the richest fields for the study of individual differences. And the attempt to get statistical control of data that could not be measured by the yard-stick was highly significant for psychology.

Galton's chief interest in the problem of imagery, as in most other problems, lay in the attempt to establish hereditary resemblances; he showed, for example, that similarity between brothers and sisters was greater than similarity between individuals taken at random. But Galton's own insight, as well as the comments of his critics, made it clear that the discovery of traits not explicable in terms of environment was no easy matter. There was no way of excluding the influence of tradition in the family. A barrister is likely to bring up his son as a barrister; and there is a legal atmosphere in the household, augmented by social and economic forces. Such environmental factors might cause resemblances even in such traits as imagery. Galton grasped the difficulty, and centred his attention upon the immensely significant fact of *twin-resemblance* in the problem of heredity.[1] Though very little of the mechanism of heredity was then understood, Galton knew that twins inherit more in common than other individuals. He collected, indeed, some remarkable anecdotes about twins who were susceptible to the same diseases, or who, though separated for some months, died on the same day. The many sources of error involved in his method seem not to have held his attention.

He was interested in the variability of human stock as a practical social problem, and the eugenics movement was his personal achievement. Eugenics, as Galton formulated it, aimed not merely at the elimination of the unfit, but at the general and systematic improvement of the race through the study and use of biological laws. Spencer had discussed the future of humanity in social and moral terms, taking practically no account of biological factors. Darwin had made it clear that evolution involved not merely changes in species, but actual elimination of some stocks and increase

[1] Thorndike, Merriman, and others have carried out Galton's original ambition of getting the intellectual resemblance of twins into quantitative terms. See pp. 361–2

in others. Galton asked whether it might not be possible
to establish a new biological foundation upon which a more
adequate social organization could be constructed. This
eugenic programme is still of small importance as far as its
social accomplishment is concerned.[1] But it has a good
deal of significance in the development of the biological
approach to the study of mental traits, because this type of
problem helped to force psychology to attain more adequate
technique for measuring such socially significant traits as
intelligence, and has impelled us more and more urgently
to determine the degree to which such traits are hereditary.

In all this work, as we have seen in several instances,
Galton was thinking quantitatively, and one step of the
greatest importance to psychology was his immense contribution to the science of statistics. Statistics may perhaps
be said to have come into existence in the seventeenth
century in connection with the tabulation of births, marriages,
and deaths, and had been greatly advanced by the discovery[2]
of methods of ascertaining the likelihood of errors of various
magnitudes. Nineteenth-century science, in pursuit of
causal relations between variables, had had to make much
use of the theory of probability, wherever causal relations of
a one-to-one type were not apparent. There existed, however, no standard procedure for stating the degree to which
two variables were causally related. The first step in the
creation of such an instrument, " the coefficient of
correlation," was the work of Galton.

Suppose he wished to find the relation between height
and weight. The relation was, of course, not one of perfect
correspondence ; there were *some* men five feet eight inches
tall who were heavier than *some* who were five feet nine.
Yet he could predict, with small risk of error, that the
average weight of a hundred men of the first group would
be less than that of a hundred men of the second. But
he sought to get the relation of such variables as height
and weight into quantitative terms. He devised a primitive
correlation method of measuring concomitant variations.

---

[1] Yet the growing disinclination to marry into stock in which some
individuals are mentally afflicted almost certainly owes something to
Galton.
[2] By Laplace, Gauss, and others.

He laid off the familiar x and y axes perpendicular to one another (as in analytical geometry) and marked off units upon both of these axes. Let us consider first an ideal case, a case of perfect correspondence between two variables. If, for instance, weight depends *solely* on height, there is a definite coefficient which measures the relation of a unit of height to a unit of weight. As the result of adding a certain number of units of height we have a directly proportional increase in weight: we have added one unit of height and one unit of weight at the same time. The recorded data when entered upon our graph give us a straight line at an angle of 45° from the x axis; this symbolizes a perfect correlation. But suppose we find, in another case, that at some points the addition of a unit of height does not add quite as much length as before. We shall then have a line which departs more or less from the 45° line, representing something between a perfect correspondence and a zero correspondence. If we find an increase in height, but no increase in weight, we record the addition of a number of units on the x axis and no units at all on the y axis; that is, there is no correlation.

But the treatment of variables like height and weight is actually more complicated. Among a hundred men there may be, for example, *several* men of the same height but of *differing* weights, and, though greater height would in *general* mean greater weight, there would be many individuals below average weight but above average height. These exceptions to the general tendency would "lower the correlation." How was the relation to be precisely measured?

Pearson, Galton's pupil, saw the application of Gauss's " theory of least squares " to this problem. He saw that in measuring a correlation we may take the products of the x and y deviations and add these products algebraically. Tending towards a positive or plus correlation, for example, is a man above average in both weight and height; tending towards a negative or minus correlation a man above average in one and below average in the other. His formula, worked out in the last decade of the century, superseded Galton's graphic method, and made possible the statement of correlations on a scale from 0 to 1·00. It permitted a quantitative statement of the degree of dependence between

any two measurable variables, or, of course, of their dependence upon some other factor or factors.[1]

Evolutionism profoundly affected also the sister sciences of
anthropology, sociology, and economics in many ways,
tending in general to bring their subject matter closer to the
interests of the psychologists, to make them more psychological. In the social sciences, as in the physical and biological
sciences, the idea of evolution was already familiar ; it had
been a current method of approach to the phenomena of
social life long before Darwin.   But Darwinism gave it a
force, a rational basis, a mass of empirical data, and hence
a prestige which it could not otherwise have attained.

Evolutionary thinking, to use the term very broadly,
appears in the work of the German travellers, Bastian and
Ratzel. Ratzel's volumes, published early in the latter half of
the century, described human customs as ways of adjusting
to various environments. This work was followed by
the world-wide assemblage[2] of data by Herbert Spencer.[3]
His work, however, was hardly inductive ; he was concerned
rather to find support for a scheme of evolution through
which he believed human institutions must pass. Spencer
held that social institutions passed through a definite series
of *stages ;* fundamental laws of development were supposed
to lie behind changes in economic and social structure.
This was the first clear evolutionary approach to anthropological data.

The work of Tylor[4] expressed a somewhat less extreme
evolutionism. Tylor's central problem, and that which
stands out as his greatest contribution, is connected with the
doctrine that religion has evolved from certain attributes
of primitive mentality. His theory of *animism* held that
primitive man universally thinks of the world as a host of
animated beings. The forces of nature, and all things
perceived, are friendly or inimical to man ; they are quasi-
personal, animate, or " besouled." No difference is made

---

[1] It does not prove *direct* causal relationship, but does measure the
" concomitant variation " which must appear (though perhaps masked)
if causal relationship exists.
[2] Through many scattered collaborators.
[3] *Principles of Sociology* (1880–96).
[4] E.g., *Primitive Culture* (1871).

between a man, a flower, a stone, and a star, as far as their animate nature is concerned. If a man trips on a stone, giving himself an ugly fall, the stone is malevolent. Or he may go fishing, and the moment he casts his net may get a large catch ; this must be due to the favour of some natural deity. He seizes upon the most obvious thing, perhaps the lake. to worship. Moreover, human and animal souls are, for primitive man, something separate from the body. Like wine which can be poured into or out of a bottle, the soul in dreams seems to him to pass into or out of the body. This animism was shown to be general among primitive people, and important in their thinking. Tylor succeeded in establishing his view ; it was widely accepted practically without change until very late in the century, when it underwent certain modifications to which we shall refer later (p. 301). It was an epoch-making contribution to psychological anthropology. Religion and magic were given a simple and universal psychological interpretation. This doctrine of Tylor was accompanied by an emphasis upon a theory of cultural development known as " parallelism," which asserted that wherever cultures are at the same level of advancement, the same customs may arise independently among different groups. Wherever the environments of two tribes or peoples are similar, the peoples tend to develop the same adaptations.

Towards the close of the century a large amount of data came to hand whose effect was to undermine this more naïve evolutionary point of view. In particular, there was evidence to show that many of these cases of " parallelism " were due not to independent adaptation of different groups to similar environments, but to borrowing or " diffusion " between tribes.[1] The possibility of diffusion necessitated a more critical and inductive approach to each alleged instance. Another factor equally important in forcing a revision of anthropological evolutionism was the discovery that no definite series of stages through which societies pass can be found · the stages are different for different societies. The use of evolutionary conceptions had its value ; its very weaknesses helped to make clear the necessity of taking account of the extraordinary variety of cultural changes,

[1] Moreover, many supposed cases of parallelism turned out on closer examination to involve only the most superficial resemblances.

and helped to give anthropology the opportunity of becoming an inductive science. The problem of parallelism and diffusion has also played its part in turning cultural anthropology towards a highly empirical and inductive programme of research.

Much the same kind of development was going on in sociology. One of the first great figures was Auguste Comte. During the second quarter of the nineteenth century he became known for a simple but definite evolutionary theory associated with a philosophy to which he gave the name of " positivism."[1] His viewpoint was, in part, a reaction against the " idealism "[2] of French philosophers, a demand for empirical methods, for objectivity and definiteness. Comte became a colossal influence in social theory, chiefly through the efforts of John Stuart Mill, who introduced his views to the British public. Through Mill's work, curiously enough, he then became an important figure in French thought, to which positivism in Comte's day had meant little. Comte's evolutionism can be summarized in a few words : there are three stages in human evolution, the theological, the metaphysical, and the positive. Social reconstruction is to be effected through the emancipation of mankind from metaphysics in favour of the habit of direct appeal to experience. Terse as the doctrine was, it was important for social theory, allying itself easily with other forms of evolutionism and helping greatly to substitute dynamic for static conceptions of society. Comte also inveighed against introspective methods very much in the spirit of modern behaviourism; if he had offered a programme of research, he might fairly be called the first behaviourist.

Another great social evolutionist was Karl Marx, a figure intermediate between economics and sociology. His *Communist Manifesto* (1847), in collaboration with Engels, and his work on *Capital* (1867) were steps in the enunciation of the " economic interpretation of history," the view that social changes result primarily from the operation of economic laws. Marx was but one among many who gave expression before Darwin to what we may call " economic evolutionism." But, popular though such systems were, they suffered the same fate as the anthropological evolutionism just mentioned.

---

[1] His first important work was *Politique positive* (1824).
[2] One aspect of the idealistic movement was the work of Royer-Collard mentioned above (p. 58).

Theories were overdriven, and the "German Historical School" of economics pointed the way to a more critical and inductive analysis of economic change.

The theory of evolution was also conspicuous in linguistic science. Max Müller stood out as one of the greatest products of the university system which, as we have seen, was the cradle of philological science in the late eighteenth and early nineteenth centuries. As an instance of German philological work in the nineteenth century may be mentioned Müller's study of the gradual differentiation of the Indo-European languages. Closely allied to such philological work was the study of the religion of early Aryan peoples, and the stages in its development, as exemplified in mythology and sacred writings.

Another social science, which concerns us more closely, is the "folk psychology" of Steinthal and Lazarus. In a journal[1] appearing in 1860, they published much material relating to the folklore, customs, and religion of many peoples. Their work presupposed the existence of differences in the fundamental psychology of races, by virtue of which, for example, the Norwegian looks at things differently from an Italian or an American Indian. The elements which go to form the aggregate of what members of a race have in common psychologically they regarded as a social mind.[2] They were concerned also with the problem of transition from one to another type of social mind, and the material which they gathered contributed its share to the vast stream of evolutionary thinking. Their work was important also as background for the "folk psychology" and "social psychology" of the late nineteenth century, to be considered later.[3]

---

[1] *Zeitschrift für Völkerpsychologie und Sprachwissenschaft.*

[2] They espoused, in fact, the theory of a "social mind" distinct from that of individuals in the social groups.

[3] Page 172, and Chap. XVIII.

CHAPTER VIII

PSYCHIATRY FROM PINEL AND MESMER TO CHARCOT

This art of medicine, if research be continued on the same method, can all be discovered.—Hippocrates.

THE development of psychiatry during the nineteenth century may be divided into the study of three types of mental abnormality : insanity (the psychoses) ; mental deficiency ; and the psychoneuroses (functional nervous disorders).

Several of the common types of insanity had been recognized and described during the seventeenth and eighteenth centuries. Our first concern is with Pinel, who succeeded near the end of the eighteenth century in greatly strengthening the medical as against the demonic view of mental disease (see p. 34). He insisted that the insane are sick, not wicked ; that insanity is a disease which can in some cases be removed through removal of physical causes. He did much to encourage humane treatment for the insane, and his work obtained immediate and wide recognition. Such views had been held before, but Pinel's authority helped to make them the orthodox or established doctrine. There was practically no demonological psychiatry after his time. Pinel was more than the advocate of a new viewpoint. He was one of the great classifiers of mental disorders, working out a fairly satisfactory rule-of-thumb classification, in which the gross symptoms of many disorders were delineated. Perhaps his greatest successor was Esquirol, who assisted in the refinement of Pinel's classification. In the meantime, Moreau de Tours[1] gave a distinctly *psychological* account of mental disorder.

During the time of Esquirol's dominance in France, German psychiatry began to appreciate the significance of the work

---

[1] *E.g., Études physiologiques sur la folie* (1840).

being done, and there arose during the second quarter of the century a number of German physicians who contributed to the problem of classification. Chief among them was Griesinger, whose work was much more elaborate and detailed. He conceived of mental disease in the definite terms of physical pathology. Throughout the remainder of the century emphasis alternated between somatic factors and psychic factors. The importance of the somatic conception lay not only in pointing to the etiology of some of the " organic psychoses," but in awakening physicians to the fact that insanity was *their* problem. In the generation which followed, new systems of classification were legion. (Of course, the classifications took account for the most part of gross symptoms rather than of etiology.) We find, for example, good descriptions of the condition known as mania : the patient is excited and agitated, talks incoherently, and is frequently elated. Such problems as the average duration of such conditions, the existence of intellectual disorder remaining after recovery from the attack, and the like, were very inadequately treated. Griesinger's work was followed by more and more subdividing of clinical types. Among his followers, the subdivision of clinical types into sub-heads bearing new names went so far that some classifications listed as high as three hundred mental disorders. In the third quarter of the century the pendulum began to swing back, and there was a tendency to emphasize a few main types. We shall see later on (p. 171) that under Kraepelin's influence, psychiatry tended to settle down to the recognition of about twenty main types of mental disorder. Remarkably enough, there was no general recognition among physicians that normal psychology had anything to offer, and no recognition among psychologists that mental disorder could teach them anything.

Another dominant element in the development of psychiatry was research on the nervous system, particularly on the brain. Many mental diseases had now been recognized as physical entities ; for example, by the middle of the century many of the gross pathological changes in the nervous system in *dementia paralytica* (general paresis) were definitely known from post-mortem examinations. In this field, as in that of classification, German work overtook the French.

Progress in neurology was paralleled by the movement for humane treatment of the insane. This was of extraordinary importance for psychiatry, because it was the chief means by which the insane were taken from the hands of jailers and almshouse-keepers, and given into the care of physicians. Before the middle of the century institutions for the insane were few and far between. Private institutions were pitifully inadequate ; and society was not sufficiently interested to support public institutions. The creation of a public conscience recognizing the obligation of society to care for the insane was chiefly the work of one person, a woman subject to long illnesses and interruptions, but a person of very extraordinary personal gifts. Dorothea Dix became interested about 1840 in the condition of prisoners, and made visits to the prisons and jails of her own State, Massachusetts. The conditions prevailing were unspeakable, one of the worst abuses being the incarceration of many insane and feeble-minded together with criminals of " normal " make-up. From this beginning her work extended into two fields, one the reform of institutions for criminals, the other the creation of public institutions for the insane. Her method was the arousal of public conscience and the persuasion of legislative bodies. Massachusetts, as a result of her efforts, appropriated funds for an institution for the insane ; nearby States quickly followed. Miss Dix travelled down the Atlantic coast and into the Southern States, sweeping everything before her ; legislature after legislature capitulated. Within thirty years twenty States had established such institutions. Always in delicate health and realizing the necessity of avoiding a breakdown, she went to England. But finding that there were no public institutions for the insane in Scotland, she proceeded to get an Act of Parliament to provide for them. " She extended her work into the Channel Islands, and then to France, Italy, Austria, Greece, Turkey, Russia, Sweden, Norway, Denmark, Holland, Belgium, and a part of Germany. Her influence over Arinori Mori, the Japanese *chargé d'affaires* at Washington, led eventually to the establishment of two asylums for the insane in Japan."[1] There are few cases in history where a social movement of

---

[1] *Encyc. Brit.*, 11th ed., " Dorothea Dix."

such proportions can be attributed to the work of a single individual.[1]

In 1798 a group of French sportsmen found in Aveyron a boy about ten years old who seemed to be as wild and uncivilized a creature as they had ever seen. He was apparently living on such things as he could pick up. He could not talk intelligibly. (About a dozen such "wild" foundlings are known to history.) He was taken to Paris, and turned over to Itard, an expert in the methods of training the deaf. Itard was under the influence of associationist psychology, particularly as represented by Condillac, whose principle, it will be recalled, was that experience is the basis of all mental capacity, and that from experience is to be explained all mental growth. Adult intelligence is built up through the accumulation of sensory experiences. Itard saw the opportunity to put the theory to the test. Here was a boy who obviously had very little intelligence, very few ideas. Perhaps if he were given more ideas his intelligence would be raised. Itard set to work, and for five years laboured most assiduously in the attempt to make a social being out of this pathetic foundling. He did not succeed, and reported sadly to the Academy that the boy was practically untrainable. The great Pinel had foreseen this outcome, predicting that Itard would be successful only if the boy were free from intrinsic mental defect. But tho Academy refused to regard Itard's work as a failure ; they were much impressed with the definite progress which he had made in helping the boy to form a number of useful habits. Itard continued to interest himself in the problem of the subnormal, until there came under his influence a young man, Seguin, who was destined to be the greatest figure in the training of the feeble-minded.[2] During the 'thirties Seguin became known for his own achievements. His emphasis was chiefly upon what he called a " physiological method," the development of the sensory and motor func-

[1] Her many other extraordinary achievements, prison reform, co-operation with Howe in the work for defectives, service as Chief Nurse of the Union Armies, 1861–1865, are described in Francis Tiffany's *Life of Dorothea Lynde Dix* (1890).

[2] The term, as used in this volume, is equivalent to the term " mentally deficient."

tions. The subject was to be educated first through stimulation by bright colours, loud noises, and the like. He was to be trained in motor control by being made to walk along lines, upon ladders, and so on. Seguin realized that there was no hope of bringing the feeble-minded to normal intelligence ; the aim must be to develop what capacities they had. In 1842 he became the head of a recently founded institution[1] for the training of the feeble-minded, but unfortunately he soon got into administrative difficulties and had to give up his position.

It so happened, however, that there was a large opportunity for his work elsewhere. Dr. Samuel Howe,[2] of *The Perkins Institution for the Blind* in Boston, found in the course of his work that blind children suffering from mental defect could not be trained by the same methods as blind children of normal intelligence. He recognized that Seguin would be a suitable person for him to bring to the United States to give instruction in methods of training the feeble-minded. Seguin accepted the call, and for two decades contributed abundantly both to the improvement of methods and to the movement for the establishment of institutions for mental defectives. Then, with the assistance of Miss Dix and other philanthropists, Howe succeeded in 1848 in getting an appropriation for the training of a few feeble-minded children. Institutions for the feeble-minded spread rapidly through the United States.

Seguin's methods remained the central feature in psychological work on mental deficiency until about the end of the nineteenth century, when we come to the modern period, with its measurement of intelligence and study of heredity (see pp. 348 and 358).

Following the lead of the French, a similar movement was spreading in Europe. Switzerland is of particular interest in this connection because of the prevalence along its southern frontier of the special type of mental deficiency

---

[1] Established at Paris, 1828.
[2] Howe is one of the most picturesque figures in our history. He took an active part in the revolution which gave Greece her freedom from Turkey ; and a few years later, while making a tour to examine European methods of caring for the blind, he tried to carry American contributions to assist the Poles in their struggle against Prussia. The latter exploit caused his arrest and imprisonment until the American Minister at Paris intervened.

known as cretinism. Napoleon had tried unsuccessfully to extirpate the malady by the transplanting of families. The serious problem of cretinism called forth the devoted efforts of a young physician, Guggenbühl, who undertook (1842) the systematic study and instruction of these defectives, in a colony of buildings constructed high up in the mountains.[1] This was the beginning of the now widespread " colonial " system of caring for defectives. It made possible the care of groups at a minimum cost, arranging them in such a way that they could be given attention without being subjected to disagreeable confinement. Guggenbühl won wide public recognition—indeed too wide, for extreme claims regarding his success led to a loss in public confidence and to the collapse of his undertaking, though not indeed of his influence.

Saegert, in charge of an institution for deaf-mutes in Berlin, encountered the same problem which Howe had had to face ; mental defectives among the deaf required special methods of training. He not only worked out methods of instruction but succeeded in founding in Berlin (1845) an institution for the feeble-minded, which led to the rapid establishment of similar institutions in many of the German-speaking States.

In Great Britain a home for mental defectives at Park House, Highgate, in 1848, was quickly followed by other publicly endowed institutions. The movement for the public assumption of responsibility for the care of mental defectives made rapid gains during the third quarter of the century and still continues. In the United States and in most of western Europe a large number of mental defectives are, however, still to be found in institutions for paupers, or without protection.

A fascinating story is offered by a history of the study of the psychoneuroses and of their treatment through suggestion. The story really begins with Paracelsus,[2] a sixteenth-century physician who undertook to show the influence of the stars on human health. Mesmer, an Austrian student of medicine, came into contact with this view of Paracelsus

---

[1] Cretinism is not found above a certain altitude.
[2] His chief importance in the history of medicine was his conception of the *chemical* nature of disease.

about 1760, and was profoundly influenced by it.[1] The conception of magnetic influences from the stars was in the background of his mind when, a few years later, he witnessed a demonstration of cures apparently effected by the use of magnetized plates. He discovered[2] that the human hand was as effective a means of magnetizing as were metal plates. The term "animal magnetism" designated this magnetic influence of the human body. He went to Paris, where, of course, as the intellectual centre of the world, all eyes were turned upon anyone who had some new idea to disseminate. He quickly attracted the patronage of patients suffering from all sorts of diseases. "Mesmerism" became a fad.

The centre of his practice was the *baquet*, a tub containing magnetized iron filings around which his patients sat. Long metal bars reached out from the tub in different directions. The magnetic influence was supposed to pass from the filings through the iron rods to the bodies of the patients. We have a few descriptions of what happened to these people. Some of them had "fits," or crises; they manifested sudden and violent disturbances. And after these crises a large number of them got well, at least well enough to keep Mesmer's prestige at a great height.

He was shortly confronted with severe opposition from the medical profession, which branded him as a quack. A royal commission was organized to inquire into the value of his work. This commission included the great chemist, Lavoisier, and Benjamin Franklin, the ambassador of the newly constituted United States. The commission, after studying Mesmer's work, did not controvert the claims of cure; they concentrated their attention upon the theory of animal magnetism. The cures, they said, were due not to magnetism but to the patients' "imagination." As a result of this negative report, Mesmer was forced to leave Paris. But the therapeutic use of magnetized metal and of the hands continued.

The chief of Mesmer's followers was the Marquis de Puységur, who made the important discovery that it was possible to throw the patient into a quiet sleep-like state,

---

[1] Mesmer's disquisition *De Planetarum Influxu* (1766) shows his early interest.

[2] With the aid of Gassner, a priest whom he met in 1776.

from which he emerged to find his condition bettered. Puységur found, at Soissons, that not only human hands, but trees, could be "magnetized." If patients stood beneath these trees, cures were effected. Then Franklin tried the experiment of telling peasants that certain trees had been magnetized. Some stood under them and were cured as effectively as those beneath Puységur's magnetized trees. This was, to Franklin's mind, good evidence that "imagination" was a sufficient explanation. The followers of Mesmer, however, went on with their work.

Shortly after 1820 another period of intense popular interest in mesmerism led to a second medical investigation. The movement had spread, in the meantime, to Germany, England, and America, and popular demonstrations were given everywhere. Mesmerism became an international problem ; from the medical viewpoint an international nuisance. The new committee spent several years studying the mesmeric methods and their results. They reported that the cures were genuine, and that, moreover, there were a number of mysterious phenomena not understood. These included the transference of thought from one mind to another without a word spoken, the reading of letters so sealed that no normal reading of them was possible, the "transposition of the senses"—seeing with the tips of the fingers, etc.—and other similar marvellous phenomena of the kind associated in the preceding century with the name of Swedenborg. The committee, however, drew no definite conclusion as to the nature of "animal magnetism." This report provoked the most violent dissent, not only because of its emphasis upon the genuineness of the cures but also because of the marvels that had been reported—telepathy, clairvoyance, and the transposition of the senses—which they regarded as cases of imposture. The easiest way to explain the cures was to say that they were all based on fraud or illusion. A third committee was appointed, which came to a conclusion more in conformity with the opinions of medical men, with emphasis upon the statement that "animal magnetism" itself was a hoax. Mesmerism fell into even more serious disrepute. It had never succeeded in getting a standing, and now it was thrown into outer darkness.

Not that it lost its popular appeal. Among British mesmerists the leading figure was Elliotson. He had such

L

faith in the mesmeric cures that he willingly submitted the phenomena to tests by skeptics.   He would " magnetize " a coin ; then the coin would be applied to the body of a patient, and the patient would feel better.   He gave a demonstration before one of the editors of the *Lancet*, who tried an experiment closely similar to Franklin's.   It was found that the only necessary condition was the patient's *belief* that a coin had been " magnetized " ;   Elliotson's " magnetization " made no difference.   But although mesmerism had fallen low, it dropped to a still lower ebb through its association with phrenology.   Since the hands had magnetic influence, it was argued that when they touched a particular part of the skull the trait having its seat at that location would be called into function.   This union of mesmerism and phrenology was defended in Elliotson's journal *The Phreno-magnet*.

A surgeon named Braid witnessed some demonstrations of mesmerism in 1841, which he could not explain as " imposture."   He later gave a vivid account of experiments with a young woman who, while in the mesmeric trance, gave ample demonstration of these wonders.   " Under ' adhesiveness and friendship ' she clasped me, and on stimulating the organ of ' combativeness ' on the opposite side of the head, with the arm of that side she struck two gentlemen (who, she imagined, were about to attack me) in such a manner as nearly laid one on the floor, whilst with the other arm she held me in the most friendly manner.   Under ' benevolence ' she seemed quite overwhelmed with compassion ;   under ' acquisitiveness ' stole greedily all she could lay her hands on, which was retained whilst I excited many other manifestations, but the moment my fingers touched ' conscientiousness ' she threw all she had stolen on the floor, as if horror-stricken, and burst into a flood of tears."[1]   Braid felt forced to recognize the strange phenomena produced by the mesmerists, but he had no use for " animal magnetism " and was determined to describe the phenomena in *physiological* terms.   He experimented with various methods of inducing the sleep-like state which mesmerists induced.   But in time his wide experience led him to see the inadequacy of the simple physiological doctrine which he had expounded.

[1] *Neurypnology* (1843), pp. 135–6.

The influence of imagination or expectation was obviously important. As his work went on, his view tended more to emphasize these psychological conceptions, inclining toward the theory of suggestion.[1] Both the theory and the experimental methods helped to put the phenomena of hypnotism on a scientific basis. Hypnotism began, shortly after the middle of the century, to be accepted by medical men. Even fifty years after Puységur's experiments, reputable physicians were few who would accept any explanation for mesmeric phenomena other than fraud on the part of experimenter or subject or both ; after Braid, the existence of a genuine physiological and psychological problem came to be generally recognized.

Another man who did much to attract the attention of physicians to the problem was Esdaile, a surgeon of Ceylon. He operated on many hundreds of natives, sufferers from many different diseases, using the hypnotic trance[2] to produce anæsthesia. It so happened that chloroform as a general anæsthetic was just coming into use (being shortly supplanted by ether). Important as Esdaile's method might have been in an earlier age, these more dependable anæsthetics made his discovery a short-lived one as far as general utility was concerned. It contributed, however, to the tendency to take hypnotic phenomena seriously.

The next great step to be made was that of Liébeault,[3] of Nancy. Following upon the work of Braid, Liébeault worked out more systematically than any of his predecessors the theory of suggestion. For Liébeault and his pupil Bernheim, suggestion was a name for the process by which ideas were accepted by the patient in such a way as to lead directly to new beliefs, attitudes and conduct. They believed that the mesmerist's, or hypnotist's, command or statement was simply accepted uncritically by the patient ; not only could temporary changes in the patient be produced, but, through belief in the hypnotist's suggestion of health, the patient seemed in many cases to be cured. Bernheim showed further that many common diseases, such as hysteria, could

---

[1] The theory of suggestion had been outlined over twenty years before by Bertrand. But he never succeeded in attracting attention to his views ; for this reason Braid rather than Bertrand is of chief historical significance.

[2] The method is said to have been familiar to native surgeons.

[3] *Du sommeil et des états analogues* (1866).

be understood through supposing that the subject is suggestible in respect to his inability to perform functions which no actual organic condition prevents ; as suggestion caused the trouble, so it could cause the cure. A man who has been in a railroad accident is amenable to the suggestion that his legs are injured ; the suggestion may be given him by another person or by associations within his own mind. Paralysis of the legs ensues. Similarly he may develop blindness in one eye or loss of sensation in one hand. The same individual, therefore, may be susceptible to a variety of suggestions. Such suggestions may go so far as to affect memory. These views were all systematically worked out by Liébeault and Bernheim, and became the corner-stone of the " Nancy School." The Nancy School developed hypnotic methods which emphasized the direct *suggestion of sleep* as a means of inducing the hypnotic trance, in place of the physiological methods associated with the name of Braid. Verbal suggestion was the chief method by which experimental study of hypnotic phenomena, as well as the treatment of patients, was carried on.

About the turn of the century the school came under the influence of the concept of " auto-suggestion." The term marked a rebellion against the assumption of the all-importance of *rapport* between hypnotist and patient, insisting that all suggestion is imposed by the patient upon himself. This conception marks the transition from the " Old Nancy School" to the " New Nancy School," of which Coué[1] was the best-known exponent.

A few years after Liébeault's work there occurred a partial return to the physiological viewpoint. Charcot, at Paris, though making constant use of hypnotic methods, advocated a conception of hypnosis which was in clear conflict with the theory of the Nancy School. Hypnosis was for him a physiological phenomenon to be understood as one manifestation of hysteria ; and hysteria was a disease of the nervous system to be compared and contrasted with various other nervous disorders. Hypnosis was, from Charcot's viewpoint, a condition peculiar to hysterics, and a method, *par excellence,* of investigating the hysterical predisposition. Charcot's eminence as director of two great hospital services

[1] *E.g., La maîtrise de soi-même par l'autosuggestion consciente; conférence faite par M. Coué à Chaumont en* 1912.

for mental disease in Paris was augmented by his introduction of clinical methods, which gave him an opportunity
to become the greatest teacher of neurology in the nineteenth
century.

Thus, a century after Mesmer's arrival in Paris, hypnotic
technique became an all-important method for this greatest
of clinical neurologists at the French capital. The position
of Charcot in French psychiatry and psychology is one of
such prominence that we shall return to him (p. 183) in
connection with our survey of French psychology towards
the close of the century.

CHAPTER IX

WE must now return to consider the progress of physiological psychology in Germany, which, in the hands of Weber, Fechner, and Johannes Müller, had made such a magnificent beginning.

Helmholtz was the son of a Prussian army officer, and was educated with a view to becoming an army surgeon. But the practice of medicine did not interest him, and he began to devote himself to physics and physiology for their own sake. Exposure to the " philosophy of Nature," on the one hand, and to the exact scientific methods of his teacher, Johannes Müller, and his contemporaries on the other hand, led to a definite rebellion against the former and an eager acceptance of the inductive and mathematical methods of the latter.

Among Helmholtz's many experimental and theoretical contributions, which dealt with physics, physiology, and psychology, three are of chief interest to us : his experiments on reaction-time, and his studies of audition and of vision.

The reaction-time problem was old when he undertook it, though new as a field for physiological experiment. It was discovered in 1795, in the Royal Observatory at Greenwich, that there was a difference between observers in the recorded time of the passage of stars across the meridian. In 1822 a German astronomer, Bessel, noticed that this held true not only for two, but for all observers. Bessel and other astronomers found this individual variation in recording the times of transit an important source of error. It became known as the " personal equation." In the 'twenties and 'thirties a number of physiologists devised simple methods by which to measure such differences. The easiest explanation of the facts seemed to be that one individual reacted more quickly than another because his nerves conducted more quickly.

Not very much more than this was done until Helmholtz

took hold of the problem. His first outstanding research (in the late 'forties) was upon the speed of conduction of nerve impulses. There had been as yet very little work upon this problem; Müller, in fact, had thought that the speed of nerve conduction was comparable to the speed of light. Helmholtz found a method by which he could determine the speed of conduction in the motor nerves of the frog. In some experiments he stimulated a point on the nerve near the muscle, and in others a point further away from the muscle. The difference between the time intervals from stimulus to muscular contraction in the two experimental series was the conduction-time from the first point to the second. This method gave him fairly consistent results, indicating a speed of about thirty meters per second.

Carrying the problem further, he undertook with human subjects the study of the complete circuit from the stimulation of a sense organ to the motor response. By varying the point of stimulation he sought to ascertain variations in reaction-time which would throw light on the speed of conduction in sensory nerves. These were the earliest " reaction-time " experiments as such. The results he obtained were so very inconsistent, showing enormous differences not only from one individual to another, but from one trial to the next in a given subject, that he abandoned the investigation altogether. What he was trying to do was to get a reliable measure of the speed of conduction in nerves. The individual differences which would have so much interested Galton were for him merely uncontrollable variables. Within the thirty years following Helmholtz's experiments more than a dozen investigators tried to confirm his work, reaching results most widely discrepant from one another and from Helmholtz's figures.

It was not Helmholtz, but Donders, a Dutch physiologist, who grasped the psychological significance of the problem. He undertook in the decade of the 'sixties, in co-operation with de Jaager,[1] a series of investigations which aimed at the discovery of the various factors intervening between stimulus and response. He realized the importance of some of those psychological factors which for Helmholtz had been a nuisance and a despair. The method of applying the

[1] *Over den physiologischen tijd der psychische processen* (1865).

stimulus and the nature of the task required of the subject were of capital importance. Donders used three methods. In the first, the subject made a specific movement as quickly as possible upon the presentation of a stimulus. This was called the " *a* " method. Next, he was shown two stimuli, and instructed to react in one way if one was presented, and to react in another way if the other was presented. This was the " *b* " method. Then the individual was again shown two stimuli ; he was to react if he saw one and *not to react* if he saw the other. This was the " *c* " method. The time in the " *c* " method (*e.g.*, reacting to red light, but withholding reaction to green light) was longer than that in the " *a* " method (simple reaction) ; Donders explained this on the hypothesis that the " *c* " method involved not only reaction but discrimination between red and green. This led later to the idea of measuring discrimination-time by subtracting simple reaction-time from that taken by the discrimination method. Finally, in the *choice* reaction between red and green (reacting, *e.g.*, with the right hand if he saw the red light, and with the left hand if he saw the green), the time was longer than in the mere discrimination reaction, so that by the same reasoning one might calculate the speed of choice. If the simple reaction was 200 one-thousandths of a second, the discrimination reaction 300, and the choice reaction 375, the discrimination-time was 100, and the choice time 75 one-thousandths. In view of the originality and ingenuity of this first attempt to measure the speed of higher mental processes, it is astonishing to see the small amount of data upon which Donders based his judgments, thirty trials or less with some of his subjects. The influence of training was disregarded. Furthermore, he failed to realize the danger of statistical errors in small samples. The validity of the method of subtraction has never been accepted by most investigators. But the work of Donders is of permanent importance in two respects : first, he showed that some of the variability of results was clearly due not to simple differences in the speed of con-duction, but to central processes ; second, he laid the corner-stone for the analytic study of the time relations of mental processes. He found also that the reaction-time for the different senses showed characteristic differences.

But to return to the researches of Helmholtz. Our next

concern is with his experiments in optics. His great book on *Physiological Optics* (1856–66) deserves a permanent place as a general treatise which brought together all the existing facts in the field, whether drawn from physics, physiology, or " mental philosophy," as well as the important new material discovered and interpreted by the author. Among the most important experiments he performed were those in relation to the external muscles of the eye, and among his important theoretical contributions was the statement of the mechanism by which the lenses are focussed by the internal eye-muscles.

A prominent aspect of Helmholtz's work in optics was his sponsoring of Young's theory of colour-vision. According to Helmholtz, the receptors in the eye which make differential response to colour are only three ; separate stimulation of these three gives respectively red, green, and blue. Each type of receptor is stimulated to a maximum degree by a certain wave-length, and to a lesser degree by wave-lengths adjacent in the spectrum. A wave-length of 526 mμ, for example, has a given stimulating effect on the " green " receptor, while wave-lengths of 500 and 550 stimulate it to a lesser extent. But these wave-lengths stimulate also to some extent the " red " and " blue " receptors. The sensation resulting from 550 is not a faint green, but a mixture perceived as a yellowish green. He showed that these three fundamental colours may be combined in various proportions to give the various colours of the spectrum ; and, when properly balanced, to give white or grey. In this scheme Helmholtz made the far-reaching assumption that there is in the brain a specialization corresponding to these three elements in the retina. There must be three kinds of activity evoked in the cortex by the activities of the three receptors ; combination is a central function. The doctrine of the " specific energies " of cortical areas (the alternative raised but rejected by Müller) was essential to Helmholtz's formulation.

The theory, of course, had serious difficulties to encounter, for example, in the problem of colour-blindness (and of partial colour-blindness). It had been discovered long before Helmholtz's time[1] that the colour-blind individual usually

---

[1] The pioneer contribution coming from Dalton, who gave a paper before the Manchester Literary and Philosophical Society in 1794, entitled *Extraordinary Facts Relating to the Vision of Colours.*

lacks sensitivity to both red and green. Why should red and green be lost together, but leave the perception of yellow ? This was difficult to account for on the Helmholtz theory. Similarly with the " negative after-image " ; why, after staring at a red patch, do we afterwards see green ? The facts of colour contrast were not for him so disturbing. The green border seen around a red spot on a grey field was due, Helmholtz thought, to the subject's judgment. For example, a small patch of white or grey is seen as if through a coloured covering. It is not distinguished as independent and colourless. But we think we see the complementary colour, since this, combined with the coloured covering, would make white the actual colour experience. Notwithstanding its difficulties the theory has kept itself alive and has in recent years served as the basis for new " three-colour theories."[1]

Helmholtz's work in acoustics[2] is both as substantial and as epoch-making as his work in optics. The brilliance and the significance of his experiments are difficult to exaggerate. We may subdivide these investigations into the study of three problems : the perception of individual tones ; the perception of combinations of tones ; and the nature of harmony and discord.

It had long been known that the pitch of a tone depends upon the rapidity of vibration of the sounding instrument. As regards the perception of individual tones, Helmholtz came to the conclusion that there is in the ear a mechanism capable of receiving all those individual variations of pitch which the hearer can discriminate. Experimentally determining the highest and the lowest audible pitch and the number of distinguishable tones between, he supposed that the rods of Corti were capable of vibrating " sympathetically" in differential response to all distinguishable tones. But the basilar membrane, lying in the inner ear in a conch-like form, was shown by Hensen to meet the needs of the theory more adequately. It was only necessary to assume that each fibre responded sympathetically to a given wave-length or pitch. For these fibres were just such as would be expected from the study of a harp, and of other instruments

[1] McDougall's theory, for example, assumes originally four primary colours, white being added to the three postulated by Young.
[2] *On the Sensations of Tone*, etc., (1862).

with strings of different lengths corresponding to various pitches.

But whereas the longest fibres in the basilar membrane are less than three times as long as the shortest, the highest audible pitch has many thousand times the vibration rate of the lowest. This point was taken care of reasonably well by Ewald,[1] who pointed out that we find frequently in sympathetic vibration a tendency for a body to vibrate not in little subdivided areas, but as a whole, and in a number of different patterns. A familiar experiment in physics, in which sand is placed on a vibrating brass plate, demonstrates that as the pattern of vibration changes, the arrangement of the sand on the plate varies, in accordance with the relative activity or quiet at each point. Similarly, instead of regarding each basilar fibre as an independent reacting mechanism, we may say that the whole basilar membrane responds in characteristic figures or patterns corresponding to all the distinguishable pitches. Ewald's work was not only theoretically sound, but empirically demonstrated on a " model " of the basilar membrane. Another objection to the theory was met by the same argument. In the loss of part of the basilar membrane through disease there is usually no loss of individual notes, but a disorder in the perception of pitch over several octaves ; it is as if many patterns were disordered. Helmholtz's theory, frequently with Ewald's modification, is still the dominant theory of pitch perception, though it has never won universal acceptance.

Helmholtz worked on the closely related problem of pitch discrimination ; and upon the " difference tones " produced by the difference in vibration rate between two tones, as well as the tones resulting from the *summation* of vibration rates. But perhaps his greatest experimental contribution was the discovery of what it is that makes the characteristic differences in *tone quality* or *timbre*. Of course, everyone knew that the vibration rate of middle C on the violin was the same as that of middle C on the piano. But the difference in qualities was not understood. Helmholtz discovered the significance of the fact that every kind of musical instrument gives off not only a certain fundamental tone, but, in addition, certain overtones with vibration rates more rapid than those

---

[1] *Pflüger's Archiv.*, LXXVI, 1899, and XCIII, 1902–3.

of the fundamental. The first of these overtones is the octave; that is, together with the fundamental, the vibrating body gives off a tone having double the fundamental vibration rate. The next overtone is the musical "fifth" above the first overtone. With the use of resonators he showed that by varying the intensity of the overtones he could produce synthetically the characteristic quality of each instrument, thus establishing the correctness of his hypothesis beyond doubt.

He went on from this to a theory of discord and harmony. Discord he believed to be due to a familiar phenomenon known as " beating "—the production of throbbing sounds resulting from the simultaneous presentation of two tones of nearly the same vibration rate. Dissonance was due to the presence of beats, either between fundamentals or between the overtones of the two tones under consideration. He believed harmony due to the absence of discord.

Helmholtz was much interested in the history of music. He showed that there had been consistent development (from Greek to nineteenth-century music) in the direction of a constantly greater complexity of relations between tones combined for purposes of harmony. To the simple octave there have been added progressively the fifth, the fourth, the major third, and the minor third ; the mathematical relation of vibration rates has become more and more complex. Apparently listeners, when adjusted to one combination of tones, are preparing for another with more complexity. Harmony has inevitably become more and more complicated.[1] The chief significance of the theory was its emphasis upon factors of habituation. The man who contributed most to the physiological approach to tone perception was not content to neglect the importance of educational and historical factors.

Several other Germans contributed largely during the third quarter of the century to the establishment of a

---

[1] Partial confirmation of the theory has been secured by H. T. Moore, who has shown that practice with simple intervals makes them less satisfying, while practice with intervals which are at first too complex makes them more satisfying. (" The Genetic Aspect of Consonance and Dissonance," *Psychol. Monogr.*, XVII, 1914.)

physiological psychology.   We shall arbitrarily select two, known for specific contributions which still form part of the working principles of psychology as a science.

It would not be far from the truth to say that Hering made it his duty to disagree with Helmholtz, or with some other authority, on everything.   Two of his counter-theories, one against Helmholtz and one against Weber, are of historical importance.

Weber had taught (p. 80) that the *rising* or *falling* of the skin temperature is responsible for the temperature sensations.   Hering attempted[1] to show that it is not the rising or falling, but the relative temperature of the skin, whether below or above its own " zero point," that determines the appearance of sensations of warmth and cold.   The familiar experiment in which one hand is immersed in warm, the other in cold water, and then both plunged into lukewarm water, can be interpreted as well on Hering's as on Weber's hypothesis.   Perhaps the skin of each hand has adapted itself to a given temperature, its temporary " zero point " ; the lukewarm water is below one zero point and above the other.

Hering concerned himself also with experiments in optics, particularly in the muscular aspects of the problem.   But he is chiefly celebrated for the theory of colour with which he opposed that of Helmholtz.   Hering did not claim originality for all aspects of this theory.   He elaborated and systematized the suggestions of Goethe[2] and Aubert,[3] and introduced improved experimental methods for the study of such phenomena as contrast, after-image, colour-blindness in the periphery of the retina, etc.   Goethe had argued that there must of necessity be four elementary colours (disregarding white and black).   If, said Hering, we take white (or grey), as demonstrated by Newton, to be due to the mixture of all wave-lengths, we encounter on any three-colour theory serious difficulty in explaining cases where *two* primary colours give the same white or grey.   If, for example, red and green mixed give white, the blue remaining should give us together with the white an

---

[1] " Der Temperatursinn," in *Hermann's Handb. d. Physiol.*, III, 1879–80.
[2] *Farbenlehre* (1810).
[3] *Physiologie der Netzhaut* (1865).

" unsaturated " blue (a tint or shade, not a pure colour). It seemed to Hering that while Goethe's hypothesis must be supplemented with more psychological detail, the four primary colours must be accepted. There must be two pairs. Red and green when mixed would give grey. Each, moreover, was the after-image of the other as well as its contrast-colour (the colour seen as a border around the stimulus-colour when shown on a grey field). Similarly, in the case of blue and yellow, Hering assumed that as a pair of primary colours which are thus related in after-image and contrast phenomena, they must, when mixed in the right proportions, give grey. Now it was known that blue and yellow when mixed do give perfect white or grey, but that many familiar reds and greens when mixed give not white, but yellow. This forced Hering into the curious problem of constructing a red and green which when mixed *would* give white. The red and green thus selected are not the red and green which seem to most subjects to be pure and simple colours. We have then red and green, yellow and blue, together with white and black. These six primary colours were regarded as having direct stimulating effect on the receptors in the eye.[1] To explain negative after-images and colour contrast, he assumed that blue and yellow light act upon one type of receptor, red and green upon a second, and white and black upon a third. In this he found an explanation for negative after-images and colour contrast. Each colour was believed to produce a chemical change in the receptor just the reverse of that produced by the other colour of its pair. Yellow light caused dissimilation or katabolism in the receptor ; blue light caused assimilation or anabolism. Thus the same receptors might serve to communicate either blue or yellow to the brain, depending upon whether the chemical process within them is one of building up or of breaking down.[2] In the same way, red

[1] The " duplicity theory," based on the work of Schultze, and enunciated by von Kries, asserted that there are in the retina receptors the stimulation of which gives colour sensations, and other receptors whose stimulation gives colourless sensations. Histology has not as yet determined whether the colour-bearing receptors (the cones) are of three types, as required by Hering's theory.

[2] It has been pointed out that this assumption of anabolism in the functioning of a sense organ is rather bold. Stimulation, as far as we know, regularly means katabolism. The doctrine of specific energies was likewise attacked by Hering's theory ; a given type of nerve fibre

and green, white and black, upset the chemical equilibrium in opposite directions. Now, of course, if any two of these opposed functions tend to take place simultaneously, we have the sensation of grey ; red and green cancel one another, leaving the grey which all light arouses through its action on the white-black substance. Blue and yellow similarly cancel. Negative after-images were easily explained. If we gaze fixedly at red we overwork the process of katabolism and break down tissue, and the reverse process sets in so that we experience green. The explanation of contrast was similar. Gazing at a red stimulus on a grey field causes katabolism in one retinal area and anabolism in the adjoining region.

One of the greatest successes of Hering's theory was its easy explanation of the fact that in colour-blindness red and green are usually lost together, as if dependent on one type of receptor. This conquest was pushed further by the experimental investigation of the zones of the retina ; the outermost zone was shown to be responsive only to white and black, the second zone to blue and yellow as well, and the central zone to all six of Hering's primary colours. The formulation of a hypothesis by which the blue and yellow, red and green, were linked together in all the main problems of their relation made it immediately acceptable to a large number of psychologists, with many of whom it is still retained without material modification. It did after all bring an extraordinary amount of order into a very chaotic field.

The theory has, however, undergone many revisions, some of which differ so much as to be designated new theories. Among these may be named that of Ladd-Franklin, which approaches the problem from the evolutionary standpoint.[1]

was accredited with two radically distinct functions. Not only the receptor but the fibre coming from it could initiate either " red " or " green " impulses.

[1] In this view, white and black were the first differentiations from a primitive sensitiveness to light. White in the course of time became subdivided into blue and yellow ; the end-organs became specialized so that either blue or yellow wave-lengths could be distinguished from those coming from the primordial " white receptors." Later on, the yellow became subdivided into red and green. This formulation had the advantage that the red and green did not need to be so selected as to give grey ; familiar reds and greens, which when mixed gave *yellow*, met all the requirements of the theory in relation to contrast, after-image, colour-blindness, etc.

The problem of colour has led to a vast quantity of research, and a great number of colour-theories has been and continues to be put forward. The significance of Hering for our purposes is not in the establishment of an unchallenged doctrine, but in the introduction of a relatively simple and suggestive hypothesis which continues to stimulate new investigations.

In the psychological work of Lotze there was an extraordinary synthesis of materials drawn from medicine and philosophy. He was in his day better known for his masterful handling of philosophical and biological problems than for the specific contribution which still bears his name in psychology. Lotze studied at Leipzig, took both Ph.D. and M.D., and became Professor of Philosophy at Göttingen (1844). He began, in a few years, to be a prolific writer. Within a decade he was well known as an author of both philosophical and medical works, especially of works which were *both* philosophical and medical. Like Bain, Lotze sought to unify physiological and psychological material in a coherent system in which justice should be done both to empirical findings and to the philosopher's demand for interpretation. Unlike Bain, he was a master of the physiology and the neuropathology of his day. He contributed to the elaboration of a form of idealistic philosophy which was destined to be of considerable significance in nineteenth-century thought. It influenced such men as Wundt, and became in time a foundation principle for many psychological schools. Lotze insisted, in the first place, on the futility of trying to find mental processes which are not related to physical processes ; in other words, he protested against those forms of idealism which sought to save a part of psychology from the encroachments of physics and chemistry. Psychology must deal with the organism. The nervous system and the mind must be seen in relation to each other. On the other hand, he maintained with equal definiteness that it was ridiculous to suppose that the mere existence of physical and chemical process was an " explanation " of mind. Exact science can give us no clue as to the ultimate nature of mental processes. In particular, said Lotze, the meanings of life, the significance of things about us, the reality of our pleasures and pains, the reality of our ideals and dreams, is not affected by the discovery of mechanical laws. Such doctrines sound like a commonplace to-day. Their importance in Lotze's time arose from the bitterness of the controversy between those who emphasized mechanism and those who emphasized human values.[1]

This approach helped to clarify the problem for the psychologist. It gave courage to those who were seeking a formulation of psychological principles based upon the natural sciences, while at the same time it cut the ground from under those who easily dismissed all problems of value as irrelevant, and those who denied to psychology a subject matter of its own.

Lotze made two specific contributions in addition to this general one. He went into the psychology of the emotions and was one of the first to give a detailed statement of the nature of the expressive functions, the way in which the face and posture, as well as the pulse, breathing, etc., behave in the various emotional states. He had, therefore, considerable influence in later formulations of the relation of emotions to bodily change (such as the James-Lange theory) and helped to prepare the way for the experimental studies of emotion which became numerous towards the end of the century.

But he is chiefly known for his theory of " local signs."[2] This was an attempt to find a compromise between the opposed views on space perception which had been constantly reiterated since the days of Kant. Herbart had made the entire spatial order the product of experience. Johannes Müller, had taught that the germ of space-perception is innate, but that the elaboration of the world of space, and its organization through the modes of perception known to the adult, come only with experience, He had advocated, as we have seen, a compromise view—that in spite of a primitive awareness of bodily extension much of the process of space-perception depends on learning. But many who rejected transcendentalism held with Kant that space-perception is purely innate. Müller's authority carried, of

---

[1] This is, of course, an arbitrary selection, for emphasis, of but one aspect of Lotze's philosophy. That he was one of the greatest of nineteenth-century philosophers is scarcely to be questioned.

[2] *Outlines of Psychology* (prepared from his lectures, 1881), Chapter IV.

course, much weight.   But he had not explained how a serial order is built up in the visual world so that each object is seen in a certain relation to each other object, above or below, right or left ; nor had the problem of tactual space been seriously considered.   These were the tasks Lotze imposed upon himself, and solved so ingeniously that the outlines of his theory still remain central in our analysis of space-perception.

Beginning with vision, Lotze conjectured that each stimulus acting on the retina caused not only a characteristic non-spatial quality such as colour, but a sensation specifically related to the point stimulated, and differing qualitatively from sensations aroused by the same object when stimulating any other point on the retina.   Each point on the retina had its " local sign."   The nature of these local signs and of their organization into a continuum, to give the world of visual space, was stated in terms of the muscular sensations aroused when, upon stimulation, the eye turns so as to bring the stimulus to the point of clearest vision.   A light striking the retina at any point causes the eye to swing reflexly to fixate the object.   But the direction and magnitude of the arc through which the eye must pass is different for each point on the retina.   Corresponding to all stimulable points on the retina there are, therefore, an immense variety of " feelings of position," forming an orderly, graded series. In the course of time each visual stimulus arouses by association memories of the muscular sensations previously excited as the eye sought its fixation point.   In this way stimuli which were at first non-spatial take on a spatial character.

There are likewise local signs in the skin.   We need only to note that in addition to the non-spatial experiences of pressure, temperature, etc., there are a variety of experiences which depend upon the region stimulated ; the tension and the curvature of the skin vary from point to point.   Each stimulus arouses, therefore, a number of distinct impressions depending on location ;   and these, through experience and association, come to form a coherent, graded series.   The order thus constituted is now associated with the world of visual space.   In the case of those born blind it is necessary to emphasize the orderly series of muscular sensations, in making contact with objects at various distances and in various directions from any given starting-point.

Both in visual and in cutaneous space the fundamental conception was that psychological space is built up from sensations which in isolation would not be spatial, but whose order of stimulation corresponds to transition of the stimulus from one point in physical space to another.   The theory was not only highly important as an application of physiological findings[1] and associationist theory to an extremely complex and baffling problem ; it marked one of the boldest and most fruitful attempts to make the muscular sensations[2] play their part in mental life.

[1] In particular, Weber's data on the two-point threshold, which Lotze interpreted as indicating that local signs change more rapidly in some regions than in others.

[2] Lotze's emphasis on the muscle sense in connection with vision was welcomed and carried even further by many, *e.g.*, by Wundt and Münsterberg, a generation later.

CHAPTER X

WUNDT was probably the most complete expression in his time of the scientific forces that were remaking psychology. He was one of those men who are great because they recognize the complicated intellectual forces that are developing about them, realize where they are tending, and undertake a synthesis of them.

We have seen that much of the psychology of the mid-nineteenth century was incorporated within *experimental physiology*. The latter included such psychological problems as sight and hearing, comparisons of " sensation-intensities " in the Weber-Fechner work, and the various studies of reaction-time. All these types of investigation were carried on in physiological laboratories, but were beginning to be coloured by a psychological cast of thought. There was in progress, on the other hand, the development of genetic method, due more to Darwin than to any other man. An evolutionary outlook had led, through Galton, to the empirical investigation of association and imagery ; evolutionism also encouraged the tendency to emphasize not only cognitive processes but affective and volitional processes as well. These various tendencies were synthesized in the work of Wundt.

Wundt took his degrees of Ph.D. and M.D. at Heidelberg, and was for a time a colleague of Helmholtz. He went in 1874 to the University of Zürich. He was shortly thereafter called to Leipzig as Professor of Philosophy, and there remained until his death in 1920.

In 1873-4 he published his monumental *Principles of Physiological Psychology*, containing the foundations of much of his later work. " Physiological Psychology " had, for Wundt, a rather special and technical meaning. It meant a psychology not only rooted in physiological conceptions, but investigated by *physiological methods*. Its emphasis was on certain aspects of the technique of the physiological laboratory. A genuinely psychological experiment involved an objectively knowable and preferably a measurable stimulus, applied under stated conditions, resulting in a response likewise objectively known and measured. But there were certain intervening steps, which were known through introspection, sometimes supplemented by instrumentation. In this formulation Wundt radically broke with the introspective psychologists from Hobbes onwards. For no matter how much emphasis had been given to behaviour, and to stimuli causing behaviour, by such psychologists as Hobbes and Hartley (and even by men who, like Bain and Lotze, were saturated with physiology), no one had grasped in its full entirety the significance of stating mental events in relation to objectively knowable and measurable stimuli and reactions. Nevertheless introspection, which had been present in rudimentary form in the experimental programme of Fechner and Helmholtz, became with Wundt the most significant tool of the experimental psychologist. To Wundt the keystone of all total adjustments of the organism was a psychophysical process, an organic response approachable through both physiology and psychology. What, then, were the relations between the psychological factors and the physiological factors ? We must, Wundt believed, study the processes by which stimuli act on the sense organs and those by which the sense organs transmit the impulses to the centres ; we must study the passage of impulses from centres to muscles as well as physiological changes in lower or high centres, in so far as all these may be known. But parallel with these central processes are the phenomena of mental life. We must, therefore, have psychology and physiology side by side, always beginning with a stimulus and following through to a response. Physiological psychology was, throughout, an empirical science ; it was a union of the long established introspective methods with methods borrowed from nineteenth-century physiology.

It is not an exaggeration to say that the conception of an experimental psychology was almost entirely Wundt's own creation. Many psychologists had insisted on empiricism, and many physiologists[1] had experimentally approached

---

[1] As well as philosophers, physicists, and others.

psychological problems. But four years after Wundt went to Leipzig, namely, in 1879, this conception of psychological method took definite form in the founding of a laboratory for psychology, independent of the laboratory for physiology. This was of no great consequence so far as its immediate technical results were concerned, but it was of infinite consequence in its effect on psychology. Shortly afterwards Wundt began to publish a periodical, *Philosophische Studien,* containing some theoretical articles, but devoted largely to reports on the problems of the laboratory. The yearly tables of contents give a fair indication of the interests of Wundt and his school. These interests, though widely varied, were for the most part identified with problems already generally known to physiologists.

We may classify Wundt's contributions under two heads: first, his work as a " systematic psychologist " ; second, his work as an experimentalist. His psychological system, his point of view and the edifice which he created, are presupposed throughout his detailed theoretical contributions, and in his organization and interpretation of experiments.

Starting with his physiological viewpoint, Wundt found a one-to-one correspondence, a parallelism between the excitation of the cerebral cortex and the various forms of experience. Sensations were ultimate or elementary forms of experience. Sensations were those experiences which were aroused when a sense-organ was stimulated and the incoming impulse reached the brain. They were classified according to their modality—seeing, hearing, smelling, etc. ; or according to intensity ; or according to other special features, such as duration and extension. There was no fundamental difference between sensations and images. These latter were also associated with local excitation within the cortex. In addition to these two groups of elements there were qualities known as feelings. Under this head were to be included all qualities of experience which did not come from any sense-organ, nor from the revival of sensory experiences. Just as there was a vast number of possible elementary sensations, one might not say how many possible feelings there might be. But they might be classified[1] into

---

[1] This classification appeared in the *Outlines of Psychology* (1896).

six main *groups:* the pleasant and the unpleasant, the tense and the relaxed, the excited and the depressed. This " tridimensional " theory of feeling may be crudely represented by three lines intersecting at one point. This point of intersection represents " zero," or an absence of all feelings. We may pass from this zero point towards greater and greater degrees of pleasantness or unpleasantness, proceeding in opposite directions along one of the axes ; in the same way we may record degrees of excitement and depression, tension and relaxation ; these would be represented by passing away from the zero point along the other axes. But whereas a feeling may be both pleasant and excited, it could not be both pleasant and unpleasant. Each term excludes not its correlates but its opposite. Of course we may have feelings that belong at the same time to two or three categories, so long as the " opposites " are excluded. It is important to note that this does not mean six different feelings, but six groups of feelings. The ultimate analysis of feelings was regarded as impossible, at least for the time being.

Another type of elementary experience was accepted by Wundt in his early work. This was the feeling of innervation, the feeling we have when we set going a nervous impulse to a muscle ; an experience to be differentiated from kinæsthetic experience (the sensations from muscles, tendons, and joints). Wundt abandoned this conception in later writings, because of the lack of introspective evidence for it. His empirical attitude was reflected in his willingness to keep changing his mind with each new volume or edition.

Sensations carry with them feeling qualities, and when sensations combine to form more complex states, a certain feeling quality results from the total. This total may again combine with another total, a new feeling resulting from this higher compound.

These feeling qualities are arranged not only in patterns, in cross-sections of experience in time (the experience at a given *instant*), but in certain *sequences ;* feelings follow certain regular orders, and these regular orders of feelings are called emotions. Emotions cannot be understood in terms of mere cross-sections at given moments ; they are characteristic sequences. In rage, for example, there is a characteristic series of feelings, giving a temporal pattern distinguishable from the patterns of other emotions.

Usually emotions lead into acts of will. Will, like emotion, is characterized by a special temporal pattern of feelings. Will, itself, is a series of feelings in which, at first, emotional elements, together with ideas, are present ; then ensue peculiar feelings of " resolution," from which the overt act follows. A particular series of feelings, therefore, constitutes the act of will. The line between emotion and will is purely arbitrary, except that volition includes some feelings never found elsewhere.

The question then arises, from our genetic viewpoint, as to which of these various processes are fundamental—reflex acts, sensations, images, simple feelings, emotions, or acts of will. Wundt approached this problem from a biological point of view, emphasizing the essentially adaptive nature of reflex acts (the term " adaptive " here summarizing the conception of biological adjustment). Acts which, ages ago, were the direct expression of the animal's wants have in time become mechanized, so that their essentially voluntary character is overlooked. Reflex acts, from the simplest to the most complicated, do, in the long run, what the organism needs to do ; therefore reflex acts were, for Wundt, " purposive."

Here we must mention the influence of Schopenhauer, who had made the will the central point in his philosophy. Schopenhauer's most important works were written early in the second quarter of the century, but it was not until past the middle of the century that his influence reached its peak. He had taught that life was essentially a struggle in which every satisfaction led to a new struggle, implying, therefore, the impossibility of attaining real or complete satisfaction except through the annihilation of desire.[1] Schopenhauer's metaphysics had a profound influence on German thought. He had also a very specific influence on psychologists through his attention to the will. With evolutionism it became easy to think of the will as the thing that adapts us to situations, that drives us when we are not adapted.[2] With Schopen-

[1] Schopenhauer's writings reflect the thought of India just as Fechner's *Zend-Avesta* reflects that of Iran ; such influences are a part of the new interest in early Indo-European philosophy and religion.

[2] Lamarck had stressed the point ; Darwin's theory, without using the concept, easily lent itself to such construction.

hauer the will was absolute and primal ; and intelligence had been evolved simply as a means to give what the will demanded.[1] Cravings were the ultimate mainsprings of conduct.

Schopenhauer had undertaken to show that will need not be regarded as a conscious function ; Wundt utilized the conception and adapted it to his own system. For Wundt the will was primal and fundamental, but in evolution its activities had, in some cases, degenerated into the mechanical reflex response. Wundt was heart and soul a voluntarist, a believer in the purposive nature of all life, from the most primitive amœboid conduct to the most abstract intellectualism. The will, though structually a *compound*, is of the very life of the organism.

We should expect to find in him just this preponderant interest in feelings and will. The feelings were indeed coming into their own in this period. Horwicz[2] had constructed a psychology upon the basis of the affective life. Bain[3] and Maudsley[4] represent the same emphasis in British thought. Wundt was not alone in his desire to get rid of the intellectualism which had dominated psychology. He was a voluntarist in the sense that he believed the will central, ultimate, genetically all-important. But the description of any experience must take account of the whole complex integration of sensory and feeling elements.

This leads to the characteristically Wundtian doctrine of apperception. Leibnitz had distinguished between obscure perceptions and those clearly apprehended or " apperceived " (p. 12–13). Psychologists had in general disregarded this observation, and had contented themselves for the most part with the study of focal consciousness (that which chiefly occupies attention) ; relatively few men had generally concerned themselves with total experience. With Kant, and with Herbart, apperception had been the process of assimilating and interpreting new impressions. Wundt used

---

[1] The conception seems to go back to Bichat's distinction between " animal " and " vital." Compare recent neurological emphasis on the priority of autonomic over central nervous structures, and the theoretical uses made of this by psychologists and psychiatrists (*e.g.*, Kempf, *The Autonomic Functions and the Personality: Nerv. and Ment. Dis. Monogr.*, Series No. 28, 1918).

[2] *Psychologische Analysen auf physiologischer Grundlage* (1872–78).

[3] See p. 110.

[4] See p. 185.

the term apperception, with slightly different emphasis, to describe the process by which the elements of experience are appropriated or laid hold of by the individual, that is, drawn into clear introspective consciousness.[1] At the same time Wundt felt the need of a term to describe the process of relating the various elements in a unity, the process of " creative synthesis."[2] Many elementary experiences— sensations, images, and feelings—are organized into a whole by the process of creative synthesis. We have in all psychological processes the following necessary steps : first, stimulation ; second, perception (in which the experience is present in consciousness, nothing more than that) ; third, apperception (in which the experience is identified, appropriated and synthetized) ; finally, an act of will which sets going the reaction. Wundt's apperception has enjoyed a prominent position in German psychology, though vigorously attacked by Ziehen and those of a more mechanistic turn of thought ; its influence was less profound and of shorter life outside of Germany.[3]

Everywhere, however, Wundt's doctrine helped to awaken psychologists to the necessity of distinguishing between focal and marginal events, in other words, to a more serious study of the nature of attention. The term apperception has in general been discarded, while many features of Wundt's description of apperception are still current under the caption of attention. Wundt's emphasis upon unity and activity represents, moreover, the same point of view that we saw in John Stuart Mill, in the reaction against his father's extreme associationism and atomism. Wundt held that it is of the very nature of human experience to give itself a certain organization.

Next we must consider Wundt's work and influence as an experimentalist. For in the early years of his laboratory it was he who set the problems for experimental psychology.

---

[1] This is but one aspect of a theory much too intricate to be expounded here.

[2] The necessity for such a relating process had been recognized by Lotze, who, in fact, described it as " creation."

[3] Though Herbartian apperception still found favour in many educational circles, James's gentle cynicism regarding all " apperception " (*Talks to Teachers*, 1897), seems to be shared by most contemporary psychologists.

Wundt, like Nestor, was "alive on the earth" with three "generations of mortal men." Born in 1832, and living until 1920, he grew up in the atmosphere of Hegel and Schopenhauer and the new experimental physiology which came to flower in the work of Helmholtz; he lived to dominate the psychology of the late nineteenth century, permanently impressing his empirical spirit upon it, and to witness in his old age the extension of his experimental methods to a range of problems vastly beyond the scope of his own experimental purview.

For Wundt believed that experimental psychology must concern itself at least for the time being with problems which had already been attacked and reduced to more or less quantitative form. He did not occupy himself greatly with *new* experiments. His task was conceived rather as the extension and systematization of studies already inaugurated.

Most of his laboratory problems may be classified under a few main heads which are already familiar to the reader. First came the psychology and physiology of vision and hearing, and, to some extent, of the lower senses; much of his work in optics (latent time of the retina, studies in eye movements and the like) represented a continuation of Helmholtz's work. A second concern of Wundt was the reaction-time experiment, as taken from Helmholtz and Donders. In this he thought he possessed a method of showing experimentally the three stages which he believed to be present in all responses to a stimulus: perception, apperception, and will. When the stimulus is presented to the subject, he first perceives it; he then brings it into the focus of attention, or apperceives it; finally, he wills to react, and from this the muscular innervation follows. Wundt's interest in the reaction-time experiment arose largely from the belief that it gave him an opportunity to verify psychological principles which were of much wider application.

But a wealth of data (gathered by Exner,[1] Cattell,[2] Ach,[3] and others) pointed to a very different conception. In

---

[1] See Hermann's *Handb. d. Physiol.*, II, ii, p. 271.

[2] *Philos. Stud.*, III, 1886, p. 452, and *Natl. Acad. Sci.*, VII, 189 p. 393.

[3] *Ueber die Willenstätigkeit und das Denken* (1905), p. 116 f.

practised subjects these stages were not clearly apparent. It seemed rather that the act of will occurred in the " fore-period " before the stimulus, while perception and apperception were to some extent prepared in advance, so to speak ; the subject knew what stimulus to expect.   In some cases certain aspects of apperception might be delayed until after the execution of the movement.   Introspective data made clear both the difficulties of Wundt's formulation and the difficulty of obtaining by introspective methods any exact knowledge as to the length of time which perception, apperception, and will may require.   Wundt devoted attention also to several other problems in the measurement of the speed of mental processes.[1]

Thirdly, Wundt encouraged in every way the experiments in psychophysics to which Fechner was still giving attention, and to which G. E. Müller had made important methodological contributions.[2]   Psychophysics, in the hands of Wundt, continued to present quantitative problems.   He did, however, disagree with Fechner on one very crucial point. It is indeed possible, he held, to say that two stimuli seem to be of equal intensity, or that one is just noticeably different from another, or that the difference between two stimuli seems as great as the difference between two others.   But he was not prepared to admit that sensations could be measured ; measurement, strictly speaking, applied only to the *stimuli*.   Instead of seeking the relation between the physical and psychical worlds, Wundt was content to regard the psychophysical method as a means of studying the relation between sensation-intensities and the process of *judgment*.   Stimuli have to differ to an extent which makes possible a correct *judgment* as to their relative magnitudes.[3] Wundt adopted a purely psychological interpretation of Weber's law, which was for him simply an example of the psychological law of relativity.

The fourth field of experimentation in which Wundt worked was the analysis of association, begun by Galton.

---

[1] Another aspect of the reaction-time experiment with which Wundt concerned himself was the distinction discovered by L. Lange in 1888 (*Philos. Stud.*, IV, p. 479), that some subjects attend to the stimulus, others to the response ; the latter were found capable in general of quicker reactions.

[2] *Zur Grundlegung der Psychophysik* (1878).

[3] For Wundt's work in psychophysical method see also p. 90*n*.

In 1880, Wundt adapted this experiment to the needs of the Leipzig laboratory. Galton had made use of single words as stimuli, but had recorded his responses in many different forms ; some were single words, others were descriptions of images of varying complexity. In the latter case a genuine classification of the responses was difficult, and their time-relations were insusceptible of exact measurement. Wundt simplified the experiment, and made it a more accurate instrument, by requiring his subjects to give each response in the form of a *single word*. In conformity with his whole conception of experimental psychology, it was now possible to examine in each case the relation between stimulus word and response word, and to measure much more accurately the time-relations involved.

Wundt and his pupils worked out devices for the uniform presentation of word stimuli in visual form. Auditory presentation was sometimes substituted.[1] Wundt then proceeded to classify the types of word-association given in the experiment. The types of association discovered when one-word stimuli were presented were classified under major and minor headings, which were to be keys to the nature of all verbal association. Since Hartley there had been scores of attempts to classify the types of association ; these were uniformly worked out so as to constitute a system intellectually satisfying to the psychologist. Even Thomas Brown, the most gifted of those among the moderns who attempted such analysis, never realized the simple wisdom of finding out inductively what the common types of association might be, in that world of heard and spoken language which plays so great a part in reflecting, if not, indeed, in the very structure of thought. Wundt recognized that Galton had hit upon a method all-important for inductive psychology.

He subdivided all word-associations into two grand categories, *inner* and *outer*. The *inner* association is one in which there is an intrinsic connection between the meanings of the two words. Definitions, for example, are inner asso-

---

[1] The desire for exact and uniform methods of presenting the stimuli, and of recording and measuring the responses, led to the use of the lip-key and of the Hipp chronoscope, and made possible a precision in time measurement which has seldom subsequently been thought necessary.

ciations ; the meaning of the response word is identical with or closely similar to that of the stimulus. Supraordination is a second type of inner association; when the stimulus *snake* evokes the response *reptile*, the subject has emphasized an aspect of the meaning of the stimulus word and has given it the form of a generalization ; similarly, subordination (*snake —viper*) and co-ordination (*snake—lizard*) involve meaningful relations ; so also do noun-adjective associations (*snake— venomous*) ; adjective-noun associations (*slippery—snake*) ; contrasts (*white—black*) ; and many others. Sharply distinguished from all these, the *outer* associations are those in which a purely extrinsic or accidental connection exists between stimulus and response. Contiguity in time and space are found here ; if the stimulus " candle " evokes the response " box " or " Christmas," the cause is presumably to be found in the subject's habits of buying candles by the box, or of seeing them at Christmas time rather than to any inherent similarity between the meanings. When the stimulus word itself, rather than its meaning, evokes the response, as in the case of rhymes, the association is classified as outer ; so also with the very common " speech-habit " group, in which the response word completes some catch phrase or ingrained verbal habit (dog-days, fire-fly). The elaboration of Wundt's system of classification was undertaken in 1883 by Trautscholdt.[1]

Among Wundt's pupils in the early days was Kraepelin, a young physician who saw the possibility of extending Wundt's experimental method to the related field of psychopathology. Not only were mental abnormalities to be studied through experiment, and their phenomena stated in quantitative terms, but mental abnormalities of the milder type were to be experimentally *induced*. The association method was applied by Kraepelin and his pupils to groups subjected to the effects of fatigue, hunger, alcohol, and other disturbing influences.[2] All these agencies increased the number of " superficial," that is, outer associations ; it was as if a disorder of attention had been produced similar to that

---

[1] *Philos. Stud.*, I, 1883.
[2] See Kraepelin's *Ueber die Beeinflussung einfacher psychischer Vorgänge* (1892). Bekhterev and his pupils were carrying on similar investigations in the same period (see Walitzki, *Rev. Philos.*, XXVIII. 1889).

observed in mania. Kraepelin's laboratory yielded also much valuable material on the curve of work, both in relation to fatigue and in relation to other factors making for increase or decrease of efficiency. These and many other investigations, such as those upon the effect of a great variety of drugs, have not only fulfilled his hope that much could be done towards the establishment of an "experimental psychopathology," but have directly furthered the course of experimental psychology itself.

Kraepelin is even better known for his systematic and substantial contributions to "clinical psychiatry," his descriptions of mental diseases being accompanied by an analysis of etiological factors. His classification of the psychoses[1] has been widely adopted. In this, one of his greatest contributions lay in perceiving a fundamental similarity underlying several types of "deteriorating" psychoses, which he proceeded to class together under the name of *dementia præcox*.

In 1894 appeared Sommer's *Diagnostik der Geisteskrankheiten*. This gave prominence to the association-test, by which Sommer thought it possible to differentiate mental disorders. In catatonia Sommer believed there appear many responses which have no real *connection* with the stimulus words—"irrelevant" responses (angel—spider, dark—triangle); in mania there are an exceptionally large number of outer associations, such as those arising from rhyme or assonance. These generalizations, though excessively broad, have in general been confirmed,[2] but their value for clinical purposes is now recognized to fall far short of Sommer's hopes; Kraepelin himself has been most cautious with reference to such sharp differences between the word-associations of clinical types.

These four experimental fields, physiology of the sense-organs, reaction-time, psychophysics, and association experiments, occupied Wundt and his pupils to an extraordinary degree; they comprised more than fifty per cent. of all the research work published in the first years of the *Philosophische Studien*.

Wundt did concern himself to some extent with child

---

[1] *E.g., Lectures in Clinical Psychiatry* (1901).
[2] See, for example, Kent and Rosanoff, "A Study of Association in Insanity," *Am. J. Insan.*, LXVII, 1910.

psychology, and to some extent with animal psychology, but he did no experimentation in these fields ; he was at his poorest in them.

To folk psychology Wundt devoted some of his best energies.[1] Believing that "cultural products" are a legitimate subject matter for psychology, he undertook a systematic psychological interpretation of the data of anthropology and history. His studies on the psychological interpretation of language are perhaps his best known contributions. He emphasized the interpenetration of psychical and physiological factors in linguistic structure, protesting against that naïve psychologism to which phonetics was a mere incident, and with equal explicitness against that merely philological approach which had sought to explain all linguistic change in terms of the laws of vocal utterance. But he gave the weight of his authority to that trend which aimed towards the understanding of each social group through the analysis of its language, believing that the very vocabulary and grammar of a people reveals its psychic constitution. Here, as in much of his vast and scholarly work in folk psychology, his conclusions were destined to be swept away by the constant advent of new empirical material. Studies in the diffusion of language[2] gradually made it impossible to think of language as an index to a cultural pattern or even to a specific mental make-up ; both the complexity and the plasticity of language seem now to call for genetic methods of analysis much more thorough than are yet available.

In consequence of his vast learning and the many problems on which he worked, Wundt gave a unity to the field of psychology such as no one else in his day conceived. Before Wundt published his *Physiological Psychology* and established his laboratory, psychology was little more than a waif knocking now at the door of physiology, now at the door of ethics, now at the door of epistemology. In 1879, it was an experimental science with a local habitation and a name. Although he was unqualified to handle many phases of the new science, Wundt tried to bring together experimental psychology, child psychology, animal psychology, folk psychology ; nothing that was psychology was foreign to

[1] *Elements of Folk-Psychology* (1900-1920).
[2] See, *e.g.*, Sapir, *Language* (1921), Chapter IX.

him.   He poured his energies into examination of nearly every corner of mental life.   And even when he failed as an experimentalist, he stimulated a great quantity of research work, which led far beyond anything he was himself capable of imagining.   It was through Wundt that the conception of an independent inductive psychology came into being. Through him, also, interchange of thought between persons working in the various branches of psychology was greatly facilitated.

Such a synthesis, and the establishment of such an experimental movement were, of course, the natural outcome of the development of the biological sciences, especially within the German universities.   Wundt was the fulfilment, not the origin, of the movement with which his name is associated.   But to bring such a movement to its fulfilment, and to outline with vigour and earnestness the conception of an experimental psychology which should take its place among the natural sciences, was an achievement of such magnitude as to give him a unique position among the psychologists of the modern period.

We have tried to emphasize the close relation between Wundt and his immediate followers, the fact that we cannot really distinguish between what Wundt himself did and what his pupils did.   When we speak of the Wundtian laboratory we have to think of a group of individuals, drawn from many nations and speaking many languages, catching the master's enthusiasm for the creation of an experimental psychology, free both from its sister sciences and from philosophy.   This viewpoint of Wundt inspired directly or indirectly a very large amount of research, and in discussing the work of individuals in the school it is a matter of opinion how far we should regard them, during their stay at Leipzig, as pursuing investigations in their own right.   Work with the association-test illustrates the point.   Some of Wundt's pupils, however, began even while still with him the study of problems which were both envisaged and prosecuted with originality and relative independence.

Cattell may be chosen as the most original and productive member of the Wundtian group.   His work brilliantly exemplified the spirit of the school.   This was partly through

N

the fact that he succeeded in winning wide respect for the point of view and methods which he had seen at Leipzig ; but he was also conspicuous for the versatility and volume of his own work, and the significance of the problems and results associated with his name.

Cattell went to the Leipzig laboratory in 1880 ; he later became Wundt's assistant. Partly on his own initiative and partly as a result of suggestions from Wundt, he performed a series of experiments which are corner-stones of subsequent research. His return to America in 1888, as Professor of Psychology at the University of Pennsylvania, marked no interruption in his life as an experimentalist. New problems were constantly attacked, and through him Wundt's methods made repeated conquests.

Of Cattell's various contributions the most elaborate in detail and most extensive in quantity was his reaction-time investigation.[1] At Leipzig he not only studied elaborately some physiological aspects of the problem, but gave close attention to introspective analysis (p. 167). Nothing could show more clearly than this that Wundt's point of view as to the nature of psychology constituted a large part of the background of Cattell's work. The study of reaction-time led to two elaborations, one the measurement of the speed of perceptual processes of various degrees of complexity, the other the use of classification-methods in the association experiment—another of Wundt's favourite children.

An important contribution to the study of the time-relations of mental processes was Cattell's investigation of the " span of attention."[2] He found that a subject could correctly name the number of lines shown in a brief exposure if the number did not exceed four or five ; the span for letters was about the same ; and it was not appreciably less for short words. For the study of the speed of perception under a variety of different conditions, Cattell made use of the gravity tachistoscope (which makes possible the sudden exposure of an object through a slit in a screen) and in conjunction with it the gravity chronometer. He measured the length of time during which a coloured stimulus must act

---

[1] *E.g., Philos. Stud.*, II and III, 1885.
[2] *Philos. Stud.*, III, 1886, p. 94. The problem had been approached experimentally by Bonnet (in the eighteenth century), and by Sir William Hamilton.

on the retina in order to be perceived as colour. He proceeded to study the speed of perception of letters and words. Problems in the latter field led to the invention of another method of exposing stimuli. This was a revolving drum behind a screen containing a slot which enabled the subject to read letters pasted on the drum ; the speed of rotation of the drum determined the rapidity of presentation of the various letters. Cattell found that in order to name the letters correctly, when they were presented one at a time as single objects, almost half a second was required. On the other hand, if he enlarged the slit so that one letter could be seen while the preceding one was being named, the time was from one-third to one-fifth of a second. In fact, as the slit was enlarged until three, then four, and then five could be seen, there was for the majority of the nine subjects a constant improvement in speed. This pointed conclusively to the factor of *overlapping :* that an individual could not only carry on simultaneously a perceptual and a motor response, but could deal at the same time with various stages in the total response to several stimuli.[1] This recognition of the measurable nature of overlapping processes is one of Cattell's most significant achievements. As we shall see later (p. 246), Bryan and Harter showed the applicability of this concept to the learning process.

These studies were part of a systematic attack on the problem of reading. Cattell presented words as well as letters, noting the variation in reading time as the words became longer and less familiar. In this work he found that the perception of whole words of moderate length took no longer than the perception of single letters ; in fact, letters frequently took longer. Here he recognized the principle that such perceptual responses need not involve the serial perception of elements present in the pattern. This principle of the organization of " higher units of response " was much utilized later in experiments on learning.

In the association experiment[2] Cattell employed the

---

[1] Cattell used the same approach in experiments on the perception and naming of colours, showing that the time required to give a colour its name was shortened if the subject was allowed to have a new colour in view before naming the preceding one ; overlapping was again present.

[2] Cattell and Bryant, " Mental Association Investigated by Experiment," *Mind,* XIV, 1889.

classification method as described above (p. 169). In his major contribution in this field there were about five hundred subjects. The responses were classified according to the frequency of each response word given. In relation to each stimulus, each response word was shown to have a certain degree of commonplaceness. This was the first " frequency table," an instrument elaborated and widely used in later investigations. Sommer[1] utilized it for psychiatric purposes, believing that the presence in a patient's associations of a large number of rare associations was characteristic of certain disorders.

The word-association method led naturally to the investigation of " controlled association," in which the subject was required to give not simply *any* one word, but a word bearing a specific relation to the stimulus word. Associationism had in general neglected the factor of control through the subject's attitude and the situation accompanying the chief or more obvious stimulus ; experimentalists like Galton and Wundt had quite naturally failed to see the importance of such control. In these experiments Cattell made use to some extent of Wundt's classification of association. He required the subject in some cases to give a contrast word, in some a supraordinate, in others a subordinate, etc. Cattell found that in general such controlled association was quicker than free association ; secondly, that some types of controlled association were regularly quicker than others, for example, supraordinates took less time than subordinates. This was apparently because the habits of classifying—passing from a species to a genus—are in general more firmly established than are connections from a genus to any one species within it. To classify " pine " as " tree " was easy and familiar ; but " tree " might arouse a variety of subordinate responses, each of which tended to inhibit all others. And just as this matter of interference delayed response so it was easy to see why free association, offering such a wide variety of possible response, was in general slower than controlled association. The same principle came out even more clearly in naming, for instance, a country to

---

[1] *Diagnostik der Geisteskrankheiten* (1894). Cattell's and Sommer's methods were carried further by Kent and Rosanoff in 1910, with 1,000 normal and 247 psychopathic subjects, using 100 stimulus words (*Am. J. Insan.*, LXVII).

which a city belonged or a city to which a country belonged. If given the stimulus word *Rome*, the subject quickly replied *Italy ;* whereas *Italy* might tend to arouse *Naples, Venice,* and so on, with almost equal facility.

Cattell found that an individual could read his own native language at far greater *speed* than other languages which he could speak and write virtually as well. Germans, even if very familiar with English, actually read it more slowly than German ; in the same way, although several experimental subjects were well trained in the classics, the speed of reading Latin and Greek was very much less than that for the native tongue. This showed that even such associations as were regarded as absolutely fixed and mechanized were capable of quantitative differentiation.

A natural outcome of all these experiments of Cattell was the tendency to pass beyond the formulation of general rules and to define quantitatively the nature and significance of *individual differences.* He had found, even in his early work, that some individuals differed markedly from others. But Wundt's concern was regularly with principles, not with questions of degree ; and it was not until the 'nineties that the field of individual differences, which had been originally explored by Galton, became, through Cattell, a prominent part of experimental psychology. Cattell's first elaborate exploration of individual differences, as aside from the determination of general laws, was in the use of the freshman (and senior) tests[1] conducted at Columbia, in 1894. This was the first battery of " psychological " tests ever given to a large number of individuals. Among these tests were measures of free and controlled association, and of simple perceptual processes, reaction-time, and memory. The improvement of statistical methods in the handling of results was much needed, and methods of studying central tendency as well as variability engaged Cattell's attention.

Another field in which Cattell saw the possibilities of a new mathematical treatment was psychophysics. This work he carried out in conjunction with Fullerton, in the years immediately after returning from the Leipzig laboratory. They devised a substitute for the Weber-Fechner law. The psychophysical work which had been commenced by Fechner

[1] Cattell and Farrand, " Physical and Mental Measurements of the Students of Columbia University," *Psychol. Rev.,* III, 1896.

had been continued in the Wundtian laboratory and elsewhere. Fullerton and Cattell collected a mass of data by a variety of psychophysical methods,[1] and proceeded to formulate a mathematical generalization which they believed nearer the truth than the Weber-Fechner law.[2] It postulated that the organic response to a stimulus must vary as the square-root of the intensity of the stimulus. Errors of observation are included among such organic responses, and as the stimulus increases, the factors which produce errors in observation increase not directly, but as the square-root of the stimulus. " The usual increase of the error of observation with the magnitude of the stimulus is accounted for in a satisfactory manner by the summation of errors." This work of Fullerton and Cattell was close enough to the general trend of psychophysical findings to be taken very seriously, but not close enough to be generally accepted.

Prominent among the later researches of Cattell were studies in the " order of merit " method,[3] the practical use of the method in the study of *American Men of Science* (1906), and the great stimulus given to methods of ranking and rating qualities difficult to determine in the laboratory, such as the " personal " qualities of individuals.

Throughout all these investigations Cattell was clearly working further and further away from the confinements of the Wundtian method. He might almost be regarded as a pupil of Galton rather than of Wundt (he enjoyed some personal contact with Galton, assisting him at the South Kensington Museum). He did, in fact, to an extraordinary extent reconcile and interweave the Helmholtz-Wundt tradition with the extra-mural psychology of Galton. Next to his versatility, perhaps the most striking of Cattell's characteristics as a psychologist has been the constant effort to reduce everything to quantitative terms, in which general principles and individual variability win equal attention.

In Germany the movement, begun by Wundt in 1879, to

[1] " On the Perception of Small Differences," *Publ. of the Univ. of Pennsylvania*, Philos. Series, II, 1892.
[2] Cattell, " On Errors of Observation," *Am. J. Psychol.*, V, 1893.
[3] " A Statistical Study of Eminent Men," *Popular Science Monthly*, LIII, 1903 ; " Statistics of American Psychologists," *Am. J Psychol.*, XIV, 1903.

separate experimental psychology from physiology, and the founding of journals to disseminate psychological material, went on apace. Most of the larger universities soon had their psychological laboratories. Switzerland, the Netherlands, and the Scandinavian countries were drawn to some extent into this development. The movement never reached anything like as great proportions in Austria as in Germany. This was due partly to the fact that there were in Austria at the time several great psychologists whose interests were chiefly philosophical; they were less concerned with experimentation. So, in thinking of German experimental psychology we must in general think more or less in terms of the German Empire.

And significant psychological experimentation was still being done in the laboratories of physiology. That is to say, in spite of Wundt's declaration of independence, the Helmholtzian tradition was going on and constantly contributing psychological data, of which psychologists had to take serious account. The exploration of the sensory functions in the skin is an important instance. At the time of the founding of Wundt's laboratory, no systematic exploration of the cutaneous senses had been undertaken. Wundt and his followers recognized, of course, that there was no such thing as a sense of touch in general, but it remained for the decade of the 'eighties to study intensively the sensations from the skin. This work was begun by Blix[1] and carried further by Goldscheider.[2] The latter is responsible more than anyone else for the existing technique for ascertaining the points on the skin which are sensitive to warmth, cold, touch, and pain. He heated a stylus and moved it from point to point, demonstrating that receptors for warmth are scattered irregularly throughout the skin. Similarly, cold, pressure, and pain had their sensitive " spots." The pain-spots were found to be more numerous than the others. Parallel with the study of the skin-senses, similar anatomical and physiological studies were published on the kinæsthetic senses, through which receptors in the muscles, tendons, and joints, enable us to determine the position of our limbs.[3]

[1] *Zeitschr. f. Biol.*, XX, 1884.
[2] *Arch. f. Anat. u. Physiol., Physiol. Abt.* 1885.
[3] See Goldscheider, *Gesammelte Abhandlungen, Physiologie des Muskelsinnes* (1909).

Whereas the work of Wundt, centring in such questions as reaction time and association tests, set the main problems for many psychologists, these studies in the lower senses, conducted outside the Wundtian school, became by the end of the century standard laboratory investigations wherever the " structural " approach, the introspective analysis of experience, was dominant. Physiologists and physicists were, in fact, contributing a great deal of important material on sensory functions. König and Brodhun[1] published, in the 'eighties, a systematic and highly important work on psychophysics in the field of light-sensations, showing that Weber's law holds for a middle range, but is quite unsatisfactory for low and high intensities.

Physiological psychology, in fact, despite Wundt's prowess and prestige, continued to be advanced by many workers who were not dependent upon him. Stumpf's *Tonpsychologie* (1883–1890), for example, and other studies of music, placed him second only to Helmholtz in the realm of acoustics. Much original experimentation was accompanied by ingenious interpretation. His theory of consonance and dissonance[2] won special favour. He emphasized the fact that tones an octave apart seem to " fuse " into one psychical unity, and that such fusion involves musical agreeableness. But when one tone is sounded together with another a semitone higher, the hearer is keenly aware of the distinctness of the two tones, and at the same time finds the combination highly discordant. The degree of fusion between tones was regarded by Stumpf as the basis for musical harmony. The fact that the increasing complexity of vibration-ratios is in general accompanied by decreasing consonance fits well with the theory ; but Stumpf's emphasis on " fusion " makes it distinctly not a physical but a psychological theory.

Another great figure in the era of Wundt, whose best work is in no sense a reflection of Wundt's influence, is Lipps. The study of optical illusions led him to the conclusion that the observing subject tends to project himself into the pattern. A vertical line, for example, gives the observer the sense of contending against gravity, while the angles and curves of many illusions make the subject expand, bend, or whirl. The theory has very important consequences for

---

[1] *Sitzungsberichte der Berliner Akad. d. Wissensch.*, 1888 and 1889.
[2] *Beiträge zur Akustik und Musikwissenschaft*, I., 1898, p. 1.

æsthetics. A man " feels himself into "[1] the material of
visual art, and the nature of the tension or relaxation which
he experiences determines many aspects of his æsthetic
response. A column, for example, must not have too large
a capital, because this would oppress the observer with an
insufferable burden ; while too small a capital would give
him the sense of great strength devoted to a trifling task.

Stumpf and Lipps are but two of many who in Germany
maintained their autonomy and continued to enlarge the
boundaries of psychology. The work of G. E. Müller, and
more clearly, that of Külpe, is in a sense a part of Wundt's
experimental psychology, but both of these students devoted
themselves to problems far, indeed, from those which chiefly
occupied Wundt. To each of these men we shall return later
(p. 197, and p. 237), in order to trace from them certain
investigations which are highly characteristic of recent
psychological work.

With regard to the experimental psychology of the
United States, it may be said without hesitation that in
the first few years of its development it was almost wholly
Wundtian in its outlook and approach. American psychology had been saturated with the spirit of the Scottish school.
It had been dogmatic in its approach, disregarding both
physiological and experimental methods. Prior to 1880, the
only important American contributions were a few articles
by William James (during the decade of the 'seventies).[2]

But now American psychology began suddenly to be
captured by the experimentalists' enthusiasm. The new
psychologists, who came back from Germany as pupils of
Wundt, carried everything before them. The first of these
in order of chronology was Stanley Hall, who was also a pupil
of several other physiologists and philosophers. Returning

---

[1] The term *Einfühlung* (" empathy ") has in fact come into general
psychological use.   See Lipps, *Raumaesthetik und geometrisch-optische
Täuschungen* (1897).

[2] The task of conquering the soil and devising means to utilize its
vast resources, the possibilities for the acquisition of land, and an
absorbing commercial activity, had kept philosophy and pure science
at a low level. America had made some significant contributions to
physical science (*e.g.*, through Franklin and Henry), but mostly in
relation to its application to industry. It would probably not be
forcing the point about practicality to recall that, whereas psychology
as a science had amounted to very little in America, the practical task
of care for mental defectives and the insane had offered through Howe
and Dorothea Dix an opportunity for American leadership.

from Leipzig, he went in 1883 to Johns Hopkins, establishing the first American psychological laboratory.[1] Hall did not carry out any important original experiments during his six years at Johns Hopkins. By founding, however, the *American Journal of Psychology* (1887), he gave the adherents of the new psychology not only a storehouse for contributions both experimental and theoretical, but a sense of solidarity and independence. When Clark University was founded, Hall was called to be president (1889). Two years later, Hall took another original step of considerable value to psychology, the founding of a journal dealing with child psychology. The *Pedagogical Seminary* contained much empirical work, but very little that was experimental ; and a large proportion of its studies of children rested upon very incomplete biographical data. But it did perform the important function of stimulating, both in psychologists and in educators, an eagerness to bring the psychology of the child within the scope of their respective fields. Hall played a leading part in founding the *American Psychological Association* in 1892.

Cattell, as the reader will recall, returned from his training abroad in 1888. Münsterberg was summoned to Harvard[2] in 1892, and Titchener began his career at Cornell in the same year. In 1894 an inquiry made into the experimental psychology of the United States revealed twenty-seven laboratories. In the same year was founded the *Psychological Review*, and in the year following the *Psychological Index*, both destined to play a very important part in the development of American psychology because of their collation and summary of widely scattered material. The laboratories and journals, and the *Association*, furnished good opportunities for the intercommunication of ideas and for personal contact. The chief factor in saving American psychology in this period from becoming essentially a branch of Wundt's laboratory was the influence of William James. American psychology, as the early journals show, was indeed interested in many problems not strictly experimental, but it was James who did most to give psychologists a broad and flexible definition of their field, in which the whole wealth of

---

[1] His pupils there included Jastrow and Dewey.
[2] Where James had done some psychological experimentation even before the opening of Wundt's laboratory.

human experience was welcomed for investigation. Before long we shall be considering James's contributions in greater detail.

French psychology, during the middle of the century, had been eclectic and sterile, except in psychiatry, to which continuous and important contributions had been made. Associationism and physiological psychology found, indeed, an able exponent in Taine,[1] but psychiatry continued throughout the century to be the field of the greatest French contributions.

Charcot began, in the 'sixties, the study of functional nervous disorders. Braid had made important theoretical and experimental contributions, outlining the theory of suggestion, which had been carried out more systematically by the Nancy school. Charcot became the head of the women's hospital for mental disorders, at Paris, also shortly afterwards head of the men's hospital for the same maladies. He first established in them the clinical method in psychiatry ; he demonstrated mental disorders before groups of physicians and students, lecturing upon them, and illustrating as far as possible the different methods of treatment.

He undertook investigations in hypnotic suggestion, to observe its relation to the phenomena of hysteria. The Nancy school had taught that hypnosis was a special case of normal suggestibility. Charcot, while conceding the great importance of suggestibility, clung to a physiological point of view. He came, as we have seen (p. 144), to the conclusion that hypnosis and hysteria were the same thing, or, more precisely, that hypnotic sleep was a phenomenon of hysteria, which could be induced only in persons of hysterical make-up. In this conception he emphasized, of course, the phenomena of " deep " hypnosis. He undertook to classify hypnotic phenomena according to various stages. The hysterical subject was put through a series of stages in which he showed a variety of symptoms, classifiable in three main groups—lethargy, catalepsy, and somnambulism. Lethargy is the state in which the patient is drowsy ; catalepsy, that in which there is loss of consciousness, inactivity of the limbs (usually with rigidity), sometimes with complete forgetfulness of the state afterwards ; and

---

[1] *On Intelligence* (1870).

somnambulism, a period in which there is a splitting of consciousness or personality into two parts, so that one part is ignorant of what the other does. Just as an individual may walk in sleep, so a person may, in what we call the waking condition, carry on for a considerable period an activity of which he afterwards has no recollection. These three states were regarded by Charcot as inevitable fixed phases through which the hypnotic subject must pass when hypnotized with proper technique. The Nancy school protested that these three stages were themselves dependent on specific suggestions—that the number of stages and the symptoms of each varied with the subjects' expectations. And they continued to challenge Charcot's identification of hysteria with hypnosis; emphasizing *light* hypnosis, many claimed to hypnotize more than eighty per cent. of all subjects.

Several of Charcot's pupils attained eminence. Among them, Pierre Janet[1] was especially interested in dissociation, the splitting of personality. This led to a systematic conception of personality as an integration of ideas and tendencies. In normal personality the integration is relatively stable and constant ; hysteria is characterized by imperfect integration, which in extreme cases may result in the cleavage of the individual into two or more " alternating " personalities. During the 'eighties and thereafter, Morton Prince[2] and others made the French work popular in the United States, while William James incorporated much of it in his writings (p. 209 f.). In Great Britain Braid had already prepared the way, and the work of the Paris and Nancy schools was easily assimilated.

A figure exhibiting the psychiatric interests of French psychology was Ribot. Though a contributor to many fields, Ribot is perhaps best known for his writings on psychopathology, especially the *Diseases of Memory* (1881), and *Diseases of Personality* (1885). He represented the fusion of two streams, psychiatric practice and mechanistic theory. The mechanistic physiological psychology of Hartley and Cabanis had made consistent headway through the adoption of much new material from neuropathology.

---

[1] *The Mental State of Hystericals* (1892); *The Major Symptoms of Hysteria* (1907).
[2] *Nature of Mind and Human Automatism* (1885).

Wundt's conception of physiological psychology, though not itself mechanistic, lent itself through Ziehen[1] and others to re-statement in mechanistic language.   British writers showing the same tendency were Maudsley[2] and Carpenter,[3] who saw in physiological psychology the possibility of achieving an empirical statement of personality, with the use of purely mechanistic concepts.   This movement, which was international in character, having its origin at no single point, but in the general trend of the times, showed itself most vigorously in the writings of Ribot, who made brain physiology and brain disease the basis of personality and its disorders.   He sought to show that personality is essentially a hodge-podge, a collection of odds and ends, conditioned upon bodily changes.   Ribot's desire for an empirical psychology, and his familiarity with the German work, made him a logical candidate for the position of director of the first French psychological laboratory, at the Collège de France, to which, a decade after the founding of the Leipzig laboratory, he was appointed.

This was followed immediately by the establishment of a psychological laboratory at the Sorbonne.   Here Binet began his career.   He was in his early years a student of hypnosis. He and Féré published a series of experiments on *Animal Magnetism* (1886), in which the chief interest lay in the investigation of hyperæsthesia during hypnotic trance.   The importance of the work lay mainly in the separation of hypnotic practice from its clinical surroundings, opening the way towards its utilization by the experimental psychologist. Binet shortly became associated with Beaunis at the Sorbonne.   One of his greatest services was as editor of the *Année Psychologique*, founded in 1895—a year later than the *Psychological Review*, and serving the same purpose.   He wrote a large proportion of the articles in its early numbers. This journal became a vitally important compendium of current psychological work.   Binet did but little experimentation, feeling that the problems and methods of the German school were in large measure futile.   But he was interested in systematic study of the thought processes ; his *Psychology of Reasoning* (1886) was followed fifteen years later by an

---

[1] *Introduction to the Study of Physiological Psychology* (1891).
[2] *Physiology and Pathology of Mind* (1867) ; *Body and Will* (1884).
[3] *Principles of Mental Physiology* (1874).

experimental study of thinking, in which his two little daughters were subjects. To these studies and to his all-important intelligence tests, we shall refer later (p. 239, and p. 348, f.).

Binet's collaborator, Féré, made two other notable contributions in this period. He discovered, in 1888, the electrical disturbances in the body associated with strong emotion, to which the name " psycho-galvanic reflex " is given (see p. 373). He conducted also important experiments on fatigue, devising the first ergograph for the measurement of muscular energy expended. The latter experiments are associated with his celebrated doctrine of dynamogenesis,[1] which emphasized the function of stimuli in liberating energy within the organism ; muscular contractions were increased even by apparently irrelevant stimuli. We may say that by the end of the century French experimental psychology was still far behind the German, but had displayed its own intrinsic genius through several men of the first calibre.

Psychology in Italy in this period was modelled to some extent upon that of Germany, and never attained proportions to make it comparable with Italian neurology and psychiatry. Not many laboratories were founded. Child study, as we shall see later (p. 281), attained popularity ; and considerable work was done on the physiology of the emotions,[2] but little that we should call experimental psychology was in progress.

Experimental psychology was received but slowly, and with little enthusiasm, in Great Britain. In spite of Galton's genius, and his marked influence upon Wundt and Cattell, British psychology made small use of his methods. It was not until the appearance of Karl Pearson that there was any Galtonian psychology to speak of ; and with Pearson and his school, Galton's *statistical* methods enjoyed much greater favour than his *experimental* methods. As a matter of fact, with the death of associationism had died much of the British physiological psychology that had accompanied it. Leadership in psychology was captured by the school of

---

[1] See, *e.g.*, *Sensation et mouvement* (1887).

[2] Though much of the work was simply of descriptive character, Mosso was one of the first to study physiological changes experimentally induced by fear and excitement (*La Paura*, 1884).

which James Ward[1] was the leading representative. This had two points of great advantage over associationism. In the first place, it emphasized the unity of human experience and behaviour, of total experience as against discrete functions ; secondly, it emphasized activity and adjustment, and began to absorb evolutionary ideas. The evolutionary point of view came in through this school as easily and naturally as through Spencer and Galton.

Toward the close of the century, nearly all British psychologists freely utilized evolutionism in relation to both man and animals ; Romanes and Lloyd Morgan devoted attention especially to mental evolution and to the concepts of instinct and intelligence. Such animal experimentation as was done was inspired more by Darwin than by Wundt. Evolutionism became, in fact, the dominant tendency.

The first British psychological laboratory was at Cambridge ; here C. S. Myers attained eminence as an experimentalist. Other laboratories followed from time to time, but their combined researches for many years did not equal the volume of work published in journals, such as *Mind*, whose chief concern was with non-experimental material.

This total picture shows rather wide geographical differences, much wider than exist to-day. Part of our problem in tracing the development of contemporary psychology is to show how international co-operation tended to demolish such extreme specialization on the part of different countries. We may say in general that German and American psychology at the end of the nineteenth century were chiefly experimental, that French psychology was chiefly psychiatric, that British psychology was to a considerable extent evolutionary and comparative. In the modern period some of these characteristics still survive, but the lines of separation have gradually faded.

---

[1] His article on Psychology in the ninth edition (1886) of the *Encyclopædia Britannica* was of great importance. " The article clearly challenged the associationists to show cause why they should continue to exist. No one wished to deny the value of the laws of Association as true for some aspects of consciousness and some of its connections ; the question here put to the issue was whether ' association ' should be regarded as the bedrock of all mental complexity and unity, or whether it was a minor affair dependant upon some larger and deeper conception of unity." Brett, *History of Psychology*, III (1921), p. 229.

PART III

Contemporary Psychology

CHAPTER XI

EARLY STUDIES OF MEMORY

We clearly understand by this what memory is. It is nothing else than a certain concatenation of ideas, involving the nature of things which are outside the body, a concatenation which corresponds in the mind to the order and concatenation of the modification of the human body.—*Spinoza.*

It was noted above that the decade of the 'eighties marked the first systematic experimental investigation of learning and memory. There had indeed been a little fragmentary investigation of memory and allied processes before that ; a close approach to experimental work on memory was Galton's comparison of childhood associations and adult associations in his own mind. There had been a little animal experimentation in the field of learning, concerned, for example, with the attempt to find out whether certain acts were instinctive or learned. There was not a sufficient mass of material to establish any general principle regarding the learning process. In general, psychologists were thinking in terms of learning *versus* forgetting, making a sharp line between what was learned and what was not learned, between what was forgotten and what was not forgotten. They were not yet thinking in quantitative terms ; they took no account of degrees of learning and degrees of forgetting.

The whole character of the problem was changed by Ebbinghaus, who (1879–84) subjected both learning and forgetting to quantitative treatment[1]. This was inspired by Fechner ; it was an attempt to do for memory what Fechner had done for sensation. For the first time, moreover,

[1] *Memory* (1885).

experimental psychology undertook, with an attempt to introduce the safeguards and precautions of scientific procedure, a psychological problem which was not simply an adjunct to physiology.[1] The great bulk of Wundt's experimental procedure had been borrowed from physiologists. The field of experimental psychology changed immediately as Ebbinghaus entered it.

His first step was the adoption of certain statistical methods through which the accuracy of observation was to be gauged by the extent to which various observations agreed (*i.e.*, the study of variability about the mean). This principle, furthermore, was stated in terms of the symmetry of the curve of errors. Such symmetrical curves, said Ebbinghaus, give us reason to believe that we are dealing with variable errors, not with constant errors. Variable errors can be disregarded ; for, if observations are sufficiently numerous, such errors in one direction from the mean should cancel those in the opposite direction. Bringing this method into psychology, he reduced psychological material to that department of the language of science which speaks in terms of averages and probable errors of observation.[2] In so doing, he atoned in part for the fact that he made use of only one experimental subject, himself. He got rid, to a large extent, of variable errors. Of course, the *constant* error, due to his own personal idiosyncrasies, remained.

His second great innovation was the elimination of another group of variable errors which may be called qualitative rather than quantitative—the *meanings* of things learned. We cannot by any possible process of analysis take account of the varieties of meaning that attach to words as they are learned and forgotten. Ebbinghaus wished to find materials entirely or at least relatively free from meaning. One can do this more effectively in German than in English ; over two thousand nonsense syllables can be constructed in German by the utilization of two consonants separated by a vowel. At one stroke Ebbinghaus solved a problem which had confused students of psychology, particularly associationists, for

[1] Psychological experiments performed outside the physiological laboratory had inevitably been amateurish and crude ; even Galton's association experiment illustrates the point.

[2] Fechner's psychophysical methods had expressed the closest previous approach to such a conception ; but Ebbinghaus borrowed not only from Fechner but from contemporary physical science.

centuries.[1] The extraordinary complexity of factors which make for meaning was in large measure excluded. These nonsense syllables were of unequal " difficulty," but when combined in groups their differences could be treated as variable errors of the type described.

Whereas Galton and Wundt had measured the time relations of the process of association initiated by a single verbal stimulus, Ebbinghaus devoted himself to the formation of *series* of connections. Instead of studying associations already formed, he investigated the steps in the formation of associations ; he presented for memorization a series containing many syllables which were to be learned in their order. An important contribution here was the standardization of the rate of presentation. This was set at two-fifths of a second per syllable.[2]

Throughout his experiments he made the general conditions of the experiment as constant as he could, experimenting at the same hours from day to day, and keeping his regimen and habits as regular as possible. The reader who takes cognizance of the vast quantity of work to which he subjected himself may well inquire whether his interest remained constant throughout.

One of his first problems was the effect of varying the length of the series to be learned, finding how the number of readings necessary for memorization[3] increases with the length of the list. He found that under ordinary conditions he could learn seven, frequently eight, nonsense syllables at one reading. This was the first systematic measurement of the " memory span." A sudden and immense increase occurred in the time required as he increased the number of syllables to nine, ten, and beyond. For example, instead of merely increasing twenty-five per cent. in passing from twelve to fifteen syllables, the labour required was considerably greater.

---

[1] " It is not too much to say that the recourse to nonsense syllables, as means to the study of association, marks the most considerable advance, in this chapter of psychology, since the time of Aristotle."— Titchener, *A Text Book of Psychology*, pp. 380–81.

[2] In spite of the many systematic variations of procedure he failed to study the effect of varying the speed of presentation, an important factor in relation to some of the discrepancies between his results and those of later experimenters.

[3] Construed in one series of experiments as memorization to the point of one perfect repetition ; in the other (earlier) series to the point of two perfect repetitions.

Ebbinghaus failed to notice one significant factor. He suffered from an intellectual blind-spot which is only comprehensible when one recalls the cardinal tenets of associationism. Associationists, with few exceptions, had disregarded the possibility that mind is anything more than a series of impressions contributed by experience, the possibility that it may *actively* adjust itself to its tasks.[1] Ebbinghaus made no distinction between mere re-reading, on the one hand, and the process of active recall on the other. He read through the lists passively until he thought he knew them ; he then forced himself to recall them, and wherever necessary he prompted himself. In some of these series he knew the list perfectly without prompting, and in other cases he might prompt himself several times. We cannot tell to what extent he made use of forced recall of material. He was saved from failure only by his statistical method, which, with so much material, presumably caused this factor of active recitation to operate (at least in most of his problems) as a variable, rather than as a constant error. It must, however, have tended in general to shorten the learning time. Not until the early years of the present century (see p. 258) was the importance of this principle of active recitation recognized.

The " memory span " experiment was a direct development of Ebbinghaus's study of the influence of varying the length of a series. In 1887, Jacobs[2] published a further investigation of the memory span with a number of subjects, the first intensive study of the problem. The method was adopted by Cattell and others, and has been in wide use ever since.

Ebbinghaus's next problem was the influence of repeated reading after the attainment of the capacity for perfect repetition, *i.e.*, the influence of " overlearning." He wished to know what happened when, after he had learned a series completely, he continued to study it. This involved his conception of memory as a matter of *degree ;* he sought to measure the *strength* of the connections established between observed items. Instead of relying upon the distinction between learned and unlearned material, he introduced the celebrated

---

[1] Herbart had, indeed, explicitly recognized *activity;* yet he failed to utilize the concept so as to draw a distinction between what is actively recalled and what is effortlessly brought back by new stimulation. For him, activity belonged to *ideas;* the distinction between active and passive *learning* was disregarded.

[2] " Experiments on ' Prehension,' " *Mind,* XII.

" saving method," which undertakes to measure how much labour is necessary to bring back what has once been known. Suppose we learn two lists of forty-eight syllables each, and then allow twenty-four hours to pass. We may find that from the first we can recall two-thirds of the syllables, but that it takes twenty repetitions to regain the whole list ; from the second list we recall the same number of *items*, but it takes thirty repetitions to complete the series. Ebbinghaus realized the possibility, in fact, the probability, that he could get a better test of retention by measuring the amount of work needed to *relearn* than by measuring the gross amount of material recalled. There is, of course, room for difference of opinion as to the best single test of memory in any given case ; in fact, Ebbinghaus's methods did much to make it clear that memory is not a single process, and that a variety of methods is needed because of the variety of problems presented.

The use of the saving method made possible also a determination of the value of various amounts of " overlearning," by measuring the relation of overlearning to saving. If it takes twenty repetitions to get the list of syllables, how many more repetitions are necessary to *retain* it twenty-four hours ? Ebbinghaus recognized that there is not only a stage just below the point of knowing the material, but a stage just *above* knowing it, so to speak. These are the convex and the concave sides of the same problem ; the formation of linkages between terms is not an all-or-none matter, but a question of degree. Now the amount of overlearning was compared directly with the amount of saving manifested in relearning. Knowing how much work would ordinarily be required after a given interval to relearn material which had been *just* learned and no more, it was possible to show how much more quickly the material could be relearned if it had in the first place been overlearned. The ratio of overlearning to saving turned out, in Ebbinghaus's data, to be roughly a straight-line relationship. Additional units of overlearning produced after a twenty-four-hour interval fairly uniform amounts of saving. With nonsense material, under the conditions stated, the number of repetitions saved was consistently about one-third[1] of the number of repetitions in overlearning. This investigation was one of Ebbinghaus's most important con-

[1] This linear relation held up to sixty-four repetitions ; the nature of the curve above that point was not ascertained.

tributions. The importance of overlearning, though slow in attaining recognition, has recently been much emphasized in education.[1]

One of the great triumphs of the saving method was the quantitative examination of the process of forgetting. From a standard mass of memorized material, decrements due to the lapse of various intervals of time could be computed. Having learned a list, for example, requiring fifteen repetitions, Ebbinghaus could find how much work it would take, say twenty-four hours later, to bring back that list to the point of perfect repetition, so that he could go through it without aid. In this way he obtained the material for his famous " curve of forgetting," which showed that forgetting was extremely rapid in the first few minutes, considerably less rapid in the next few hours, and even less rapid in the next few days. It became at last almost a straight line, asymptotic to the x-axis upon which time intervals were measured. This method established definitely a quantitative basis for the study of forgetting, and therefore of retention. The curve was extremely simple mathematically, stated in a form of very general validity. The exact form of the curves of forgetting, plotted by Ebbinghaus for his own data with himself as subject, has not, of course, proved adequate for other data and for other observers. These qualifications do not, however, affect the general form of the curve, which has been abundantly verified—an initial drop, gradually becoming less steep in asymptotic form.

The method was capable of application to meaningful material, and Ebbinghaus later compared this with nonsense material in order to determine whether the form of the curve still held good. He memorized many stanzas from Byron's *Don Juan*, and ascertained the amount of material retained after varying intervals, using the saving method. The same *general* shape of the curve was found for the meaningful as for the nonsense material, though the fall was less rapid throughout. Twenty-two years later he relearned many of these stanzas, having in the meantime completely forgotten them so far as his introspective memory or capacity for recall was concerned. Comparing these with the new stanzas memorized, he found an appreciable difference in learning

[1] The work of Book on typewriting (1908) was important in redirecting attention to overlearning (see p. 247).

time.   The saving method revealed some retention over the twenty-two-year period.[1] This result could scarcely be explained on the basis of mere familiarity with particular words in the text.   For in another connection Ebbinghaus directly attacked the question whether the familiarity of elements in memory material interfered with the curves or not.   He made up lists in which each syllable was familiar to him, and found that the lists were just as hard to learn as lists of equal length containing unfamiliar syllables.   It seemed to be the *connections* which were significant in the learning process.   It appeared then that connections established in meaningful material enjoyed very long life.

Another contribution which has been recognized and used on a large scale was the study of the most effective distribution of working time ;   the question whether a given amount of time yields a larger return when given uninterruptedly to the memorizing of nonsense or meaningful material, or when broken up into shorter periods with rest intervals between. Is it better, for example, to give an hour all at once to incessant repetition of a task, or to break it into periods of two half-hours separated by an interval, or into four fifteen-minute periods ?   Ebbinghaus found that " spaced " repetition was decidedly to be preferred to continuous and " unspaced " repetition.   He did not ascertain the optimum interval between work periods ;   but such evidence as we have indicates that the twenty-four-hour interval, which he used, was a good choice.[2]

Now we come to what is by no means the most conclusive, but in some ways the most dramatic, of all his findings.   He sought to answer the question whether associations are ever formed according to any other pattern than A-B-C-D, the letters representing items learned, and the dashes associations or linkages.   Hartley had asserted that if a series of elements, A-B-C-D, is learned, there is a tendency for A to recall faint images, b, c, and d, which are memories of the original elements.   Now, said Ebbinghaus, we know from Herbart's work and his mathematical formulæ (which Ebbinghaus almost alone of all psychologists took rather seriously) that there are associations not only from A to B, but also from

[1] *Grundzüge der Psychologie*, I (1905).
[2] Perkins, " The Value of Distributed Repetitions in Rote Learning," *Brit. J. Psychol.*, VII, 1914.

A to C and from A to D. There are ideas rising into consciousness and disappearing again ; there may be several present above the threshold at once. There may be in the process of learning more than two items undergoing linkage at a given moment ; several terms, A, B, C, D, may be in consciousness at once, and many linkages may be in the process of formation. At a given moment A may be about to disappear from consciousness, while B is, so to speak, at its zenith ; C is rising into clear consciousness, while D is only vaguely present. A moment later A has disappeared, B is declining, C is at its zenith, and D is rising. Any two items present in consciousness tend to form linkages. Hence there may not only be connections such as A-C and A-D but backward associations such as D-C and even C-A. Ebbinghaus undertook to find out empirically whether connections would actually be formed as the theory demanded. He devised a great variety of nonsense material for the purpose. Taking lists which had once been learned, he constructed, from these, *new* lists in which every *second* syllable was used, A-C-E-G, etc. Similarly, lists were formed by taking every third item' of a learned list, A-D-G, etc., and so on to the point of selecting every eighth syllable. Now he found that he could learn the new list (made up by skipping every second syllable, etc.) more rapidly than comparable nonsense material that was new. For him this proved that when he had originally learned the list A, B, C, D, he had actually formed associations not only from A to B and from B to C, but from A to C, etc. Herbart was vindicated. Psychologists smiled and waved Herbart aside ; but the results were interesting. By the saving method Ebbinghaus showed that the linkage of A with C was more effective than that of A with D ; and that the strength of the linkage consistently decreased with the number of syllables skipped, until, with the skipping of seven syllables, the curve approached the base line.

Similarly, he constructed lists of nonsense syllables in an order the reverse of the one used in the original learning. He found that he could learn these more quickly than comparable material which was new, thus apparently showing that when learning the list in the first place he had established connections also from B to A, from C to B, and so on. And he constructed lists in which both backward association and skipping were to be tested—such as E-C-A. Even these lists were more effectively learned than was new material.

Various objections have been raised, and subsequent experimental work has shown that such results may, in some cases, be attributed to the tendency to revert unwittingly to syllables several steps earlier in the series, or, in successive repetitions, to anticipate syllables which are still several steps away. But some of this work, utilizing meaningful material, can scarcely be said to count against Ebbinghaus's findings with nonsense syllables, and it is by no means certain that these objections dispose of the problem. It seems in general agreed that the whole problem of skipping and backward association calls for further investigation.

Ebbinghaus's memory work inspired a great variety of further investigation. G. E. Müller, working now with one and now with another collaborator, improved some of the methods of Ebbinghaus, and attacked many new problems. Müller and Schumann, for example, devised a method for the uniform presentation, upon a revolving drum, of nonsense syllables for memorization, so that the rate of presentation could be systematically varied. This instrument, with modifications, is still in use. An " exposure slot " makes it possible for the subject to observe one syllable in one unit of time. Another improvement in Ebbinghaus's methods was the devising of lists of nonsense syllables which were found in practice to be of approximately equal difficulty.

While such modifications in method were being made, Müller and many others contributed new experiments and results. It was found by W. G. Smith[1] in 1896 that early and late syllables were fixated much more quickly than those in the middle of a series. Steffens discovered[2] shortly thereafter a principle which has been much utilized. She demonstrated the futility of trying to break up long passages of meaningful material into short passages for memorizing ; material was found to be better learned when read through from beginning to end than when learned in parts and pieced together. The task of fitting together the different parts

[1] " The Place of Repetition in Memory," *Psychol. Rev.*, III.
[2] *Zeitschr. f. Psychol.*, XXII, 1900.

when learned separately was very wasteful of time.   The
experiment has been repeated by many students, the majority
of whom have confirmed the reality of this advantage of
" whole learning " over " part learning " in most individuals.
It was pointed out, however, shortly thereafter,[1] that it is
sometimes worth while to stop and repeat more difficult parts
of the list.   And it naturally made a difference whether the
individual had to memorize a *list* so that it could be recited
without prompting, or whether his task was simply to recall
as large a number of elements as he could.   With the latter
procedure, the method of "retained members," the advantage
of " whole learning " was not apparent.

It was discovered also that the rate at which the individual
learns depends on his attitude or purpose.   The task which
the individual undertook determined the manner of learning ;
if, for example, the syllables were simply read through without the purpose of learning them, very little connection
between them was formed.[2]

One of the most important of these extensions of Ebbinghaus's procedure consisted in the study of individual connections or linkages ; emphasis was withdrawn from " serial "
learning and given to association between pairs of elements.
To this end, Calkins[3] devised a method of presenting, both
visually and auditorily, *pairs* of items, the items having no
obvious meaningful relation ;   for example, a pair might consist of a word and a number.   Her first use of the method was
to study the influence of primacy, recency, frequency, and
vividness.   By demonstrating the influence of these factors
in assisting her subjects to recall the second item of each
pair, she gave experimental confirmation to some of those
" secondary " laws of association which Thomas Brown had
enumerated three-quarters of a century before (p. 61).   Pairs
early and late in the series were compared with those in the
middle ;   frequently-presented pairs were contrasted with
those less frequently shown ;   variation in size and colour of
type gave to some items special vividness.   The method was
shortly afterwards adopted and developed by Müller and

---

[1] Pentschew, *Arch. f. d. ges. Psychol.*, I, 1903 ; Ephrussi, *Zeitschr. f.
Psychol.*, XXXVII, 1904.

[2] Müller and Schumann, *Zeitschr. f. Psychol.*, VI, 1894 (see also below,
p. 260).

[3] " Association," *Psychol. Rev., Monogr. Suppl.*, I, 1895–96.

Pilzecker.[1] Performance was measured in terms of the number of cases in which the second term could be recalled when the first term was presented. Whereas Ebbinghaus's method failed to obtain qualitative analysis within different parts of a series (yielding only gross scores covered by statistical checks[2]), the new method of " paired associates " was applicable to a study of many sorts of variables appearing with each association to be formed.

We may summarize the history of memory-investigation during the twenty years which followed the experiments of Ebbinghaus by saying that research was dominated by his concepts, and concerned primarily with the extension of his methods. And Müller and his collaborators had the advantage over Ebbinghaus not only in improved methods, but in the use of many individuals as experimental subjects.

Nevertheless, one main result of the long series of memory studies, especially those of Müller, has been to reveal the great variety of devices spontaneously adopted by the memorizing subject to facilitate his difficult task. Rhythmical and other groupings, similarities and other relationships observed, even in nonsense materials, and meanings of all sorts read into the material, make the memorizing process very different from a passive or receptive establishment of contiguities. It has been urged (as by Poppelreuter[3]) that all memory experiments have really been examining " higher " or more complex processes than the simple formation of associations.[4]

The era of memory study called necessarily for all available data on the neurological functions involved in learning. By the beginning of the present century, in fact, a general tendency prevailed to think of learning in terms of certain current neurological doctrines ; these doctrines became in many quarters even more popular than the new memory methods. We must take account here of certain striking neurological advances made during the latter part of the nineteenth century, which were of great importance to physi-

[1] *Zeitschr. f. Psychol., Ergänzungsb.* I, 1900.
[2] Ebbinghaus himself later introduced the " prompting method " for this purpose (*Grundzüge der Psychologie*, I, 1905, p. 648). The subject is prompted whenever he falters.
[3] *Zeitschr. f. Psychol.*, LXI, 1912.
[4] This much-needed paragraph was added by R. S. Woodworth.

ological psychology in general and to the theory of learning in particular.

In the middle of the nineteenth century, in spite of the work of such men as Bain and Lotze, relatively little detailed information regarding the physiology of the nervous system was available for psychological purposes. The hope of a physiological psychology, repeatedly uttered in the eighteenth century, had so far resulted in but meagre data of a type really useful in the explanation of specific psychological events. But from about 1860 onwards there occurred a series of discoveries in neurology, which by the end of the century had exerted important influences on psychology. It will be recalled that Broca had published during the 'sixties his famous generalization as to the motor speech centre (p, 98). In 1870 work was published by Fritsch and Hitzig[1] on the localization of motor functions in the cerebrum of the dog. Stimulation of the region immediately in front of the Rolandic fissure was found to elicit movements of the limbs.

During the period of the 'seventies and 'eighties this work of mapping cerebral localization was carried on extensively. One of the most significant contributions was that of Ferrier,[2] who succeeded in working out the localization of motor functions in the brains of monkeys ; this proved to be similar to that found for the dog. Ferrier did more than explore the motor area in order to find out how the subdivisions of the motor cortex were arranged ; he and others began to contribute much to the localization of *sensory* functions. Not content with the mere tracing of sensory fibres through their devious paths to the cortex, they made use of the technique of cutting sensory fibres and determining whether the visual, auditory, or other functions were affected. In this work, in general fairly accurate, Ferrier made some errors, in the localization, for example, of the visual centre ; where pathways are so intricate, it was but natural that errors should result from unwittingly interfering with fibres considerably removed from the point chosen for the incision. A number of experimentalists were soon in the field, and such errors were rapidly corrected.

A number of changes in technique were now being made, as

[1] *Arch. f. Anat. u. Physiol.*
[2] *Functions of the Brain* (1876).

by Grünbaum and Sherrington[1] in relation to the mapping out of the motor cortex. Instead of applying to the cortex two electrodes separated by only a short distance (which seemed to cause a wide flaring of the electrical current) they applied a single electrode to the cortex, the other being applied at some distant region. In this way relatively little irradiation was supposed to occur (the relative merits of uni-polar stimulation are still under discussion). Such changes in method made possible a closer examination of earlier results (rectifying the common mistake of supposing the motor area to extend dorsally across the Rolandic fissure) and the extension of the work to the field of comparative anatomy, with the study of the similarities and differences between the ape, monkey, and other mammals. Grünbaum and Sherrington were the first[2] to explore the brains of anthropoid apes.[3]

This kind of research made it possible to say in a general way that there are regions in the cortex which have specific functions. The whole problem of cortical localization stood in a new light as compared with the middle of the century. By 1885 or 1890 the main cortical centres for sensation and (voluntary) movement were worked out for mammals to the general satisfaction of most critics. Partly by the use of analogy, but chiefly through clinical studies and anatomical research, similar localization within the human brain won general acceptance. It became a matter of agreement that the area immediately in front of the fissure of Rolando is uniformly motor and the post-Rolandic area specialized for the " general senses " of warmth, cold, touch, and pain. The visual centre was assigned to the occipital lobe and the auditory to the temporal lobe. A region near the olfactory bulb was recognized as the " olfactory lobe." The centre for taste was not (and has not yet been) clearly determined. The evidence indicated that simple sensory and motor functions are performed by both hemispheres, symmetrical areas having like functions. The results from tracing fibres and those obtained from the extirpation and cutting of fibres

---

[1] E.g., Transactions of the Pathol. Soc. of London, LIII, Part I, 1902.

[2] A summary of this work appears in Sherrington's Integrative Action of the Nervous System (1906).

[3] Though one orang had been studied by Beevor and Horsley (Philosophical Transactions of the Royal Society of London, 1890, B., p. 129).

were consistent, so that textbooks written in the 'nineties described the cortical localization of sensory and motor functions approximately as it is given to-day.

Many writers carried cortical localization much further. Wernicke[1] and others helped to define the types of aphasia on the hypothesis that there is a specific cortical localization for each type (disorders in reading, in writing, in talking, and in understanding spoken language). They described, for example, patients who had lost the ability to read, that is, to *understand* printed symbols, without manifesting any other language disturbance. This disorder was attributed to a specific lesion so circumscribed as to leave the rest of the brain unaffected. Hinshelwood[2] among others believed that the centres for visual memory are distinct from those for visual sensation. Destroy the visual centre, and the patient still has visual memories ; destroy the visual memory region, and the patient may have the capacity to see, without recognizing what he sees. While in general rejecting this simple localization of memory functions, many neurologists and psychologists came to the conclusion that certain lesions can disturb perception without affecting sensation. Hence the doctrine that perceptual functions are carried out, not by the sensory centres themselves, but by regions adjacent to them. This fitted in well with the theory that co-ordinating or integrating centres for motor functions lie adjacent to the motor area in the pre-Rolandic region. Many clinical and anatomical[3] studies were being made in this period, which seemed in general to confirm the view.

A closely related problem was the task of tracing sensory fibres through the spinal cord and brain-stem to the cortical sensory areas. Pathological cases helped greatly to clarify and interpret anatomical research ; injuries to the nervous system could be directly compared with losses of specific sensory functions. Animal experimentation also added much ; if certain fibres in the cord were cut and certain functions were consistently lost, it was possible to say with fair certainty what functions the fibres served. The discreteness of these

---

[1] *Der aphasische Symptomencomplex* (1874).
[2] *Letter, Word, and Mind Blindness* (1900).
[3] The evidence from post-mortem examination was scarcely definite, in view of the extraordinary irregularity of lesions and the scarcity of " pure " aphasic types.

functions seemed to call for the discovery of separate " pathways " serving their respective functions.   Pain and temperature pathways, for example, were satisfactorily traced.

Another field of research important for psychology was the
intensive study of the general anatomy and physiology of
nerve-cells.   Histological methods, such as the staining of
normal and injured nerve-tissue, made possible not only the
tracing of fibres but the observation and classification of
many types of cells previously unrecognized.   One of the
most important steps taken in this direction was the method of
staining used by Golgi, in Italy, in the 'seventies.   A common
view that the various parts of the nervous system are all
anatomically connected did not seem to be confirmed by the
evidence from staining, and from other methods utilized
during the 'seventies and 'eighties.   Staining methods seemed
to indicate that nerve-cells are anatomically distinct from one
another ; there appeared, at least in higher animals, no clear
cases of fibres passing from one cell into another.   This led
students of the subject to gravitate toward the view that each
nerve-cell is in some way connected physiologically, but not
anatomically, with other nerve-cells.   Cells are capable of
influencing one another, but each cell carries on independently
such functions as nutrition and self-repair.   Other
evidence to the same general effect was obtained from the
embryological researches of His.   The problem of His was
to determine whether the nerve-cells arise, so to speak, from
one another, or whether each one pursues from the beginning
an independent development.   He showed that each nerve-
cell is from the time of its appearance until completely developed an *individual*, not sharing in the life of the other cells
except in deriving its nutrition, etc., from a common source.
This was important in confirming the belief that the most
significant relation between nerve-cells was to be found, not
in their anatomical interconnections, but in the ways in which
they might influence one another in function.

These various lines of evidence were brought together and
worked into the " neurone-theory " by Waldeyer, in 1891.[1]
This was one of the most important neurological contributions for the history of psychology.   It brought together
numerous evidences as to the nature of nervous physiology

[1] *Deutsch. Med. Wochenschr.*, XVIII.

which psychologists could use.   Its central conception was the anatomical independence of nerve-cells, and their physiological interconnection at junction-points or " synapses."

We may best understand the influence of the theory upon psychology by considering briefly the kind of neurophysiology upon which psychologists had been relying.   Many psychologists had exploited the nervous system as an explanatory principle for mental life, but explanation of the part played by the nervous system in *specific* mental processes had inevitably been extremely vague.   We may choose, for illustration, the work of one French and one American psychologist. Ribot (in 1881) regarded *Diseases of Memory* as the product of disordered brain functions.   But he thought in terms of gross *lesions*, not in terms of the disorganization of microscopic or ultra-microscopic elements, such as connections between one nerve-cell and another.   Even the concept of the difference between organic and functional psychoses was at that time impossible ; the importance of gross injuries to the brain was overemphasized, simply because the significance of ultra-microscopic changes could not be clearly stated.

Similarly, a comparison of William James's chapter on Habit (in his *Principles of Psychology*, 1890) with statements of the physiology of habit current a few years *after* the acceptance of the neurone-theory, shows how great has been the revolution in the theory of learning.[1]   James was trying to think in neurological terms, and had very little to work with.   He sought to find how it was that a series of connections could be made between different parts of our bodies, one movement leading to the next; but he worked without any clear conception as to the mechanism by which one nerve-cell influences another. The same lack of definite neurological concepts with which to work is apparent in James's theory of association.   In his chapter on " Association," he offered a theory as to the neural functions involved in all the sequences of mental life. He suggested that, if any two points in the cerebral cortex are simultaneously active, the two centres tend to " drain " into each other.   Pathways are thus established, which later

---

[1] James borrowed a great deal from Meynert. Meynert's scheme postulated that habit was based upon the interconnection of brain areas, without making clear the mechanism of such connection.

are traversed when either centre is excited. If we *see* a man and at the same time *hear* his name, a linkage is established, which later enables either experience to recall the other. *Successive* association was explained in similar terms, an hypothesis being added to the effect that when one area is excited immediately *after* another, the energy drained from the first to the second is greater than the quantity drained from the second to the first. His theory has undergone many revisions, but has served as a useful instrument to explain how a sensation may set going a series of associations which continue until a prominent new stimulus intervenes. It presupposed, of course, an " irradiation " of energy in the cortex which need not involve motor discharge ; it was, therefore, a necessary supplement to James's theory of " habit." But it did not tell *how* the disturbances in one nerve-cell could affect another nerve-cell.

The neurone-theory gave both the theory of learning and the theory of association a much more definite and usable form. According to this theory each nerve-cell is an individual which carries on its own life as regards nutrition and other metabolic functions. The connection between one nerve-cell and another is, as we saw, by means of the synapse, or junction-point. The synapse is not a fibrous connection, but a point at which the nervous impulse is relayed from one nerve-cell to the next. But the terminal or end-brush of a neurone may be in close proximity to the receiving organs, or dendrites, of *many* other neurones, so that the actual pathway followed depends upon the resistance of the synapse.[1] There may, of course, be synaptic connections so intimate that they cannot be broken by anything. Such would be cases of reflex action so firmly established as to be practically unmodifiable. Some of the reflexes of the spinal frog would, perhaps, represent the extreme of unmodifiability. At the opposite extreme, or limiting case, there may be synapses in which there is an equal predisposition for the impulses to go in any one of a great number of directions, the choice between the alternatives depending on slight and momentary factors such as variations in the blood supply. These conceptions make possible the theory of learning in terms of modification of the

---

[1] The functions of the synapse have been much studied. A mass of data has come to hand which testifies to the fruitfulness of Waldeyer's conception (see p. 401).

P

synapse, as the result of the lowering of synaptic resistance in one direction and the increase of resistance in all others. Between these two extreme cases there are assumed to be behaviour-patterns less rigid than the one, and less plastic than the other, so that an original disposition may have sufficient plasticity to permit the reorganization of nervous pathways as the result of experience. This view makes possible the formulation of the learning process in terms of the building up of resistance at certain points and the breaking down of resistance at others. These aspects of the neurone-theory, developed and systematized by many physiologists and psychologists, seemed to be of immediate value for the psychology of learning and in many other problems. They were rapidly accepted and came into general use in the first years of the twentieth century.

CHAPTER XII

WILLIAM JAMES

WHILE succeeding to an extraordinary extent in bringing together the work of the Scottish, English, French, and German schools, William James gave to each a colour and a reinterpretation through which a sort of unity was achieved. But thorough as his scholarship was, the man rather than the schools spoke through his pages in the delineation of a psychology which was not so much an interweaving of traditions as it was a new creature.

In spite of his early bent toward philosophy, he was drawn to the study of medicine and became a teacher of anatomy in the Harvard Medical School. His work involved no sharp line between anatomy and physiology; in fact, his earliest researches dealt with problems in sense-physiology. He introduced psychological problems into his laboratory in 1875.

After a few years of occupation with medical studies he began to drift toward psychology. The journal, *Mind*, which was founded in 1876, contained in its first volume an article from his pen. In the next ten years a series of articles under his name appeared in this and in other magazines. Much of this material was destined to be incorporated later in his *Principles of Psychology* (1890).

From these studies it is not hard to see what major forces were acting on his thinking. He was a voracious reader, attaining a very unusual degree of erudition and range of information. He was deeply absorbed in the Scottish as in the associationist psychology, and in that mixture of the two which flourished in Great Britain in the middle of the century. Here, as elsewhere, his philosophical and religious[1] nature seized what it could use; without such religious

---

[1] His father's devotion to Swedenborg profoundly influenced him; a curious combination of personal mysticism and New England matter-of-factness is apparent throughout his work.

leanings James could not have been so much influenced by the Scottish tradition.

There were also various German influences, which aroused in James both enthusiasm and revolt. German experimental work influenced James enormously, in spite of his animus against what he called "brass-instrument" psychology. Notwithstanding his feeling that the laboratory method was a mere dissection of dead minds, he devoted nearly two hundred pages in his *Principles* to the experimental findings of the school of Helmholtz and Wundt. However, in his *Talks to Teachers* (1899), James said that in his opinion there was "no 'new psychology' worthy of the name" (p. 7). (Wundt was given full credit for the founding of experimental psychology.) It is clear that James regarded the Leipzig movement as a source of much usable material, but not at all, as the Wundtians considered it, as offering a new Constitution for Psychology. Of the three figures, Helmholtz, Fechner, and Wundt, he was least partial toward Fechner. He was deeply appreciative of Fechner's *philosophy*, but he held the upshot of his experimental work to be "just nothing." The methods of Helmholtz and Wundt interested him enough to cause him to invite Münsterberg, a representative of the new experimental psychology, to become his colleague at Harvard. In spite of James's acknowledged prejudices, he sought empirical material wherever he could get it. One has the feeling that as he adopted the German methods and results a sense of duty impelled him. The chapter on the "Perception of Space" reads like the work of a man who finds a disagreeable task to be done and "faces the music." It was for him the kind of experimental problem which could hardly have been undertaken in a country "whose natives could be bored."

Other German influences, such as the Hegelian movement and other idealistic trends, may be said to have influenced James profoundly through the very fact that his lack of sympathy with them led to strenuous and prolonged protest. His reaction to them was not a compromise but open rebellion. To him they seemed wordy and without substance; they represented the "thin" rather than the "thick" in philosophy.[1] German philosophy influenced

---

[1] *A Pluralistic Universe* (1909), p. 136.

him by way of greatly accentuating the inclination
towards "radical empiricism" which was apparent
even in his early work. His psychological outlook was
a protest against both German and British "absolute
idealism."

The same reverence for factual material which James
showed in relation to German psychology was liberated and
given new life by French psychology. He thought something really important had been discovered by French
psychiatric research. He was deeply interested in the
work of Charcot, Janet, and others who had studied hysteria,
hypnotism, and dissociation ; he believed that such studies
had something fundamental to teach about the structure of
personality. He gave much attention to Janet's evidence
that there may be parts of personality functioning unknown
to our introspective consciousness.[1] This discovery seemed
to James to be of great moment, indicating that personality
is not the little circle of events upon which the light of
introspection is thrown, but represents various levels or
strata which may be as genuinely psychological as the
superficially apparent. He felt that dissociation, or splitting
of personality, made it possible to study at different times
elements in personality which take their turns in controlling
individual conduct. The mental events which go on outside
the patient's consciousness might as a rule be regarded
as "secondary personalities," real selves distinct from the
self which is at the time in control. Strangely enough
there are, nevertheless, James believed, *some* mental events
outside of personal awareness which are not a part of any
self. After stating that consciousness tends to be *personal*,
James proceeded to quote, with sympathy, Janet's hypothesis
that there are organic memories, isolated mental states
having no selfhood.

To explain James's position, we may roughly designate
three possible interpretations of these "dissociated" processes. We may insist that whatever is not present in
personal awareness is not mental at all, but merely physiological. This is the explanation which most psychologists
have favoured. Secondly, we may say that these dissociated states, if they are to be reckoned mental, must

---

[1] *Principles of Psychology* (1890), I, p. 227 f.

as a rule belong to some secondary personality. Thirdly, we may conceive of mental states which are not personal at all, a sort of " mental dust." James was inclined to accept and to emphasize the importance of both the second and the third of these conceptions.

Now we must consider a number of points that are crucial for James's scheme or " system " of psychology. Perhaps the term " system " is misleading ; for, just as Wundt was the systematic psychologist *par excellence,* so James might be called the *un*systematic psychologist *par excellence.* He was very much less occupied with the problem of creating order and system than with the task of giving the reader something to feed upon. The chapters of the *Principles* possess little, if any, internal harmony.[1] To look for it would be like looking for one clear-cut and consistent meaning evident in all of Blake's poems. We can tell which chapters were borrowed from British sources (we have mentioned, for example, the relation of Bain and Carpenter to James's chapter on " Habit "[2]). The three chapters on " Perception " (perception of " Time," " Space," and " Things ") were taken largely from German sources. The chapters on " Emotions," " Will," the " Stream of Thought," and " Necessary Truths," while utilizing contemporary material, were in large part original.

Having emphasized the fact that the chapters do not set forth a true " system," we shall not have to ask regarding the *elements* out of which, according to James, the mind is composed ; he was not interested in such a question. Wundt had informed us that experience is composed of three main types of elements : sensations, images, and feelings, three categories which survive in the psychology of most structuralists. But the term " feelings " meant for James anything we feel like making it mean. We have certain feelings as we look at our watches. We have other feelings as we are told we shall die to-morrow, or when eating our dinners. James neither classified nor minutely analysed such feelings.

The analytic method, in fact, seemed to him to be unwarranted ; experiences simply are what they are, and not groups of elements which we can constrain ourselves to

---

[1] That James was fully aware of this is clear from his Preface.
[2] See p. III.

detect through introspection.[1] The introspective discovery
of discrete elements does not prove that they were present
before their observation occurred. This view was not
entirely original. Some of the associationists, notably
Tucker[2] and John Stuart Mill,[3] had made much of the
fact that a combination of elements may give an entity
which is psychologically new, and by no means a mere sum
of the elements which went into the combination. James
slightly reworked the theory and gave it a neurological
interpretation.

For Locke, the father of structuralism, the taste of
lemonade (for example) would have consisted of sourness,
plus coldness, plus sweetness, plus tactual sensations from
the tongue, and so on. Even for Wundt (in spite of " creative
synthesis ") there were several distinct afferent neural pathways, which brought in the various sensations, one by one,
so that the sensory elements appeared separately in consciousness and were combined into a percept. James taught
that this was a thoroughly distorted picture. The psychologist, he thought, reads into an experience what he thinks
should be there. Suppose a tea-taster trains himself to
discriminate, in a flavour, elements which to most observers
are fused into an unanalysable blend. From James's viewpoint, the fact that this individual taster can analyse his
experience does not prove that the separate analysed
elements are present in the consciousness of everyone who
tastes the compound. Moreover, the fact that an individual
can train himself to recognize the separate elements of flavour
does not prove that the total experience before training was
a psychological *sum* of such elements. Experience really is
just what it seems to be ; all such arbitrary analysis is vicious.
What really happens is this : what the different neural pathways bring in undergoes co-ordination before anything
appears in experience. Experience results, to be sure, from a
neural pattern, but there is no reason to suppose that each
afferent element is represented in consciousness by a separate
experience. Such vague terms as John Stuart Mill's
" mental chemistry " were replaced by the view that percepts
must be regarded as units, their only defensible analysis
being on the neurological level. If, in fact, we analyse

[1] *Op. cit.*, I, 157 *f*   [2] See p. 26.   [3] See p. 109.

experience, we obtain something different from the experience as it stood.

Another epoch-making doctrine, probably of even greater importance for James's influence on modern psychology, was his insistence that the attempt to subdivide consciousness into a series of temporally distinct phases is unwarranted. We cannot talk about one thing leading by association to the next, as one clock-tick succeeds another. There is, on the contrary, a continuous flow, a "stream of thought," and each of the entities ordinarily studied by psychologists is nothing more than a cross-section arbitrarily taken out of the stream.   James Mill, Spencer, and Bain had all emphasized the constant flux of consciousness, believing that it was quite impossible to describe a momentary cross-section of experience except in terms of the stages just preceding it.   Bain had written : " To be distinctly affected by two or more successive impressions is the most general fact of consciousness.   We are never conscious at all without experiencing transition or change."[1]   James, accepting and elaborating this view, held that the process of analysing experience into temporal pigeon-holes is just as absurd as the type of analysis discussed above.   It is just as artificial to cut mental life up into temporal bits as to say that it consists of A plus B plus C.   Mental life at any point is a unity, a total experience, and from this flows, as in a stream, another total experience.   Temporal subdivisions are purely a matter of convenience.   But a span of a few seconds' duration may be grasped as a unity, the " specious present."

We are bound to recognize that a great deal in this stream of consciousness is not easily grasped in introspective terms ; much of it is vague, incoherent, intangible.   A large part of it is marginal.   James made much of what he called *transitive* as opposed to *substantive* states.   Thought contains not only stopping-places which are easily observed, but transitional states so vague and fleeting that they have escaped the attention of most psychologists.   Psychologists have taken cross-sections of the stream of thought at the substantive points ;   they have neglected the vague, the fleeting, the indefinite.   If, for instance, we should say :

---

[1] *The Senses and the Intellect* (2nd. ed.), p. 325.

" Substantive states do not constitute the entire subject matter of psychology," probably the word " of " would not, under ordinary circumstances, attract attention at all. But it would be part of the total experience. James said that one of his tasks was to restore to psychology the vague, indefinite, and unsubstantial. But he was not alone. The same conception was apparent in other revolts against structuralism (to which we shall soon devote attention), and soon became a subject for experimental study.

One of the most brilliant pieces of descriptive work in James's *Principles* is his account of the will, and his classification of the types of decision.[1] " The first may be called *the reasonable type*. It is that of those cases in which the arguments for and against a given course seem gradually and almost insensibly to settle themselves in the mind and to end by leaving a clear balance in favour of one alternative, which alternative we then adopt without effort or constraint. . . . In this easy transition from doubt to assurance we seem to ourselves almost passive ; the ' reasons ' which decide us appearing to flow in from the nature of things, and to owe nothing to our will. . . . In the *second type* of case our feeling is . . . that of letting ourselves drift with a certain indifferent acquiescence in a direction accidentally determined *from without. . . . In the third type* . . . it often happens, when the absence of imperative principle is perplexing and suspense distracting, that we find ourselves acting, as it were, automatically . . . in the direction of one of the horns of the dilemma . . . ' Forward now ! ' we inwardly cry, ' though the heavens fall.' " The fourth form of decision " comes when, in consequence of some outer experience or some inexplicable inward charge, *we suddenly pass from the easy and careless to the sober and strenuous mood.* . . . The whole scale of values of our motives and impulses then undergoes a change. . . . All ' light fantastic ' notions lose their motive power, all solemn ones find theirs multiplied many-fold." In the fifth " we feel in deciding, as if we ourselves by our own wilful act inclined the beam. . . . The slow dead heave of the will that is felt in these instances makes of them a class altogether different subjectively from all the three preceding classes. . . . Whether it be the dreary

[1] *Op. cit.*, II, p. 531 f.

resignation for the sake of austere and naked duty of all sorts of rich, mundane delights, or whether it be the heavy resolve that of two mutually exclusive trains of future fact, both sweet and good, . . . one shall forevermore become impossible, while the other shall become reality, it is a desolate and acrid sort of act, an excursion into a lonesome moral wilderness."

The will is, moreover, for James, a crucial point at which all mechanistic interpretation fails. His disbelief in the possibility of a purely mechanical statement of personality was very apparent, as was his belief in the substantial reality of psychic forces which could not be stated in neurological terms. James has been accused of inconsistency regarding the mind-body relation. It is true that he repeatedly asserted that psychologists must dispense with the soul as a datum for their science; but on the other hand we find him saying[1] that there seems to him some integrating and organizing force beyond the separate experiences, which looks like personality or soul, holding in cohesion and in integrated action the many disparate functions. The inconsistency is in fact quite apparent if we contrast the treatment of the " Stream of Thought " with the discussion of the " Will." In the former, thought is, so to speak, self-propelling, the self appearing as an experienced entity but not necessarily as a reality beyond experience. In the latter, volition exhibits in certain cases the intervention of an entity not statable in terms of the elements preceding the decision.[2] James's heart was plainly in the doctrine of interaction between soul and body. He is in reality to be regarded as a psychologist who tried most of the time to think in monistic terms, using a neurological terminology, but one who did not believe such an approach to be ultimate. We shall see later, in connection with studies of religious experience, other instances of his disbelief in the finality of mechanistic, or, in fact, of any rationalistic methods.

The most famous of James's theories (and he was prolific in theories) had to do with the emotions. Since the time of Lotze's *Medicinische Psychologie* (1852), a great

---

[1] *Op. cit.*, I, p. 181.
[2] His position was more fully stated in his essays, " The Dilemma of Determinism " and " The Will to Believe," in the volume bearing the latter title (1897).

quantity of descriptive work on the psychological aspects of emotion had been published. Such descriptions were inevitably rather sterile, being neither based on carefully controlled data nor collected with reference to any distinct and verifiable hypothesis. Little critical thinking had been done as to *what emotions were :* popular terms like " fear " and " rage " served as starting points for detailed description of what various parts of the body do in such states. The first critical endeavour to determine the relation between what was called emotion on the one hand and its physiological expression on the other hand was that of James. In 1884 he published, in *Mind,* an article on this problem, which was included six years later in his *Principles of Psychology.*[1] In this article he undertook to bridge the gap between emotions and the expressive movements which attend them ; he sought, in fact to show that emotions have no existence whatever apart from such physiological changes. Each emotion, he held, is nothing but a product of the reverberation of physiological changes in the body. This was a flat contradiction of the common assumption that emotion precedes physical expression. Whereas it is customary to think that " we lose our fortune, are sorry, and weep ; we meet a bear, are frightened, and run," James maintained that we lose our fortune, cry, and are sorry ; see the bear, run, and are afraid. And not only does the arousal of physical responses precede the appearance of the emotions, but our feeling of bodily changes as they occur *is* the emotion. In other words, emotion is a name for certain feelings which are produced by bodily changes. In James's first statement of this he was unfortunate in stressing the *somatic* muscles, particularly the gross changes involved in such acts as running when we are afraid ; but his whole treatment showed that he meant to include and to emphasize visceral changes. (In most of the many elaborations of the theory by other writers, visceral factors have been given great prominence.) James urged that if we analyse out the various bodily reverberations in emotion, the tension of muscles, the fluttering of the heart, the coldness of the skin, and the like, there will be nothing left of the emotion. His view was epoch-making, not only in that it reversed the order in which emotion and physiological changes were said

[1] *Op. cit.,* II., p. 449.

to occur, but in its radical insistence that emotion is just as much a bodily feeling as is the simplest sensation.

He sought in clinics and in hospitals the evidence which might tell decisively in favour of his view, and found a few cases in which a disorder of visceral processes did indeed present anomalies of emotion. But the evidence was not satisfactory. The problem was taken up twenty years later by Sherrington,[1] who attempted to obtain direct experimental evidence. He undertook to sever in the dog all afferent pathways from the viscera to the cortex. The behaviour of the dog did not indicate any loss of emotion ; the characteristic indications of rage, for example, remained. This seemed to count against James's theory, but we cannot be sure that all afferent fibres were really severed. Nor is it certain that the dog was really enraged (subjectively enraged, of course ; for the subjective approach was a part of James's whole conception). Another line of attack on the theory has arisen in recent experimental studies in endocrinology, which have shown that the endocrine and other physiological changes manifested in fear are very similar to those present in rage and intense pain.[2] Much discussion has ensued as to the possibility of differentiating fear, rage, and intense pain, by any purely physiological technique. There are many attempts to meet this objection. Some contemporary writers assert that genuine physiological differences between these states do exist, but that they cannot at present be detected ; others believe that human subjects may differ widely in their labels for their emotions, one describing as " fear " what another would call " rage " (see p. 376). Objectors to the James theory run into the hundreds ; but we have here a view destined to be of enormous influence among psychologists, the starting point for nearly all modern theory regarding the emotions, as well as the stimulus to much research.

In 1885 a strikingly similar view was independently offered by the Danish physiologist, C. Lange,[3] who described the physiology of fear, rage, etc., and arrived at the conclusion that emotions are based simply and solely upon such physiolo-

---

[1] *Integrative Action of the Nervous System* (1906).
[2] See, *e.g.*, Cannon, *Bodily Changes in Pain, Hunger, Fear and Rage* (1915).
[3] *Om Sindsbevaegelser* (1885) ; *Ueber Gemüthsbewegungen*, etc. (1887).

gical changes.[1] For him the nineteenth-century distinction between mentally aroused and physically aroused emotions was meaningless ; in fact, it was difficult to find any emotions which were not " physically aroused." Bodily changes, especially those of the vascular system, not only gave rise to, but wholly determined, the nature of each emotional state. The general similarity of this to James's view led to the habit of designating as the " James-Lange theory " the assertion that emotions are simply the mental correlates of complex physiological changes.[2]

Another significant contribution of James, though not so well known, was his notion of the perception of space. The question of nativism *versus* empiricism still occupied the centre of the controversy regarding space perception. James maintained that each sensation intrinsically carries with it a certain spatial volume, or, as he put it, " crude voluminousness " ; each flash of light, each sound, each touch upon the skin has a certain volume. The arrangement of the spatial order comes, he believed, through association ; but the intimate spatiality of experience provides the substance out of which the complex spatial order is built. This has much in common with Johannes Müller's theory. It is, on the other hand, a particularly vivid and definite way of re-asserting, through a direct appeal to experience, the claims of a doctrine which associationism in general, and Lotze's analysis in particular, had undertaken to banish for ever.

James's theory of memory is likewise historically important. There had been two dominant theories of memory in the field since the seventeenth century. The first was the faculty psychologists' notion that memory is an ultimate power of the soul or mind. The second, that of the associationists, held that memory is simply a name for the process by which experiences are reinstated, through re-excitement of their physical basis in the brain. In the faculty psychology memory was one unitary function ; in the association psychology memory was a loose name for an indefinite number of separate events by which an indefinite number of experiences might be reinstated through

---

[1] Lange's theory was in large part derived from Malebranche (*Recherche de la vérité*, 1674), who was in turn indebted to Descartes.
[2] Changes, of course, outside the cerebral cortex, *i.e.*, changes which affect the cortex through the afferent pathways.

association. James suggested a view intermediate between these extremes. Retentiveness, he suggested, is a general property of brain structure, and varies from one individual to another. On the other hand, retention of a given item depends on a *specific* brain pathway. And he conducted a series of experiments to find out whether the memorizing of certain kinds of poetry would improve the memory for poetry in general—whether the practice of some memory functions would aid others. He came to the conclusion that general retentiveness cannot be improved by training ; practice in learning one sort of material was of no value as preparation for the learning of any other material except in so far as methods of studying were carried over from one to the other. James's conception exerted great influence. This pioneer investigation of the " transfer of training " was followed shortly by a variety of similar inquiries (p. 254 f.), the great majority of which supported James's contention that there is, in the strict sense, no such thing as general memory training. The problem as to the unity or multiplicity of memory functions had been brought to clear focus. This was the only historically important experimental investigation which James carried through.

One contribution which has not received much attention, but is interesting as an illustration of the hold which evolutionary principles had taken upon James's psychology, appears in the last chapter of the *Principles*, entitled " Necessary Truths and the Effects of Experience." In this he maintained that there are two ways in which experience may give us what we call knowledge. Some things are imposed upon us arbitrarily ; in the strict sense, we " learn " them. We learn, for example, that water freezes at 32 degrees Fahrenheit. It might as well be 28 degrees ; in fact it *does* vary from one region to another. Such facts are arbitrary. They are dinned into us by their regularity and inevitableness. The child has to collect such knowledge step by step. On the other hand, there are many things which " have to be " so, because of the very structure which evolution has given our minds. Geometrical relations and logical principles are of this sort. The logical structure is what it is because of the structure of the universe, and the nature of the minds which have developed in creatures living within it. This points to a fundamental cleavage in our mental processes between those constructed in the evolution of the race and those constructed in the lifetime of an individual. The necessary truths that seem to us so inevitable are inevitable only because our minds cannot transcend their biological constitution.[1] They are not inevitable in any absolute sense. Here is evident the effect of the evolutionary teaching that mind is the product of adaptation to environment. James works out here for us in some detail the view that our minds are biological weapons, given to us because through countless ages our ancestors were selected by virtue of their possession of certain modes of reaction to the universe. But for truths which are not thus " necessary " a plastic nervous system is needed, which will enable us to learn the arbitrary facts of every day. James did not, perhaps, fully realize the implications of his point of view. Non-Euclidean geometry had been under construction for over half a century, and both from it and from new movements in physics and logic have arisen in recent years grave questions as to just what these " necessary truths " are. That mind is biological seems true enough, but just what limits are set upon it by this fact it is extremely difficult to define.

Symptomatic also of the evolutionary point of view was James's catalogue of instincts. The first catalogue of human instincts and reflexes made on a careful empirical basis was that of Preyer (1881, see p. 280). James accepted and greatly extended Preyer's list of human instincts. He included such widely separated things as hiccoughing and hunting. Protesting against the view that man, by virtue of his reason, is but poorly equipped with those instincts that impel animal life, James asserted that man has more instincts than any other animal. In the years since James's list of instincts was presented a great number of similar catalogues have been compiled.[2]

We cannot attempt here a further account of the great variety of brilliant passages of description and analysis given in the *Principles*. We shall, however, return to James's work from time to time as we consider recent developments which owe much to him. Some of his interests lying outside

[1] The reader will note a curious similarity to the pre-Darwinian views of Fries (see p. 54).

[2] A new era in the problem was marked by McDougall's *Introduction to Social Psychology* (1908) ; to this recent development we shall return later (p. 337).

the field of psychology, as ordinarily defined, may be briefly considered here.

In 1882 was founded in England the *Society for Psychical Research*, which was to investigate alleged supernormal psychic phenomena, such as telepathy and communication with the dead, hauntings, premonitions, and so on. James played a large part in the founding in the United States of an organization for the same purpose (1884) ; he was active for many years in the examination of evidence for communication with the dead, and acquainted himself at first hand with a great variety of psychic manifestations. This interest, which absorbed his eager attention throughout his life, resulted in some of the most earnest writings which he ever penned ; few, indeed, of his philosophical or psychological writings surpass in vigour and personal self-realization his *Report on Mrs. Piper's Hodgson-Control*[1] and his review of Frederic W. H. Myers's *Human Personality and Its Survival of Bodily Death*.[2] He was early convinced of the reality of telepathy, or communication from one mind to another by other means than the mediation of the senses.[3] Whether we can have communication with the dead remained with him a purely open question, while he constantly insisted on the legitimacy of the inquiry.

Now, though it is still too early to do the subject justice, we must take some account of James's influence. During his period of service as Professor of Psychology at Harvard until 1897, and during the following years, in which his chief energies were given to philosophy, he enjoyed as pupils a large number of those who have become eminent as psychologists in the present century.[4] A significant feature of his teaching came in consequence of his interest in pathology. He took pupils to hospitals for the insane, endeavouring to make the phenomena of mental disease throw light upon everyday problems of personality. His psychology was, as we have seen, largely based upon Scottish and English work, but he paid much more attention to psycho-

---

[1] *Proc. Soc. for Psychical Research*, XXIII, 1909.
[2] *Proc. Soc. for Psychical Research*, XVIII, 1903–04.
[3] See, *e.g.*, " What Psychical Research has Accomplished," in the volume *The Will to Believe* (1897).   The article is a compilation of three previous papers.
[4] Among his pupils were Angell, Calkins, Healy, Sidis, Thorndike, Woodworth, Yerkes, and many others whose names are familiar.

pathology than any psychologist[1] in the English or Scottish schools. He was much interested, for example, in anomalies in the consciousness of self, which he found among patients suffering from severe visceral disturbances, and laid emphasis upon the part which " organic sensations " play in the ordinary consciousness of the continuity of our personal identity. He felt that material from psychopathology offered much more that was important for psychology than did experimental psychology. Despite his unwillingness to align himself with the new experimentalism, he served twice as President of the *American Psychological Association* (being the only man to hold the office twice in the first quarter-century of its existence). His personality, with the direction it gave to psychology, still remains a considerable force, as through his pupils and his printed pages it speaks to a generation whose interests and problems are in large part foreign to his own.

A few words about James's philosophical interests, particularly in relation to their influence on psychology. Some of his most influential studies dealt with the analysis of the ultimate basis of knowledge, how it is that our minds can know anything, how we can get in touch with reality. The popular notion of the correspondence between an external and an internal world seemed to him misleading. He found at various times three different solutions to his problem. He became identified with three schools of thought, all of which have ventured upon a theory of knowledge, and have had something to say also of the mind-body relation. His *Pragmatism* (1907) and *The Meaning of Truth* (1909), though expressly representing a compilation and revision of earlier teachings rather than a new school, mark the beginning of that flourishing contemporary " pragmatist school " which places its emphasis upon the relativity of knowledge, the impossibility of obtaining absolute truth, and the essentially adaptive nature of all thought. Another school which is heavily indebted to James is neo-realism. In his essay, " Does Consciousness Exist ? "[2] James puts forward the view that the world, in so far as we can ever know it, consists

---

[1] It was, in fact, not until the work of James that psychology took full account of the trend exhibited in the writings of such men as Maudsley.

[2] *J. Phil., Psychol., and Sci. Meth.*, I, 1904.

simply of things that are perceived; mind is not an independent function which knows these things, but comprises the same entities. Mental events and physical events are distinguishable only through the fact that the order in which events are perceived depends not simply upon the events at a given point in space but upon the life of the organism. This view, already sketched by Mach,[1] offered no escape to those who had admitted Mach's premises; it followed that " consciousness " does *not* exist, but is simply a loose name for the fact that events are related not only to time and space but to the life of the experiencing organism. Experience gives no data which are not already present in the physical event, nor does any relation of " consciousness of " events change their character. As we read a book, there are not two things, the book and the perception of it. All we mean by experience is a particular selection among events. If two persons stand near together and observe the same event, there are not three distinct events, but one event. But usually two persons take part in different events, and in this their personal identity consists. Neo-realism, which arose chiefly among a group of American philosophers early in the present century, has developed these conceptions to take account of many corollaries which James was disposed to neglect. Among the difficulties which have engaged closest attention are the problem of error (especially in relation to hallucinations, illusions, and delusions), and the analysis of mental events which do not at first blush seem to be identical with physical events, *e.g.*, feeling and will. Behaviourism, as we shall see (p. 269), naturally found in this doctrine much that was congenial. Holt[2] succeeded in defining consciousness itself in terms of an adjustment of the organism, and in subsuming both cognition and volition under the head of muscular response. The behaviourist's dismissal of all " mental " events was most easily supported by the adoption of the neo-realist contention that there really are no events to be added to the events of which physical science takes account. While behaviourism has in general declined to enter into discussions of epistemology, it has often tacitly,[3] and sometimes explicitly,[4] affiliated itself with this form of psychophysical monism.

[1] *Contributions to the Analysis of Sensations* (1886).
[2] *The Concept of Consciousness* (1914).
[3] See Watson's *Psychology from the Standpoint of a Behaviorist* (1919).
[4] Holt, *The Freudian Wish* (1915).

Another solution for the mind-body problem was offered by James in the form of a new variety of dualism.[1] The interaction of soul and body had been recognized in the *Principles*. The brain, he suggested, may be not the *basis* for mental life, but merely the agency which *transmits* psychic realities into the terms which organisms use in their relations to their environment. The idea that psychic events had a genuine domain of their own, not explicable through biological concepts, appears again, as we shall see, in his discussion of mysticism (p. 305). He felt that something of immense value could be learned from phenomena which appeared to him to indicate that the organism comes into contact with super-biological forces. The relation of man to reality seemed to include much that was not to be found in the biological structure of personality. Of the various philosophical positions with which James worked, the dualistic was perhaps the most precious to him. Its influence, however, is probably of less significance than either of the others.

[1] *Human Immortality* (1898).

CHAPTER XIII

STRUCTURAL AND FUNCTIONAL TYPES OF PSYCHOLOGY

At all events [say the Stoics] an image is contemplated in a different light by a man skilful in art from that in which it is viewed by a man ignorant of art.—*Diogenes Laertius.*

DURING the closing years of the nineteenth century there began a definite cleavage between those psychologists who were interested chiefly in the analysis of mental structures, and those who, abandoning this preoccupation, turned their energies to the study of processes or functions.

Probably the most typical, as well as the greatest, of contemporary structuralists was Titchener, whose system and whose experiments have been generally recognized as constituting him the spiritual successor to Wundt. Completing his training at Leipzig and coming to the United States, he became at Cornell in 1892 the presiding genius of a psychological laboratory which, even more than that at Clark, has served as a model in the study of those " qualitative " and " quantitative " problems which Wundt had attacked. The qualitative problems, however, have been more intensively cultivated.

Titchener's " structuralism "[1] is quite similar to Wundt's. Mental states are made up of sensations, images, and feelings. But the only " simple " feelings are pleasantness and unpleasantness, other feeling states being in reality compounds or " sense-feelings." " Apperception " is discarded, but " attention " is the process by which sensations or images take on greater " clearness." " Meaning " is simply the context in which a mental structure appears ; if it has any further signification, the problem concerns logic and not psychology. Among the main problems of such structuralism are : the elements and their attributes, their modes of composition, the structural characteristics of familiar types of compounds, the nature and rôle of attention.

[1] *E.g., A Textbook of Psychology* (1909-10). Titchener's psychology came later to be designated " existential."

Nearly all the work of Titchener's laboratory, though constantly inspired and directed by his interests, has been published under the names of his pupils ; the list of Titchener's personal publications gives, therefore, no suggestion of the wealth of material produced. A few of his specific problems may serve to indicate the range of his interests and contributions.

He was much interested in the question of " mixed feelings,"[1] the question whether pleasantness and unpleasantness may exist in consciousness at the same instant. Here, as elsewhere in his work, he took seriously only the testimony of subjects *trained* in introspective technique (that is, the ability to observe and describe accurately the mental states experienced). Reviewing various investigations in which such individuals were subjected to stimuli which could be relied upon to produce affective states, he decided emphatically that the evidence indicated the rapid alternation of feelings, but that genuine mixed feelings did not occur.

Another problem attacked by Titchener's pupil, Geissler,[2] was the examination of the various degrees of clearness involved in attention. Is there in attention a gradual transition from maximal to minimal clearness, or are there a number of definable " steps " ? The reports of some subjects indicated two distinct levels, focal clearness and marginal clearness. Other subjects reported several levels of clearness.

One of the most ingenious of the Cornell experiments dealt (in part) with the relation of percept to image. Perky[3] seated her subjects in a dark room before a screen. She asked them in some experiments to " project " upon the screen images of familiar objects named to them, such as apple, banana, knife. Unknown to them, in some experiments she threw a faint picture upon the screen, by means of a stereoptican lantern. The subjects were usually unaware that a " real " picture had been added ; some of them made the comment, in such cases, that their imagery was especially good that day. In another series of experiments, a stereopticon picture was presented, and the subjects were asked to observe it. Unknown to them, the illumination of the faint image was some-

[1] *The Elementary Psychology of Feeling and Attention* (1908).
[2] " The Measurement of Attention," *Am. J. Psychol.*, XX, 1909.
[3] " An Experimental Study of Imagination," *Am. J. Psychol.*, XXI, 1910. The experiment described is preliminary to a comparison of memory images with those of imagination.

times reduced to zero, so that no objective picture remained. Nevertheless, most subjects continued to " see " the picture, quite unaware that no illumination came to them from the screen. In fact, not one of twenty subjects could consistently differentiate between images and faint sensations. The introspectionist's desire to find clear points of difference between sensation and image[1] must apparently be tempered by the recognition that under special conditions the two phenomena may be indistinguishable.

In contrast to such emphasis upon the problems of mental structure, there has arisen a widespread demand for a more intensive study of problems of function. We have seen that James was unsympathetic toward the attempt to analyse states of consciousness into fragments. He was but one of a large number who in the closing years of the nineteenth century expressed the feeling that " mind " should be not a structural but a dynamic concept. Many psychologists began to shift their emphasis from states to processes. In fact, the change of emphasis was followed by a change in the whole conception of what psychology is. In place of the analysis of experience many sought to substitute statements of the ways in which the mind functions, especially in relation to the life of the whole organism. So many individuals toward the close of the century exhibit these tendencies that we can give only a kaleidoscopic view of the transition, arbitrarily selecting elements from the writings of several whose systems are widely divergent.

A few years before the publication of James's *Principles of Psychology* there had appeared Höffding's *Outline of Psychology* (1887). Höffding's chief point of deviation from the existing structural psychology, as expressed in the works of Wundt, was his use, as keys to psychology, not of ultimate *states of experience*, but of primary *types of mental activity*. This was, in a sense, a return to faculty psychology. The faculty psychology has been buried repeatedly and has come from the grave, put on its apparel, and gone on again. For faculty psychology is in essence a method of stating mental processes in a few main categories. But an important dis-

[1] See, for example, Read, " On the Difference between Percepts and Images," *Brit. J. Psychol.*, II, 1906–08.

tinction must be made. For convenience we say that we remember, we decide, we judge, we compare ; but these may be either names for ultimate and distinct functions or merely useful labels for complex activities which require further analysis. This points to one important respect in which Höffding's psychology differs from the faculty psychology of earlier centuries, especially mediæval and early German psychology. Höffding was content to lump together many specific acts under one common name, and did not presuppose a formal potency by virtue of which the acts described took place. But for him there existed the same three kinds of activity which had been so frequently named by the faculty psychologists—knowing, feeling, and willing. Each type, instead of being part of the personality (as the associationists had it), was a way in which the whole personality acted.

His treatment of cognitive functions was the least inspired of his contributions, and the one from which we derive least that is original ; we can pass over it with the statement that the experimental methods and results of examination into sensory functions were accepted and sympathetically treated. The study of feeling and willing are more significant. Höffding gave descriptions of complex affective processes such as those relating to religion and ethics, but gave them in terms of physiological as well as of introspective psychology. These complex processes were approached genetically. His treatment of the will was quite original. Superficially it seems based on Wundt's concept of the will ; but there is an important difference. Wundt, taking an evolutionary viewpoint, had made the will a central and primordial reality ; but in his hands it had nevertheless suffered the inevitable fate of reduction to a series of feelings. He made the will a structural concept, a concept to be understood only when more elementary constituents had been classified. With Höffding, however, we find that the will cannot be analysed into more elementary forms of experience. The will is, in fact, an elementary and ultimate way of *acting*. Höffding undertook to go back to the beginnings of the will, as shown in the study of the evolutionary series, beginning with the lowest organisms. Will, as a mode of action, may show itself first in simple approaching or withdrawing, becoming more and more complex as the situations arousing it are more and more complex. The genetic approach appears also in the study of the individual child's growth from blind reflex activity (here we may be reminded of Biran's doctrine) to developed consciousness, where a great variety of impulses are integrated into orderly conduct, many elements being brought together in a conscious decision. Both in the phylogenetic and in the ontogenetic series, will was shown to be a process which can not intelligibly be described as a mere series of states.

Perhaps the most ingenious of Höffding's contributions was his theory of the subconscious. Here we find a definite resolution to abandon the quest for a structural knowledge of what goes on outside of consciousness, together with a clear and forceful description of the significance of *processes* which lie outside of consciousness. In our discussion of James's theory of the subconscious (p. 209) we had occasion to describe three common ways of looking at the subconscious ; that is, three structural statements of what the subconscious may be in relation to the conscious, or three assumptions as to what may become of mental states when they lapse from the introspective field. Subconscious states may be regarded as *identical in nature* with conscious states ; or as *conscious but impersonal ;* or simply as brain states, *with no mental counterpart.* This whole attempt to find the intrinsic structural quality of the unconscious is foreign to Höffding's outlook and method. For him the subconscious is essentially a name for a group of processes of which we are not aware. These processes may frequently approach or recede from the margin where they would be introspectively clear, although not changing in their essential functions. It is what they accomplish, what part they play in the course of mental events, that chiefly matters. For instance, an idea may lapse out of mind, and yet the attitude we had when it was in mind may remain. For Höffding the essential thing about the subconscious is that it exists as a real group of activities ; these activities may at times rise to the introspective level or lapse from it, without in any sense changing their dynamic character. The subconscious is a name for all activities which do not happen at the moment to be in the field of introspection, but which, in or out of it, do not change their dynamic character. As to the question whether things outside of consciousness are the *same* as they are in consciousness, assuming that the process is the same, Höffding adopted a complete agnosticism. The important thing, he felt, is the fact that mental events often follow the same course as if they were present structurally ; and whether their structural nature is the same we have no way of knowing by our present methods of observation.   We can, to be sure, discover introspectively many degrees of consciousness, from the most definite to the most obscure.   Similarly, it may well be that, from the threshold or most indefinite region of consciousness all the way down to the purely mechanical process, there may exist degrees of consciousness which we cannot observe. All this, however, Höffding regarded as unverifiable.

Stout's *Manual of Psychology* (1899) illustrates the same division of mind into a few main ways of acting rather than a few main types of experience ; the process of cognition, for example, overshadows the analysis of cognitive *states*.   Stout gives a discussion of memory in many ways similar to that of Herbart and Beneke, emphasizing the *disposition* of experiences to return into consciousness after a period of eclipse. When material has been memorized, the appearance of the first item in consciousness creates a disposition for the others to recur.   Emphasis is not upon the structural similarity of an experience and its reproduction, but upon the tendency of experience to reinstate itself.   As we have seen, associationism had suffered decline and fall largely because of the structuralism inherent in it.   Stout is representative of the general tendency in late-nineteenth-century British psychology to make mental activity, rather than the analysis of consciousness, the central problem.   Stout's emphasis upon conation, an emphasis shared by many other leaders in recent British psychology, is perhaps an even clearer indication of the trend towards dynamic conceptions.

The same tendency is strikingly apparent in the schools of physiological and experimental psychology.   Münsterberg, who came to the United States in 1892, formulated an ingenious theory as to the nature of psychological events, in which an ultimate type of process, rather than an ultimate type of structure, was emphasized.   Höffding and Stout had taught that we must look upon mind as a group of functions, but did not tell us what physiological processes to seek as correlates for mental acts.   The " action theory " of Münsterberg[1] was a clear-cut doctrine as to the physiological unit which corresponds to the simplest act in experience.   The theory states

[1] *Grundzüge der Psychologie*, I (1900).

that when the stimulation of a sense-organ leads to a conscious event and a motor response, the sensation arises not in connection with the mere excitement of a sensory area of the brain, but with the passage of the neural impulse from sensory to motor regions. Structuralists had in general assumed that the neurological counterpart to our psychological elements is the excitation of particular points in the cortex. The experience of pain when the finger is burned had been correlated, for example, with specific local excitement in the general sense area of the cortex. In visual hallucination we may perhaps suffer from something acting directly on a point within the visual area in the cortex, although neither the sensory nor the motor neurones of the usual neural pathway have been brought into action. Münsterberg asserted, in contrast to this, that all life is impulsive, tends to action. We know nothing about sensory experiences of a purely passive nature. Says Münsterberg, every experience means not simply the excitation of a sensory region in the cortex, but the passage of that excitation through the motor centres and out to the motor response-mechanisms. The more open the path for motor discharge, the more clearly conscious the sensation (or other experience). Münsterberg insisted that consciousness occurs only when there is a *complete circuit* from sense-organ to motor response. This theory does not necessarily exclude a structural approach to consciousness ; but logical consequences are not the same as historical consequences, and the view was one of many which turned attention from states to activities, seen as a part of the behaviour of the whole individual. Many whose conception of psychology differed radically from Münsterberg's have made abundant use of his emphasis upon the whole sensori-motor arc as the true physiological unit for each mental event.

Serious objections were immediately offered to that part of the theory which stated that the more open the pathway, the more conscious must be the mental process attending it. Münsterberg's neglect of reflex action was serious ; for these pathways, as especially " open," ought, according to the theory, to involve definite consciousness. Another serious objection was the fact that the passage of the impulse becomes easier and easier as a habit is formed. Something which requires much effort, and is at first very clearly conscious, becomes gradually easy and smooth-running, but less and less conscious. The action theory would demand the reverse. On the other hand, the theory contained the germ of something enormously important.

Montague[1] has suggested that the degree of consciousness is not in direct but in *inverse* ratio to the openness of the pathway from sensory to motor elements in the cortex. This position is strengthened by a study of reflexes and some autonomic functions, which, while unconscious, appear to involve pathways of low synaptic resistance.

A compromise between these two positions has been offered by Washburn. She suggests that "consciousness accompanies a certain ratio of excitation to inhibition in a motor discharge. . . . If the amount of excitation either sinks below a certain minimum or rises above a certain maximum, consciousness is lessened. . . . The kind of consciousness which we call an ' image ' or ' centrally excited sensation,' such as remembered or imagined sensation, also depends on the simultaneous excitation and inhibition of a motor pathway. The ' association of ideas ' depends on the fact that when the full motor response to a stimulus is prevented from occurring, a weakened type of response may take place which we shall call ' tentative movement '."[2] From such conceptions, Washburn has built up a " motor psychology," which while making abundant use of introspective material,[3] is of a consistently dynamic character.

We may briefly note the recent appearance of several views which are in outline similar to the action theory, though it is difficult to tell to what extent Münsterberg (or James's theory of association) did in fact influence them. Holt[4] outlined a view to the effect that consciousness is simply a name for a specific kind of sensori-motor adjustment to an object. To be conscious of an apple is to adjust one's eye-muscles, etc., to it. Consciousness is the bringing of an object into a particular relation with the subject (that is, the organism) and this specific relation is one kind of adjustment

---

[1] "Consciousness a Form of Energy," *Essays Philosophical and Psychological in Honor of William James* (1908).
[2] *Movement and Mental Imagery* (1916), pp. 25–6.
[3] This hypothesis did not in any sense involve an *attack* upon structural psychology ; Titchener himself was not averse to such physiological hypotheses.
[4] *E.g., The Freudian Wish* (1915).

of the muscles to it.   This view derives from the neo-realist belief that objects outside of consciousness have the same qualities as those within consciousness ; cognition does not *create* the qualities which appear in experience, but simply relates them to the life of the organism.   Consciousness is not something " rolled up in the skull."   This concept is perhaps   more   radically   dynamic   than   any   heretofore named.

These are but a few illustrations to indicate that the increasing emphasis on *motor discharge*—of which Münsterberg's action theory was an early expression—contained enough dynamite to lead to a great many explosions.

The emphasis on process as opposed to structure became very evident not only in theory but in the experimental laboratory.   Külpe, trained in Wundt's methods, early came to the conclusion that the relatively simple type of conscious association to which both British associationists and Wundt had given emphasis was not sufficient to explain the great variability in the types of volition found in the same individual from one experiment to another.   The subject's behaviour in the experimental situation was found to depend not only upon elements in consciousness, but upon adjustments or attitudes, which might   operate   decisively although   not present to introspective analysis.   These findings regarding the reality of unconscious determinants to action undermined to some extent the structural assumptions which had come down from associationism.   Even in relation to the mere reproduction of learned material, such a view was significant ; but in relation to the task of adjusting to a new situation, the discovery that the course of mental life could not be understood in terms of its predecessors in the introspective consciousness was of great importance.   It involved the necessity of admitting as a real problem for psychology the study of processes outside of consciousness, and, inevitably, a shift of emphasis to more dynamic conceptions.   Simply because in many cases they could not be introspectively analysed, attitudes had to be treated as functional units.

This doctrine of Külpe's led to very important consequences in the field of systematic psychology in the twenty years which followed.   From it followed the experimental study of both the conscious and the unconscious aspects of " attitudes," with a view to determining to what extent the language of structuralism can describe, analyse, and classify them. This field of investigation was explored in Külpe's laboratory at Würzburg by men whose training and outlook were essentially structuralistic ; and many of their findings were accepted and utilized as enrichments to structural psychology. But in accepting these findings, structuralism itself tended, so to speak, to become more functional; statics already had begun to give way to dynamics.[1] And this new department of introspective psychology, while analysing the elements of thought, showed very clearly the need of a more adequate knowledge of the functional relations subsisting between these elements.

Shortly after Külpe's first recognition of the rôle of adjustment in volition came the development of the " functional psychology " of the United States. The sources of the movement are quite complex. A factor of importance had been the emergence of John Dewey[2] in the 'eighties and 'nineties. Borrowing from the general revolt against associationism in the late nineteenth century, and most of all from William James, he turned his attention chiefly to the organism's ways of adjusting to environment.[3] At the University of Chicago in the early years of this century Dewey came into contact with a group of psychologists, the most eminent of whom were Angell and Judd. With the help of kindred spirits, a distinctive school was developed, whose chief contribution lay in emphasis upon adjustment, and specifically, in a genetic treatment of attitudes.[4]

It happened that the revolt against the all-sufficiency of structuralism was waged on many different fronts at once. We may note the essential kinship of all these shades of opinion by comparing the functionalism of Höffding directly

---

[1] A summary of the newer conception of structuralism is given in Titchener's *Experimental Psychology of the Thought-Processes* (1909), in which sensation itself is treated genetically. And Titchener insists (p. 27 f.) that his psychology, like Wundt's, differs from the psychology of the associationists in making sensations *processes* rather than *states*.

[2] *Psychology* (1886).

[3] *E.g.*, " The Reflex Arc Concept in Psychology," *Psychol. Rev.*, III, 1896.

[4] The treatment of motor phenomena in Judd's *Psychology* (1907) gives a summary and classic statement of the doctrines of the school. Mental processes were brought into relation with muscular adjustments which were stated not in introspective but in functional terms. The whole question whether such muscular adjustments *can* be introspectively approached will be present with us in the next chapter.

with that of Judd. Höffding had taught that in order to understand the will we must regard it as a *process* to be approached through a genetic treatment. Judd maintained that we cannot understand attitudes by analysing them introspectively, but only through a genetic understanding of the functions represented by the attitudes; and motor phenomena were held to be of vital importance for the understanding of mental processes.

CHAPTER XIV

THE THOUGHT PROCESSES

Shall we not, then, as we have lots of time, retrace our steps a little, and examine ourselves calmly and earnestly, in order to see what these images in us are ?—*Plato*.

WE have given some attention to the revolt against the fundamental tenets of that structuralism which had begun with Locke and had been perfected by associationism. Another phase of the revolt must now be considered.

Among many rebellious figures one of the great pioneers was Brentano,[1] who built up a psychology in which the " act " rather than the content of experience was central. His distinction between the content of any experience and the act of experiencing, a distinction stated in a few words, is really quite involved ; and to grasp it we must go back at least as far as Leibnitz's doctrine of apperception (p. 12), the process by which we become conscious of our experiences. Kant and Herbart, though with personal additions to the theory, had emphasized the *activity* of mind in taking hold of the elements of experience which would otherwise have no relation to the self ; we may have experience without cognizing the fact that the experience is there, and the quality of the experience is distinct from the act by which it is recognized. In Brentano's hands this conception took a more radical form. Instead of drawing a distinction between an experience and the act of recognizing that we have the experience, Brentano held that the distinction is to be made between the experience as a structure and the experience as a way of acting. For example, in the case of sensation there is a difference between the quality " red " and the *sensing* of red. Now the true subject matter of psychology, said Brentano, is not, for example, " red," but the process of " experiencing red," the act which the mind carries out when it, so to speak, " reddens." We should have to substitute verbs instead of the

---

[1] *Psychologie vom empirischen Standpunkte* (1874).

nouns heretofore characteristic of psychology. The experience as we look at a red object is a way of behaving, and this way of behaving is to be distinguished from the quality of redness as such, which is a purely passive thing. This is rather closely related to the tendency we were discussing above in relation to Höffding, the change of emphasis from structure to process. Brentano's is one of the most influential systems of psychology which have evolved outside of the laboratory in the last seventy-five years. It was bound to produce an effect on other psychologists desirous of finding more dynamic concepts.

Another who, though a structuralist, contributed to the same movement, was Mach.[1] He held that the world of physics and the world of psychology are the same world, but that psychology must take account of certain sensations which correspond not to individual physical objects but to relations obtaining between them. If, said Mach, we see three separate spots, to each of which we react by perception, there is in our experience something more than one spot plus another, plus a third.[2] There is a relation present, and that spatial relation is just as much a quality of experience as any of the independent spots before us. In fact, the spatial quality by which we get triangularity is just as observable introspectively as any of the other elements. This can be illustrated by arranging the dots in different ways and noticing that we get different " sensations of space." Mach was structural in his way of thinking, but his emphasis was on the inadequacy of the traditional categories of sensory experience.

Following upon Mach came the work (in 1890 and thereafter) of Ehrenfels[3] and the school of *Gestaltqualität* (a word which we may roughly define as " the quality conferred by a pattern "). This school maintained that in all perception qualities appear which are something more than separate sensory entities, something added by the subject ; namely, the quality of the configuration or form or pattern presented. For example, the quality of triangularity or the quality of squareness given in the above illustrations is typical of *all* perceptual reactions ; all percepts involve

---

[1] *Contributions to the Analysis of Sensations* (1886).
[2] The point had been made by Laromiguière nearly a century earlier.
[3] *Vierteljahrsschr. f. wiss. Philos.*, XIV, 1890.

qualities dependent on the way in which sensory elements are integrated. This doctrine was in contrast to the Wundtian systematic psychology. Wundt had, indeed, recognized " creative synthesis," but the products created had to be stated in terms of the synthesis of the elements assumed in his system. The school of *Gestaltqualität* was concerned to show that the process of meeting a situation is more than the sum-total of the elements presented by the separate parts of the situation ; it has a quality given by the form of perception.

Now, none of these contributions in the 'seventies, 'eighties, and 'nineties was expressly experimental. It remained for Külpe, as head of the experimental laboratory at Würzburg, to subject some of these viewpoints to an experimental analysis. Külpe himself had contributed[1] to the analysis of factors which steer or drive volitional processes ; these factors might be either conscious or unconscious[2] (this is the concept now often called the " mental set "). Külpe's school began, at the beginning of the present century, a series of epoch-making experiments which contributed much to the anti-structuralist movement which we have just sketched. His laboratory at Würzburg became a centre for research on an array of problems which the structuralism of Wundt's school had disregarded.

There were first of all the studies of Marbe.[3] In these a situation was offered to the subject requiring him to form a judgment (as in determining which of two weights was heavier) and also a full introspective report on the processes inter-vening between stimulation and report. The decision was statable in terms of verbal report or overt act, which could be characterized by the experimenter as right or wrong ; but attention was given to the thought processes which preceded the act.

Next came a method, introduced by Watt[4] and Messer,[5] of utilizing the association-test to find out what thought

---

[1] *Outlines of Psychology* (1893).
[2] His view had in several respects been foreshadowed by others. See Titchener, *Experimental Psychology of the Thought-Processes* (1909) p. 162 f.
[3] *Experimentell-psychologische Untersuchungen über das Urteil, eine Einleitung in die Logik* (1901).
[4] *Arch. f. d. ges. Psychol.*, IV, 1905.
[5] *Archiv. f. d. ges. Psychol.*, VIII, 1906.

R

processes occurred between the presentation of a word and the word-response.   These (and similar) investigations led to very random, scattered, and incoherent masses of introspective material in which there constantly appeared evidences of preoccupation with elements of experience that to the subjects did not seem statable in sensory terms.   This mass of introspective material, though heterogeneous, indicated in a general way the existence of a kind of experience very closely similar to the transitive states which James had discussed in the chapter on " The Stream of Thought " ; something to be contrasted with the substantive, the relatively discrete and independent bits of experience.   Now these rather vague and indefinite experiences which were found to occur in the thought processes were given a name[1] which we may roughly translate " conscious attitudes " (*Bewusstseinslagen*).   These states of consciousness were not reducible to simple sensations or images or feelings.   Here we have then, very early in the Würzburg work, the emergence of elements of experience which appeared to have been disregarded by the entire school of experimental psychology under Wundt's leadership, and whose existence as a matter of fact had been generally ignored ever since the structuralism of Locke.   They bore a certain resemblance to the " imageless thoughts " which Stout[2] had mentioned in 1896.   These conscious attitudes included, for example, experiences of doubt and of certainty, of affirmation and of dissent.   Watt emphasized also the *Aufgabe* (task or problem) which, though not necessarily present *in consciousness*, exercises a controlling influence upon the judgment or act of thought.

The Würzburg school advanced, however, to new problems. Ach[3] proceeded to analyse the process by which decisions are reached, classifying individuals into " decision types " on the basis of their introspections.   He found that there are, in addition to the conscious attitudes preceding a decision, many predispositions which, although outside of consciousness, operate to control the course of thought, influences which steer toward a decision.   This discovery seemed a verification of one of Külpe's conceptions which we mentioned above (p. 232), and called attention, in the field of volition, to entities

---

[1] The word was suggested by Marbe.
[2] *Analytic Psychology.*
[3] *Ueber die Willenstätigkeit und das Denken*, etc. (1905).

very similar to the *Aufgaben* found by Watt in the study of judgment. To these agencies, so important in the process of volition, Ach gave the name " determining tendencies." Recognition of such determining tendencies was closely related to the theory of meaning. Ach outlined a theory to the effect that consciousness of meaning may be carried entirely through unconscious mechanisms. If a given imaginal content of consciousness is meaningful, it is because a number of associated ideas are subexcited, though not actually brought into consciousness. Meaning itself depends on such subexcitation of associated ideas. In addition to consciousness of meaning, Ach recognized consciousness of *relation*, and certain intermediate stages between these two groups of non-imaginal experiences.

Research upon the thought processes had in the meantime been carried on independently by Binet in France and by Woodworth in the United States. Binet's attack on the problem was not a " bolt from the blue " ; he had been interested in the thought processes for twenty years. In 1886 he had published a work on *The Psychology of Reasoning*. Its chief significance lay perhaps in the attempt to show that perception and reasoning are reducible to the same ultimate processes. The treatment was rough ; he brutally battered off, so to speak, the edges of the reasoning process, so as to state it substantially in terms of association. If within a perceptual pattern we devote attention to a marginal element, thus making it focal, new marginal elements appear, constituting a new constellation. This is the reasoning process. Reasoning is nothing but the shifting of attention which takes place as the different processes of perception go on. In 1903 he published a study of the thought processes,[1] a report of experiments in which his two little girls had acted as subjects. He had asked them to solve simple problems, and then to report on the mental steps taken. They told him what thoughts passed through their minds. He came to the conclusion that there was in their experience much which could not be reduced to simple sensory terms.

Woodworth, in a series of experiments published three years later and continued several years thereafter, came to

---

[1] *L'étude expérimentale de l'intelligence.*

the same general conclusion.[1]   Woodworth's chief emphasis
was upon the reality of thought which was not of imaginal
structure, and upon " feelings of relation."   Not contenting
himself with the statement that the experiences were not
reducible to the traditional structural terms, he emphasized
the reality of two distinct forms of meaningful consciousness,
forms closely similar to those described by Ach.

There followed a new period in the Würzburg school,
beginning in 1907 with the investigations of Bühler.[2]   These
were not essentially different in purpose from Woodworth's.
In fact Bühler used a method already employed by Woodworth—that of stating a question which required reflection
before an answer could be given, and recording the steps
involved in reaching the answer.   The important thing for
Bühler was the reality of non-sensory *thought* processes, a
finding which had been hitherto only an aspect, not the
essential purpose, of the Würzburg investigations.   Bühler's
work necessitated a very long period (say 5–20 seconds)
between problem and answer, so that introspective reports
were necessarily subject to much error.   It was largely on
this score that Wundt attacked such work, as undeserving of
the   designation   "experimental."   But   an   important
difference between Bühler's work and similar Würzburg
investigations lay in the fact that the shock of conflict with
the Wundtian methods and concepts came out much more
clearly.   It was Bühler, more than anyone else, who served
to bring out the apparent evidence for the existence of items
of experience which are not sensory.   It may be hard to see
why this should have been provocative of such a storm, in
view of the fact that the school of *Gestaltqualität* had long
emphasized the relational elements in experience.   But there
is a new feature in Bühler's work.   For all the previous
psychologists the relations, after all, were only relations.[3]
Even in the case of Mach's quality of " triangularity," a
sensationist could say that such a spatial relation is simply
a logical name for the way we react, not a name for a new
quality of experience ; or he could, in fact, accept Mach's

[1] See *e.g.*, "Non-Sensory Elements of Space Perception," *J.
Phil., Psychol., and Sci. Meth.*, IV, 1907.
[2] *Arch. f. d. ges. Psych.*, IX, 1907.
[3] Some of them were, in fact, identified with some of Wundt's " feelings."

description of these as *sensations of space*. But Bühler asserted explicitly that psychology must take account of new kinds of structural elements, namely, thought elements. He was trying to import into the precincts of introspective consciousness elements whose credentials had repeatedly been refused. Furthermore, these were vital elements and served in large measure as the content of the process of thinking.

In 1909 came Titchener's series of lectures incorporated in his book *The Experimental Psychology of the Thought-Processes*. The position here taken is of very considerable historical importance. The Würzburg school had been very much on the defensive as a result of Wundt's scathing denunciation. Every student was alert to hear what a scholar of great erudition, and long experience with introspective method, had to say. His verdict was that the defendants were innocent as regards their activities in relation to determining tendencies,[1] but that on the charge of introducing methods and terms which could never form a part of systematic psychology, they were guilty. There is, said Titchener, no such thing as an element present in consciousness, which is other than sensation, image, or feeling. There is no such thing as an imageless thought. Moreover, the "conscious attitudes" of the early members of the Würzburg school, and the thought elements of Bühler, which had been expressly stated to be non-sensory, were reduced to the familiar terms of structuralism. The "conscious attitudes" were classed as highly complex integrations of sensory components, which faulty introspective technique had failed to recognize, and in so far as non-sensory meaning-elements were really found, they were the concern of logic, not of psychology. Titchener did, as a matter of fact, repeat Woodworth's experiments, finding that his own subjects did not confirm the statements of Woodworth's subjects; the experience of Titchener's observers was described in the accepted language of structuralism.

Titchener maintained that when introspection yields no clear result the only way to get at obscure states is through a genetic study—an inquiry as to how they arose. If we go back to the earliest experience of the individual to find how

---

[1] He went so far as to commend in the highest degree their ingenuity, versatility, and inventiveness.

conscious attitudes and thought elements began, we find that they arose largely from muscular adjustments, and hence are of kinæsthetic quality. Our muscular sensations or images may be difficult to recognize, but they are all-important for the psychology of thought. The genetic approach is legitimate as an adjunct to analytical method. The muscular nature of many attitudes is apparent if we study an individual who confronts a strange object for the first time. Attitudes and thought elements are really the last vestigial form of groups of kinæsthetic and organic sensations.

The effect of Titchener's verdict was naturally to centre attention on the main point of difference between his own and the Würzburg positions. The Würzburg school interpreted Titchener's lectures as indicating that they had not given enough evidence that there were such mental states as they had described. They must redouble their efforts to make the evidence more conclusive. They rallied to the defence of what they had come to regard as their cardinal doctrine. The very hopeful approach made in the early years toward the study of a variety of mental functions did not yield as rich a return as was expected. We shall see, however, that the problem of the thought processes took, in other hands, another direction, freeing itself from these controversial discussions and emphasizing the processes rather than the structures of thought.

An instance of the labours of the Würzburg school to defend their position was the examination by T. V. Moore[1] of the relation of meaning to image. He presented a series of words both visually and auditorily to nine subjects. In one presentation, he gave the instructions that the subject was to lift his hand from a telegraph key as soon as the given word evoked meaning. In other experiments, the subject was to lift his hand off the key as soon as an image appeared in response to the word. Except in the case of one subject, it was found that the meanings came more quickly than the images. The time for evoking images averaged nearly a second, that for meanings about half this period. Moore concluded that meaning and image are distinct psychological elements. He therefore proceeded to postulate a structural psychology in which there were not three but four independent

[1] "Temporal Relations of Meaning and Imagery," *Psychol. Rev.*, XXII, 1915.

elements—sensation, image, feeling, and *meaning*—in consciousness.

A few words must be added about the subsequent history of the Titchenerian method. For Titchener this structural viewpoint and the exclusion of meanings became, as the result of the Würzburg investigation, even more vital than before. It became acutely necessary for him to instruct his pupils to distinguish between immediate experience (sensations, images, and feelings) on the one hand, and meanings or interpretations on the other hand. The subject must avoid the "stimulus-error," namely, the tendency to talk about the object which is stimulating him rather than to describe the observed content of experience. The subject must not say he is "angry," for this is but an interpretation of his mental state. A true description would deal simply with such elements as the kinæsthetic sensations experienced, and the feelings accompanying them. The all-important distinction made by Titchener and others between experience and meaning was elaborated with the use of the German technical terms *Beschreibung* (description) and *Kundgabe* (meaning).[1]

The continuation of the Würzburg movement by German psychologists has been chiefly the work of Selz[2] and other exponents of contemporary *Denkpsychologie*. Not only the elements, but the processes and forms of thought have been carefully examined. German concern with the more complex problems of perception and thinking has, however, taken another direction as well. In 1912 Wertheimer[3] reported experimental evidence to indicate that the perception of movement is not to be structurally understood as a series of sensations excited by the stimulation of different retinal points. Movement is perceived *as movement*, not as a sum of sensations. He, together with Köhler, Koffka, and others, proceeded to develop a *Gestaltpsychologie*. Each *Gestalt* (configuration, pattern, or form) is a type of organization, and the mode of organization is all-important if any experience is to be understood. The school of *Gestaltqualität* had already contributed the idea that the complete description of a percept must include not only the separate sensory data but

---

[1] The terms were proposed by von Aster, *Zeitschr. f. Psychol.*, XLIX., 1908.
[2] *E.g.*, *Zur Psychologie des produktiven Denkens und des Irrtums* (1922).
[3] *Zeitschr. f. Psychol.*, LXI, 1912.

the qualities which result from their mode of organization. The school of *Gestalt* went much further. Not only must such qualities be taken into account, but all the elementary parts of a percept must be regarded as dependent upon the whole *Gestalt* in which they appear. The whole is not the sum of its parts ; on the contrary, each detail in a perceptual pattern is determined by the nature of the pattern. The school has not only contributed much experimental work, but has given new colour to existing methods and results. For example, it had long been known that animals respond in some cases not merely to " stimuli " but to relations between stimuli.[1] With Köhler,[2] studying the behaviour of apes, the fact took on a new construction. The animals were trained to find their food in a grey container, B, darker than another container, A. Now when A was removed, and the animals were confronted with B and a still darker box, C, they chose C. They did not respond to the specific item which had always brought them food ; on the contrary, they responded to the whole situation characterized by the relation "darker than." So, in a host of other experiments, the school has contributed to the movement already discussed in so many of its aspects, namely, the tendency to distrust purely analytic methods.

The *Gestalt* school has, however, proceeded far beyond these premises. It has attempted to show that learning is no mere trial-and-error process, but conforms to definite *Gestalten ;* that " imitation " and " insight " are forms of perceptual activity which grasp situations in other terms than those imposed by the blind elimination of false starts. Judgment and reasoning, again, have their *Gestalten.* Thought can never really be " analysed," though its patterns can be grasped.

This brief sketch, designed to show some of the relations of the *Gestalt* movement to other aspects of recent investigation in perception and reasoning, is supplemented by a much fuller and more adequate treatment by Dr. Klüver in Chapter XXV.

---

[1] See, *e.g.*, Washburn and Abbott, " Experiments on the Brightness Value of Red for the Light-adapted Eye of the Rabbit," *J. An. Beh.*, II, 1912.
[2] *Abh. d. Preuss. Akad. d. Wiss.*, 1918, Phys.-math. Kl., 2.

CHAPTER XV

EXPERIMENTS ON THE ACQUISITION OF SKILL

The first beginnings of our volitional education are of the nature of stumbling and fumbling.—*Bain.*

IN the closing years of the nineteenth century and the opening years of the twentieth, vigorous study was given to the problem of the acquisition of motor skill. Memory, as Ebbinghaus had conceived it, had proved amenable to quantitative examination, but it now became apparent that other forms of the learning process could be approached in the same experimental spirit as the functions of memorizing and forgetting syllables and words.

Bryan and Harter[1] undertook in 1897–9 a study of the stages in learning to send and receive telegraphic messages. Curves of learning were constructed, indicating the stages of progress towards mastery of the task over a period of many months. The " learning-curves " thus plotted indicated that progress was more rapid at first than later. Progress being measured in terms of the number of units which could be handled in a unit of time, an expenditure of time and effort yielded gradually less return as the task went on. But they found the learning process to be not a regular, even progression, but a series of jumps. Learning to receive telegraphic messages was frequently interrupted by periods of no progress ; in these intervals the learning curve presented very roughly a horizontal line, to which the name " plateau " was given.[2] No uniform duration of the plateau nor uniform interval between plateaus was apparent.

Following the principle of " diminishing returns " noted above, the learning-curve was found also to reach a point where no further gains were apparent ; practice merely kept

---

[1] " Studies in the Physiology and Psychology of the Telegraphic Language," *Psychol. Rev.*, IV and VI.

[2] Such plateaus were not clearly demonstrable in the curves for " sending."

the subject up to his acquired standard.   This last stage was entitled the " physiological limit."   But the horizontal line of the physiological limit seemed to differ psychologically from the plateaus; the plateaus did not appear to be genuine periods of *no progress*.   They appeared to be periods in which the subject had reached the maximum attainable *with a given method ;* but after practice had continued for a time, he was able to take advantage of a new and more efficient type of response, for which he would previously have been unprepared.   But just what is being practised during a plateau ?   In one instance the subject has learned how to receive each letter of the alphabet ; he handles each word as the sum of the letters composing it, interpreting the symbol for one letter, and then, after a brief pause, the letter which follows.   He is in the " letter-habit " stage.   When the letters have been practised long enough, the subject passes rather rapidly to a new system of habits in which words are grasped and received as integrated units.   The subject has entered the " word-habit " stage, and the learning-curve again rises.   The word is a " higher unit," similar to the higher units discovered by Cattell (p. 175) in his investigation of word perception.   When the word-habit has been mastered, the subject may pass to the phrase-habit or even to the sentence-habit.   Some expert telegraphers were found to follow more than two-hundred clicks behind a message to which they listened ; they were taking in great masses of material in the form of higher units.

In immediate connection with this matter of higher units or organization into groups or wholes, the work of Bryan and Harter showed that two or more responses might go on at once, in such a way that the first " overlapped " the second. This had been found also by Cattell in the reading of letters and words ; a word might be perceived before the previous word had been enunciated, etc.   So, in receiving a message and transcribing on a typewriter, experts were found to follow from six to twelve words after the message ; higher units and overlapping were present in conjunction.   The messages were received and typed, not letter by letter, but phrase by phrase, or even sentence by sentence.   The subject could begin a new activity while waiting to complete a higher unit.

Similar studies in the acquisition of skill were made within a few years by Swift[1] and Book[2]. While in general confirming the conclusions of Bryan and Harter, and discovering similar plateaus, their interpretations of the significance of the plateau showed significant differences. Swift pointed out that higher units may be in the process of formation even during the plateau. Book, studying the acquisition of skill in typewriting, found that subjects frequently showed loss of interest at the beginning of the plateau, and, further that physiological observations (*e.g.*, pulse) indicated a lax or depressed state, which in itself seemed sufficient to account for the absence of progress. Book suggested that the plateau, far from being a period of hidden progress, was actually wasted time. Book's plateaus, similar to those of Bryan and Harter, seemed to correspond to the passage from lower to higher units.

One of Book's most important contributions related to the process of overlearning. Ebbinghaus had shown that additional memorizing, beyond the amount needed for a perfect recitation at the time, has a marked effect in facilitating the task of relearning ; in fact, that the whole curve of forgetting for overlearned material falls off much more slowly than that for just-learned material. Book's subjects, after acquiring considerable skill in typewriting—in which, of course, a great many reactions were overlearned—dropped the problem for four months. Upon resuming practice they regained in a few days the same level of skill which had at first cost them several weeks. Book concluded that something had occurred which illustrated James's maxim that we learn to skate in the summer and to swim in the winter ; the period of disuse was credited with " the disappearance, with the lapse of time, of numerous psycho-physical difficulties, . . . interfering habits and tendencies, which, as they faded, left the more firmly established typewriting associations free to act " (p. 80). Though this conclusion has not commanded universal assent, the data did at least clearly demonstrate the vast importance of intensive overlearning. In terms of Ebbinghaus's " saving method," the loss during four months of no practice was exceedingly slight.

[1] " Studies in the Psychology and Physiology of Learning," *Am. J. Psychol.*, XIV, 1903 ; " Memory of a Skilful Act," *Am. J. Psychol.*, XVI, 1905, etc.

[2] " The Psychology of Skill," *Univ. of Montana Publications in Psychology*, 1908.

While these investigations were going forward in human
learning, similar work was in progress in the field of animal
behaviour. But the methods and concepts developed in
animal investigations were in many ways quite different, and
proved in time to contain much that was new and important
for human psychology.

A word must be said about the animal psychology of the
late nineteenth century. The great bulk of animal experimentation was being done by physiologists, German work
being especially abundant. The physiologists were concerned
with part-functions, relatively little with total adjustments.
Studies in tropisms, reflex action, and secretory functions
were numerous. Some experiments dealing with perceptual
and instinctive functions were performed by British[1] and
American students. In 1875 Spalding[2] sought an answer
to the question whether swallows fly instinctively, or *learn*
to fly. Swallows were placed in a small cage as soon as
they were hatched ; when liberated at the normal flying
age, some flew without assistance. But perhaps the most
conspicuous studies of animals were those of Lloyd Morgan,[3]
pursued, for the most part, by the method of collecting
observations rather than by controlled experiment. Galton,
too, familiarized himself with the ways of wild animals,
threading his way to a vantage-point where he could observe
them without attracting attention. Among his most striking
observations are those relating to the " gregarious instinct."
Describing the life of the wild ox in relation to its herd, he
says : " If he be separated from it by stratagem or force, he
exhibits every sign of mental agony ; he strives with all his
might to get back again, and when he succeeds, he plunges
into its middle to bathe his whole body with the comfort of
closest companionship . . . To live gregariously is to become
a fibre in a vast sentient web overspreading many acres ; it
is to become the possessor of faculties always awake, of eyes
that see in all directions, of ears and nostrils that explore a
broad belt of air ; it is also to become the occupier of every
bit of vantage ground whence the approach of a wild beast
might be overlooked."[4] Galton's observations are deeply

[1] See, *e.g.*, Lubbock, *Ants, Bees, and Wasps* (1882).
[2] " Instinct and Acquisition," *Nature*, XII, 1875.
[3] *E.g., Animal Life and Intelligence* (1891).
[4] *Inquiries into Human Faculty* (1883), Section on " Gregarious and
Slavish Instincts."

imbued with the evolutionary spirit, and are one of the most obvious reverberations of Darwinian influence on psychological thought. Animals, he held, are equipped with innate mechanisms of reaction which make possible their adaptation to environment. But in most of this work there was no quantitative analysis of instinctive behaviour, very little experimental isolation of variables, and no thorough analysis of animal learning.

It is therefore no exaggeration to say that Thorndike awakened psychologists to the conception of an experimental animal psychology. His work was begun in 1897 while he was a graduate student at Harvard, studying under James. But James offered only incidental inspiration ; the general plan and the specific methods were Thorndike's. Not that Thorndike was uninfluenced by German physiology. British students, especially Lubbock and Lloyd Morgan, offered much. Perhaps, even so, the animal studies of the late nineteenth century offered Thorndike less than did the general conception of experimental psychology, as the new German and American laboratories expressed it. His first experiments were upon chicks, dogs, and cats. Shortly afterwards he improvised an animal laboratory at Columbia, where, under Cattell's supervision, the work continued. The problem most extensively studied was the nature of the learning-curve in animal behaviour.[1] A cat was placed, for example, in a cage which could be opened only by striking a latch or button, and a piece of fish was placed outside. Biting, clawing, and scurrying ensued, followed at last by the accidental movement which released the animal. On a later trial the same general behaviour followed, and so on in each new test. However, the total time required to get out, though fluctuating, showed a consistent tendency to decrease. When the number of practice days was indicated on the x-axis and the number of minutes required to complete an act on the y-axis, the learning-curve was found to fall rapidly at first, then more and more gradually, until a limit, a horizontal line, was reached, indicating the animal's complete mastery of the task. Such a curve, plotted from time units, obviously corresponded to the newly-constructed learning-curves for telegraphy reported by Bryan and Harter ; the latter, though measuring in terms of

[1] " Animal Intelligence," *Psychol. Rev., Monogr. Suppl.*, II, 1897–9 (whole No. 8).

accomplishment per unit of time, rather than in terms of time per unit of accomplishment, had pointed to the same conclusion, namely, the principle of diminishing returns with practice. Both curves were, in respect to this principle, similar to Ebbinghaus's curves of forgetting.[1] Though there were of course irregularities in the individual curves, and frequently great variations from one performance to the next, there were nevertheless no clear-cut plateaus such as those discovered in learning to receive telegraphic messages.

It appeared clear from Thorndike's curves that sudden insight into the nature of the task was rare or indeed entirely absent. There was no sudden and permanent drop in the curve indicating that the cat had "solved" the problem. The cat started with random movements, which were gradually eliminated as practice went on ; the time taken to strike the latch necessarily decreased. Thorndike saw (as had Spencer and Bain[2]) the importance of such "random" movements in leading to the discovery of the "right" movement ; for this kind of behaviour the term "trial and error" was soon in general use.[3] Even in the monkey, learning was of this general type ; Thorndike found no clear cases even of the process of "imitation."[4]

Thorndike's theoretical interpretations were perhaps nearly as important as his experimental findings. He introduced a change in the current theory of learning. The process of learning had been regarded, by most authors since Hobbes, as essentially the formation of connections ; those who interested themselves in physiology emphasized especially *brain-connections*. Thorndike saw the significance of stating learning in terms of functional connections between external stimuli and externally observable responses.[5] The

---

[1] All were, moreover, logarithmic curves, at least up to the physiological limit ; this limit, however, seemed genuinely rectilinear rather than asymptotic to a horizontal line.

[2] See p. 111.

[3] See Lloyd Morgan, *Animal Behaviour* (1900), p. 139, for an early use of the term.

[4] "The Mental Life of the Monkeys," *Psychol. Rev., Monogr. Suppl.*, III, 1899–1901 (whole No. 15). "Imitation" has been reported by subsequent workers. No general agreement prevails as to the definition of imitation nor as to the explanation of the cases reported.

[5] Hartley had emphasized motor elements in association ; movements could be associated with one another as with ideas. Thorndike's view was almost identical with this doctrine, but was enriched by data from a century and a half of neurology, and by the evolutionary theory.

units were for Thorndike the bonds between stimuli and responses. Nevertheless, the nature of these bonds was to be understood in the light of the " neurone theory."

This general conception was utilized in the formulation of a variety of " laws of learning." These were offered in his *Elements of Psychology* (1905), and elaborated in his *Educational Psychology*[1] (1913-4). The " law of exercise " stated that the use of a given connection between stimulus and response strengthens the bond (while disuse weakens it) ; such factors as recency and frequency are subheads under the law. The " law of associative shifting " stated that, if two stimuli are presented simultaneously, one of these eliciting a certain response, the other later acquires the capacity to elicit the same response. Another was the " law of effect," which stated that the *satisfaction* following from an act strengthens the bond and leads to its repetition, while *annoyance* tends to weaken the bond and hence to eliminate the act.[2] All these laws had long been assumed and used, of course, *e.g.*, by animal-trainers ; but their clear formulation was significant.

The first decade of the twentieth century brought a great number of experimental studies of animals. The mechanism to which Thorndike gave the name of associative shifting was being studied under other names (see p. 264), and was shown to be present even in very lowly forms of life ; on the other hand, this mechanism, rather than reasoning or insight, seemed to account even for relatively complicated types of learning.

During the time of these early investigations in learning there was a strong suspicion in the minds of psychologists that there might be some significant connection between the learning process and the thinking process. There was, on the one hand, good reason to believe that human beings learn in ways not characteristic of animals, that something different happens inside of them. On the other hand, it was natural to look for similarities between animal and human learning,

---

[1] Part of Vol. III is a revision of his book, *Educational Psychology*, which appeared in 1903.

[2] Satisfaction and annoyance were conceived in terms of synaptic functions ; when a pathway was ready to conduct, the process of conduction was satisfying, while annoyance might result either from the failure of a ready pathway to conduct or from the forced conduction of an unready pathway.

and to utilize as far as possible those conceptions which had proved helpful in animal experimentation. Both problems were greatly clarified by the appearance of a number of volumes (such as Mach's *Erkenntnis und Irrtum*, 1905, and Dewey's *How We Think*, 1910), which represented the thinking process as a *trial-and-error* mechanism in which human subjects manipulate situations mentally without the need for *overt* random movements.

Importance must be attached to the experiments of Ruger[1] (1910), who offered partial confirmation of the trial-and-error theory of thinking, and made extensive use of the German and American studies of "attitudes" mentioned in the last chapter. He studied the process of solving mechanical puzzles, in which the subject had to disentangle and remove some part through a complex series of manual movements. In this process it was usually necessary for the subject to go through random movements or trial-and-error activity similar to that shown by Thorndike's cats. Ruger found in his twenty-five subjects much of this random exploratory behaviour—in fact, such an extraordinary amount of it that a large proportion of the first solutions were genuinely accidental. Further, the subjects' reports showed that, in addition to such *overt* behaviour, much trial-and-error activity was going on *mentally*. But he found that there was frequently a sudden and permanent drop in the learning-curve, corresponding to a successful lead which the subject grasped clearly and continued to utilize. Such sudden drops were often due to his noticing the *locus*[2] of a difficulty. In other cases the drops corresponded to much more complex instances of analysis of the nature of the problem. Ruger had, then, obtained experimental evidence, even in a very complex intellectual process, of a thorough-going similarity between reasoning and ordinary "blind" learning, as found even in the behaviour of very lowly animals.

Ruger was really more interested in those complex mental states where the process of "analysis" occurred, that is, recognition of similarities and differences, observation of the relation between movements hitherto disconnected, and the

---

[1] "The Psychology of Efficiency," *Arch. of Psychol.*, No. XV.
[2] The same fact, in chimpanzee learning, had been noted by Woodworth in 1902–3. See Ladd and Woodworth, *Elements of Physiological Psychology* (1911), p. 552–3

like. The effectiveness of analysis was found to depend largely on the subject's attitude. The conception of attitudes, while specifically borrowed from the Würzburg experimentalists, was not, as with them, that of a new kind of *structure*, but that of a way of facing the situation. Among the attitudes discovered, by far the most effective was the problem attitude, in which the subject forgot his self-consciousness and the desire to make a good showing, and became interested in the problem itself. The problem attitude was the one most favourable to the emergence of sudden and useful insights. Even here, however, Ruger's data showed that such insights were apt to come clearly in consequence of similarities between the new task and a previous task successfully mastered. In other words, they were transfers from situations which resembled the one in which the subject was now working. Sudden insight, far from overthrowing the trial-and-error conception, seemed, at least in a large proportion of cases, to arise from the reappearance of a response-tendency which in a previous situation had given successful results. There were, to be sure, some cases in which it was very hard to see what in the past experience caused the particular flash of sudden insight to occur, and agnosticism and suspended judgment are still in order ; but at least much of the mysteriousness of thought was dispelled.[1]

The reader will recall that Binet had shown certain striking similarities between perception and reasoning (p. 239). Ruger and others had now ventured in the same direction. The reports of Ruger's subjects, as well as those of the Würzburg school, had, in fact, revealed many processes which might be classified equally well under perception, reasoning or learning. The traditional distinctions seemed to be shaken. In the case of the German investigators the new tendency took the form of reducing the reasoning processes, in some instances, to sequences of "attitudes." Ruger, and the American "functionalist" school, made attitudes equally important for reasoning and for perception.

---

[1] Rignano (*The Psychology of Reasoning*, 1920) has not only accepted the notion of *mental experimentation* as the essence of reasoning, but has worked out a systematic biological formulation of the reasoning process, in terms of the affective life and of attention.

S

We must next consider some theoretical and some experimental studies of the learning process which threw such light on perception and reasoning as to make both processes seem classifiable as subheads under learning.

Perhaps a good place to begin is the study of the transfer of training. The earliest careful study of transfer in motor functions[1] was made by Scripture and his collaborators,[2] who in 1894 trained subjects to carry out various movements with the right hand, and measured the degree of improvement in the same movement with the left hand. They found a large degree of transfer in such " cross-education." Thorndike and Woodworth,[3] in 1901, trained subjects in such tasks as the estimation of geometrical areas and of the magnitude of weights. When larger areas and weights were substituted for those used in the practice series, the effects of " transfer of training " were slight. Such effects as did appear were interpreted as due to " identical elements " present in the practice and in the final series ; these identical elements included specific habits and attitudes involved in adjustment to the task. Conclusions were stated in terms of the absence of general training in the functions involved ; the elements trained were specific habits which played a part only because of the close similarity between the situations encountered. This interpretation was in accordance with Thorndike's stimulus-response psychology, and in particular with his view that learning consists in the alteration of specific bonds. Much discussion of the whole conception of identical elements ensued.[4] Ebert and Meumann[5] undertook an experiment closely similar to that of James (p. 218), testing the effect of a practice period of memorizing upon the efficiency of memor-

---

[1] Fechner had reported that learning to write with one hand facilitated the process with the other hand (*Berichte d. k.-sächs. Ges. d. Wissensch., math.-phys.*, Kl. X, 1858, p. 70). Volkmann had shown experimentally that the reduction of the " two-point threshold " in certain regions through training lowered the threshold in other regions (*ibid.*, X, 1858, p. 38).

[2] Scripture, Smith, and Brown, *Studies from the Yale Psychological Laboratory*, II.

[3] " The Influence of Improvement in One Mental Function upon the Efficiency of Other Functions," *Psychol. Rev.*, VIII.

[4] Bair (" The Practice Curve," *Psychol. Rev., Monogr. Suppl.*, V, 1902–3 (whole No. 19) found that the curve of a skilled act showed, from its beginning, the influence of practice in another skilled act which had some elements in common with it.

[5] *Arch. f. d. ges. Psychol.*, IV, 1904.

izing other material. Their results seemed to show decided improvement as the result of memory-training. It was pointed out by W. F. Dearborn[1] that sufficient account had not been taken of the influence of the test material given before the practice period commenced ; in fact, repeating their initial and final tests without the practice period, he found a high level of attainment in the final tests, which was attributable to the effect of the initial test. Since the initial and final tests were similar, there was nothing to contradict the explanation of transfer in terms of the use of identical elements. The implications of all this for the theory of " formal discipline " were clear ; " perception " and " reasoning " seemed scarcely likely to be general functions capable of direct training, but names for very complex groups of activities, each activity being understood in terms of specific habits acquired by the individual.[2] Perception and reasoning were no longer clearly separable from the learning process.

Very significant was the work of Fracker,[3] who succeeded very well in getting rid of obvious similarities between practice material and test material. He presented to his subjects a series of musical tones in groups of four. Immediately afterward, before allowing them to reproduce what they had heard, he gave four more tones, and asked them to reproduce, in order, the first group of four. Of course there was much interference, which involved the necessity that each subject should find a mnemonic device, some scheme by which to fixate the tones so as to permit recall. The individual differences were considerable ; nevertheless, most of the subjects showed themselves capable of learning to reproduce the first series in spite of interference from the second. This result made possible the statement that the subjects improved in their performance by virtue of the acquisition of some specific " trick " or technique, and not as the result of formal memory training. This finding was confirmed by the fact that when the subjects turned to a new task, such as memorizing poetry,

---

[1] " The General Effects of Special Practice in Memory," *Psychol. Bull.*, VI, 1909.

[2] For an example of the experimental evidence indicating some transfer from one school subject to another, when closely related, see Dallam, " Is the Study of Latin Advantageous to the Study of English ?" *Ed. Rev.*, LIV, 1917.

[3] " On the Transference of Training in Memory," *Psychol. Monogr.*, IX, 1908.

they manifested no clear gain from their previous practice in memorizing ; they could not utilize their previous mnemonic devices. The work of Ruger, previously discussed, indicated that transfer was attributable to similarities between situations. Many other studies of transfer have served to confirm the Thorndike-Woodworth conclusions as to identical elements—conclusions which have now won general acceptance,[1] although strong opposition to the view has been a prominent feature of the *Gestalt* psychology (p. 244 and p. 426 f.).

Another field of investigation, usually treated in the same spirit, is " interference," or the decrease in efficiency which is observable in some activities in consequence of participation in other activities. This interference was manifest in the work of Müller and Pilzecker.[2] They found that when a given pair of items, A and B, had been learned in conjunction, and an attempt was then made to link A with C, the connection A–C might prove peculiarly hard to establish, because of interference from B. This was a statement of the problem of interference in terms of specific connections or linkages. Similar interference has been found in the study of overt motor acts. Münsterberg[3] conducted the simple experiment of changing his watch from one pocket to another and noting how many times a day he put it into the " wrong " pocket. He and subsequent investigators have reported that imperfectly formed habits tend to interfere with one another, while more thoroughly practised acts cease to do so.

An aspect of interference which has engaged much interest is " retroactive inhibition."[4] If immediately after a learning-period the subject is confronted with a new task, his recall of the learned material is appreciably less efficient than is his recall of material followed by a rest period. The amount of interference depends on the similarity between the learned material and the task which immediately follows, but all tasks exert some inhibitory effect.[5]

But evidence came to hand early in the present century to

[1] See, for example, Sleight, " Memory and Formal Training," *Brit. J. Psychol.*, IV, 1911. It must, however, be remembered that the term " element " is still hard to define.
[2] *Zeitschr. f. Psychol.*, Ergänzungsb. I, 1900.
[3] *Beiträge z. exp. Psychol.*, I, 1892.
[4] Müller and Pilzecker, *op. cit.*
[5] See, *e.g.*, Robinson, " Some Factors Determining the Degree of Retroactive Inhibition," *Psychol. Monogr.*, XXVIII, 1920.

show that the learning process could not be regarded *merely* as a relation between stimuli and responses. The internal condition of the organism was of major importance. Müller and Schumann[1] showed that the reading of nonsense syllables need not result in learning their *order*, but that when the subject's attitude is altered through the instruction to learn the syllables in order, rapid learning follows. The new attitude was called[2] the " will to learn." This suggestion vied with Külpe's movement in sweeping away the débris of the associationist tradition. The trend in all recent work is in the direction of showing the significance of the attitudes taken, the " control " or the " mental set " determining the formation of associations.

A fertile field of research has been the problem of " incidental memory," that is, memory for material which has never been consciously learned.[3] As early as 1895 this was investigated by Cattell.[4] He gave a series of questions to Columbia undergraduates as to what they had seen under a variety of situations, to determine how much in their everyday surroundings had failed to be sufficiently noted to make possible an answer to questions. He pointed out the extraordinary unreliability of casual everyday observation, showing that many things frequently seen had failed to make an impression definite enough to permit of successful recall. Moreover, individuals were frequently certain of much which had no basis in fact. This experiment was repeated by Jastrow[5] with confirmatory results. Binet,[6] using suggestion, obtained corroboration for Cattell's thesis. The study took quantitative form in the work of Stern,[7] who ascertained the increase or decrease in the number of items reported, with the lapse of time after the presentation, and found a decrease in the accuracy of testimony as time elapsed. He was interested

[1] *Zeitschr. f. Psychol.*, VI, 1894.
[2] By Ebert and Meumann, *op. cit.*
[3] The problem has generally been so defined as to include many questions which have only one thing in common, the search for mental connections established without deliberate purpose.
[4] " Measurement of the Accuracy of Recollection," *Science*, N.S., II, 1895.
[5] Reported by F. E. Bolton, " Accuracy of Recollection and Observation," *Psychol. Rev.*, III, 1896.
[6] *La Suggestibilité* (1900).
[7] *Zeitschr. f.d. ges. Strafrechtswiss.*, XXIII, 1903. See also *Beiträge zur Psychologie der Aussage*, I (1903–4), in which the decrease of suggestibility with age was demonstrated.

in the " psychology of testimony " as a practical problem ; hence not only defective memory, but the tendency to fabricate unwittingly material to take the place of what was forgotten, was important. Claparède[1] found that with the lapse of time there was a tendency to neglect the unusual and the contingent and to testify in the direction of the " probable." Following the observations of Thorndike and Woodworth on the inability of subjects to report accurately on their everyday surroundings, Garry Myers[2] offered evidence which showed the marked incapacity of most observers to report on situations to which they had been frequently exposed. For example, the vast majority of his subjects gave grossly inaccurate estimates as to the size of a dollar bill or a postage stamp.

But all these studies leave open the question whether the results are due to failures of recall or to the failure of human beings to *notice*[3] items in their surroundings. The question frequently appears to be not how good a man's memory is, but whether items were observed in the first place.

But traditional associationism was to suffer even more serious rebuffs than these. In 1907 Witasek[4] discovered that the mere passive reading and re-reading of printed matter was decidedly less efficacious than reading followed by " active recitation," in which the subject forced himself to recall what he had read. This statement was reduced to clear quantitative form by A. I. Gates,[5] who not only confirmed Witasek's conclusions, but showed that both the rate of learning and the amount retained were increased by devoting larger and larger percentages of the learning-time to recitation ; even the use of eighty per cent. of the time for recitation was more effective than smaller percentages. It was clear that learning was at least something more than the indiscriminate formation of linkages ; the ways in which such linkages were formed called aloud for investigation.

---

[1] " Témoignage collectif," *Arch. de Psychol.*, V, 1906.
[2] " A Study in Incidental Memory," *Arch. of Psychol.*, XXVI, 1913.
[3] Whatever bugbears arise when " attention " is mentioned, it would appear that the understanding of these results can come only through further investigation of the functional significance, if not, in fact, of the nature, of attention. We need to know not only the relation of attention to learning, but to the entire curve of forgetting in the case of material learned with varying degrees of thoroughness.
[4] *Zeitschr. f. Psychol.*, XLIV, 1907.
[5] " Recitation as a Factor in Memorizing," *Arch. of Psychol.*, XL, 1917.

Another experiment necessitating a revision of association-ism was the study of the rôle of the image in relation to the fixation and recall of complex visual stimuli ; in other words, the question of the extent to which we remember by virtue of mental pictures or other reproductions of the sensory content once experienced. The experiments of Judd and Cowling[1] were designed to find how much of a picture could be recalled after it had been exposed for a short interval. They found that the subject made definite attacks on the task ; he would look at different points and immediately afterward recall those details that he had noticed. Each time the picture was presented, he would name a few more things observed. But never at any time was the thing photographed on the mind so that he could " read off " from his mental image what he had seen. There was no process by which he mentally saw the picture all at once, and then read off from his " mental picture " a series of details. The results indicated simply specific observations and specific reports. Results equally damaging to the interpretation of memory in terms of simple imagery were obtained by M. R. Fernald.[2] She put before her subjects an arrangement of letters in both vertical and horizontal lines so as to form a square (Binet letter-square). Having asked her subject to get a complete visual image of this letter-square, she removed the letters. The letters could then, indeed, be named by some subjects ; but when instructions were given to read, for example, from the lower right-hand corner vertically to the upper right-hand corner, or to read letters from right to left, confusion and error resulted. The subject might be able, by rehearsing the whole series, to perform even such tasks, but one thing which he evidently was not doing was reading from a clear memory image. The contrast between the reproduction of the letters in the *order learned* and the reproduction of them in any *other* order was so great as to indicate that the square was not recalled in terms of mental images at all. The visualizer may, indeed, " see " individual letters, but he can scarcely make good his claim that he continues to see the square. The question as to the number of items which may be simultane-

---

[1] " Studies in Perceptual Development," *Psychol. Rev., Monogr. Suppl.,* VIII, 1907 (whole No. 34).
[2] "The Diagnosis of Mental Imagery," *Psychol. Monogr.,* XIV. 1912–3.

ously visualized remains open; it is sufficient to note that some memory processes which had in general been attributed to imagery were discovered to have no such foundation. Adherents to the theory of imageless thought found here much comfort.

Into the chaos of theories of thought and memory resulting from such studies came a definite and illuminating suggestion, in Woodworth's Presidential Address before the *American Psychological Association* in 1914, " A Revision of Imageless Thought."[1] This served as a historical summary and a new theory for the interpretation of scattered data on perception and memory. His view can be stated most simply in functional terms, and when the implications are grasped, a structural formulation may be offered. Woodworth described perception as a form of response ; the " perceptual reaction " theory postulated a process above and beyond the arousal of a group of sensations or images. In fact, it supposed that brain areas outside the sensory regions react *to* the separate sensory items in a way which the items themselves could never determine. It is true that in every perceptual experience there are sensory elements, but they do not constitute a percept unless the organism makes such a perceptual reaction. This perceptual reaction is not the sum of the constituent parts, but a relation which the organism bears to the various stimulating elements.

Woodworth described an experiment to show how this principle operated in the case of standard memory material, " paired associates." He had read aloud to his subjects a series of words, instructing the subjects to learn them in the usual manner, in such fashion that the first word of each pair would, when presented, recall the second. But he presented the stimuli at a constant rate ; the interval between A and B was identical with that between B and C, despite the fact that A-B and C-D were to be learned as pairs. Associationists from Hartley onward would expect that the linkage from B to C would be as firmly established as the linkages A-B and C-D. Association by contiguity throughout its various revisions had implied that any two parts of a situation presented successively form connections which later cause the presentation of the first to bring back the second.

[1] *Psychol. Rev.*, XXII, 1915.

But Woodworth reported that the tendency for the first term of a pair to recall its second term was eighty-five times as great as the tendency of the latter to recall the first term of the next pair. Clearly he was dealing with something more than mere contiguity. The connection between B and C, between D and E, etc., was, in fact, so slight that it was not definitely attributable to the contiguity-factor at all. Attention might, in some cases, have wavered so as to make B-C and the like appear in consciousness so as to be perceived as pairs. The experiment not only seemed to refute the law of contiguity, but in Woodworth's opinion it indicated that the *perception* of A and B as a pair served as a basis for the connection between them. Not their proximity, not merely the formal will to learn, not any special attitude, but the act of perception itself established the connection. Perception was interpreted not as a state within which sensation exists, but as a reaction which the sensations arouse.

Now for the structural implications of this point of view. " Imageless thought " may appear whenever a perceptual experience is revived without the revival of the sensory constituents. When the perceptual reaction has taken place, the brain patterns may be reinstated in such form as to bring back the thought without the images. Meanings are not, so to speak, brothers and sisters of images ; for images depend on the re-excitement of sensory areas, while meanings depend upon activity in regions not comprised within the sensory areas. The coming and going of images may leave the meaning unaffected. The meaning, nevertheless, must be regarded from a structural viewpoint as present in consciousness.

Another word about the neurological implications. We have in the visual cortex a number of elements which, when stimulated, produce individual sensations or images. The seeing of an object involves the excitation of a pattern within this visual area. But it involves, Woodworth suggests, something more—a process outside this sensory projection area. This outlying region is the physical substrate for recall of perceptual patterns. The importance of such perceptual patterns is apparent in illusions. Things may be " wrongly " perceived, not through the admixture of misleading images (as structuralism would in general assert), but through the transfer to a new situation of a perceptual response which was useful in a previous situation. When one is reading proof, one may fail to note misprints, not because images are misplaced, but because a firmly established perceptual habit comes into play. This doctrine may readily be harmonized with the widespread opinion (p. 202) that in addition to sensory areas in the cortex there are, so to speak, interpreting areas, the disorganization of which may produce gross damage to perception, as in the case of " word-deafness " and " word-blindness."

One more radical departure from Hartleyan associationism must be noted in the emphasis upon total experience and its " redintegration " rather than mere serial arrangement of *items* of experience. Hamilton's doctrine (p. 105), adopted and used by Bain and James, and undergoing various vicissitudes in the hands of Bradley[1] and Semon,[2] has served as the starting point for much modern discussion of learning. H. L. Hollingworth[3] uses the term " redintegration " to describe not the process by which an element *brings back* its context, but the process by which it *functions for* the situation of which it was once a part ; the part acts for the whole. It is evident that association (or " associative shifting ") is not the *key* to such a process, but rather a special case of a principle of wide application.[4]

[1] *Principles of Logic* (1883).
[2] *The Mneme* (1904).
[3] *E.g., The Psychology of Functional Neuroses* (1920), Chapter II ; *The Psychology of Thought* (1926), p. 92 f.
[4] Hollingworth interweaves this principle with the doctrine of the " psychophysical continuum," to the effect that the only difference between the subjective and objective worlds lies in the greater uniformity of our experience of the latter ; and indicates transitional orders between the two extremes.

CHAPTER XVI

BEHAVIOURISM

Dismiss therefore every idle fancy and foolish conjecture of those who confine the intellectual activity to particular locations in the body.—Gregory of Nyssa.

WE have sought to indicate how the thought processes were subjected to an experimental analysis which showed their close relation to problems in learning and in perception. Another field of investigation contributed to the fusion of these traditionally distinct problems. This new movement arose within the field of animal psychology, but soon spread to include a systematic restatement of nearly all the problems of human psychology.

Late in the nineteenth century began a series of animal studies by German physiologists who are loosely designated the "German Objectivists."[1] This group endeavoured to interpret animal behaviour without reference to any mental events whatever. Even sensation was excluded. They objected, for example, to the use of the term "ear," because the ear is the organ of hearing. We have, they thought, no right to assume that organisms hear ; let us use, they said, the term "phonoreceptor." Similarly, we have no right to assume that an animal sees ; let us use the term "photoreceptor." No one could be more drastic in the exclusion of conscious events than the German Objectivists.

The same spirit breathed in the work of the Russian physiologist, Pavlov. At the beginning of the present century he was engaged at the (then) St. Petersburg University on a programme of research upon the physiology of digestion. He gave attention for a long time to the salivary reflex, and became interested in the fact that the reflex could be elicited by other means than direct stimulation of the tongue. Having devised a technique for the observation and measurement of the influence of a variety of factors upon

---

[1] Among their leaders were Bethe, Beer, and von Uexküll.

the salivary secretion, he noticed that stimuli which bore originally no known relation to the salivary reflex might elicit the response, if they had been present simultaneously with gustatory stimuli which caused the flow of saliva. He was thinking in objective and in *quantitative* terms ; he determined how much saliva was produced by each stimulus. He sounded a tuning-fork simultaneously with the application of a given quantity of powdered meat on a dog's tongue, and repeated this procedure at intervals until the tuning-fork alone, without the meat, would produce not merely the flow of saliva but the *same number of drops* per unit of time which the meat alone had originally produced.

His early technique involved merely the use of a fistula in the cheek, to collect the saliva. Later he used a more elaborate method : a rubber tube connected with a fistula directed the flow upon a delicate platform resting on a spring. Each drop which fell upon the platform caused a movement which was transmitted to a delicate marker upon a revolving drum, so that it was possible to record not only the number of drops but the moment at which each drop fell. This made it possible not only to state the total amount of saliva emitted in a half-minute, but its variation in ten-second intervals, and so on. The saliva meanwhile was collected as it fell from the platform. This whole quantitative viewpoint was essential to Pavlov's " conditioned reflex " method ; the reflex was *conditional* upon the fact that a given stimulus had been presented together with one which was originally adequate to elicit it.

During the first years of the present century a great number of investigations were undertaken at St. Petersburg, to study the number of repetitions needed to build up such conditioned reflexes in the dog under different conditions, the variation of the time interval between original and conditioned stimulus, the influence of other stimuli in inhibiting a conditioned reflex, and kindred problems. Among these studies, some of the most interesting deal with the variation of the time interval between the " conditioned " stimulus and the " original " stimulus. Reflexes may be conditioned to a *time interval, e.g.*, saliva begins to flow ten seconds after the conditioned stimulus is given. Among these investigations a group of considerable importance deals with the influence of inhibition. If the conditioned stimulus A has come to cause a flow of saliva, but if now an irrelevant stimulus B is presented together with A, to what extent does the stimulus B augment or decrease the reaction ? The Pavlov school found evidence that such irrelevant stimuli tend to inhibit the response, the effect varying with the nature and intensity of the new stimulus. This led to the formulation of quite complicated problems ; for example, those relating to the " inhibition of an inhibition." The conditioned reflex method offered such extraordinary possibilities, a means of answering objectively such a host of fundamental problems in behaviour, that it seemed to some investigators almost a high road to Paradise.

Early investigations of " discrimination "[1] are illustrative. Pavlov's pupils undertook to determine how well the dog discriminates tones, in terms of a *differential salivary response* to tones separated by small intervals. Suppose a tuning-fork at 256 vibrations per second is sounded simultaneously with the presentation of meat, so that, in time, the fork alone elicits the full salivary response. Then a fork of a higher or lower pitch is sounded ; saliva flows, but the dog is not fed. Whenever the original fork is sounded, food is given ; when the other fork is sounded, food is withheld. Rapidly the dog exhibits a differential response ; the salivary reflex disappears in response to the pitch which has not been attended by food. Now, continuing the use of the 256 fork together with the feeding, other forks are used whose pitch approaches closer and closer to that of the original one, until at last a pitch is found at which the full salivary response occurs ; the difference between such a pitch and that of the fork vibrating at 256 measures the interval in which pitch-discrimination is lacking. In the early years of the school Orbelli[2] obtained with this method indications of very remarkable tone-discrimination, a few vibrations per second proving sufficient to cause not merely the decrease but the total disappearance of the salivary response, the number of drops falling off

---

[1] The term here describes an objective process. Pavlov warned his students to beware of the psychologists ; in everything they did they were to keep their methods purely physiological.

[2] " The Orientation of the Dog to Sound " (1905) ; " Contributions to the Study of Reactions of the Dog to the Auditory Stimuli " (1907). See Yerkes and Norgulis, " The Method of Pawlow in Animal Psychology," *Psychol. Bull.*, VI, 1909.

sharply, as the vibration rate rose to 258, 260, etc. In a similar experiment on colour-discrimination, Zeliony[1] reported evidence for colour-blindness in the dog, hues producing identical responses so long as brightness and saturation were kept constant. Within recent years Pavlov's pupils have reported confirmation of Orbelli's results, with greatly improved technique, together with much new material based upon this discrimination method.

A good deal of skepticism prevails as to all this type of experimentation. H. M. Johnson,[2] for example, using another method, has failed to find any such capacity for tone-discrimination in the dog ; and in relation to the discrimination of visual materials it is generally known that the dog is extraordinarily near-sighted. Furthermore, much of the early Russian work is subject to the criticism that the dog's responses may have been elicited by other stimuli than those controlled by the experimenter. In recent years much has been done to exclude such interfering factors ; not only is the experiment room rendered highly sound-proof, but the apparatus and experimenter are placed outside, observations being made through a periscope. In spite of these improvements, many students of animal behaviour are averse to the claim that the conditioned response method can so easily solve such complex problems.

Pavlov's antipathy to subjectivism was shared by Bekhterev, who as early as 1907 outlined an " objective psychology."[3] This represented human nature in objective terms, the conditioned response being given a prominent place in the mechanism of learning. The symptoms of psychoneurotics were, for example, to be regarded as responses transferred from one situation to another by virtue of conditioning. More recently Bekhterev and his co-workers have attempted to formulate a complete characterology or science of personality[4] in terms of behaviour ; even the term " psychology " seems to Bekhterev to savour of the mistakes of the past.

Of course, animal psychology had been using a concept

[1] " Conditioned Reflexes Resulting from Optical Stimulation of the Dog " (1908).
[2] " Audition and Habit Formation in the Dog," *Beh. Monogr.*, II, 1913.
[3] *La psychologie objective* (trans. 1913 ; German trans. also 1913).
[4] *Allgemeine Grundlagen der Reflexologie des Menschen* (3rd. ed.1926).

closely similar[1] to that of the conditioned response ; its literature had been rich in illustrations of the attachment of responses to new stimuli. But the Russian work had made the conception more definite, and had in particular offered an objective approach to the discrimination problem.

The salivary-reflex method soon attracted the attention of American experimentalists. Its use, however, did not by any means carry with it Pavlov's scorn for subjective analysis, nor eliminate from American work the discussion of the subjective side of the animal's responses. Washburn, in *The Animal Mind* (1908), devoted considerable attention to the analysis of the probable conscious states attending observed behaviour. Yerkes, the most prolific in research among American experimentalists in the first years of this century, while making use of the conditioned response method, employed many introspective terms, discussing, for example, " ideational " behaviour.[2]

Now, in the spirit of the " German Objectivists," and in harmony with Pavlov's ban upon all reference to consciousness, an independent movement began in the work of J. B. Watson.[3] Watson was impelled, on the one hand, by his recognition of the fertility of the many new objective methods of animal psychology, to explore more and more into the nature of the learning process as a problem in the modification of *behaviour*. And on the other hand, he was much disgusted

---

[1] Identical, except for Pavlov's quantitative conception. And the quantitative aspects of his work have been so generally disregarded that we shall here use the term " conditioned response " to designate simply a response attached, as described, to a substitute stimulus. Loeb had clearly described this mechanism in 1900 (*Physiology of the Brain*), calling it " associative memory," and describing it quite objectively. Hobbes, Locke, and Spencer, among others, had described some cases of association in terms nearly objective enough to pass for descriptions of conditioned responses.

[2] " Ideational Behavior of Monkeys and Apes," *Proc. Nat. Acad. Sciences*, 1916.

[3] His formulation of the behaviourist programme in 1913, " Psychology as the Behaviorist views it," *Psychol. Rev.*, XX, was followed in 1914 by his *Behavior: An Introduction to Comparative Psychology*, in which a programme was outlined for a psychology which should be based solely on the biological sciences, rigidly excluding every reference to conscious states or processes. Watson believes that Thorndike stimulated him much more than did the " Objectivists," whose " parallelism " he contrasts with his own monistic system (See the Preface to the Second Edition of the *Psychology from the Standpoint of a Behaviorist*, 1924.)

by the inability of introspective psychologists, such as Titchener, Angell, and Woodworth, to demonstrate a finality with respect to imageless thought. There seemed to be great unreliability in the testimony of human subjects as to their imagery, and this seemed to give grounds for doubt as to the possibility of using the image as a datum for psychology. Watson decided to throw overboard the entire concept of mind or consciousness, and to make both animal and human psychology the study of behaviour. Modifications of behaviour were to be studied in terms of stimulus-response situations, not at all in terms of conscious concomitants or neurological assumptions.

The "law of effect" was early a centre for Watson's attack.[1] Thorndike had maintained that if an animal does something which brings about *satisfaction*, the result is an improvement in the conductivity of the neural connections leading to the performance of the act. Acts which cause *annoyance* involve a decrease in neural conductivity tending to the elimination of the act. Watson objected not only to the concepts of satisfaction and annoyance, but to the claim that there was here a factor not taken account of by the principles of frequency and recency. If a cat obtains food immediately after the movement of releasing the bolt of a puzzle-box, this movement is the *last* act of all that occur in the cage. Furthermore, whereas unsuccessful movements are legion, there is but one successful movement ; over a number of trials the successful movement will therefore be repeated more *frequently* than any other. To this Thorndike retorted that in many cases one successful movement was promptly learned, while an unsuccessful movement, though repeated *several times in the same trial*, was eliminated.[2] Experimental evidence on the point was not decisive. No technique has as yet been offered which can definitely close the question as to the functional importance of satisfaction and annoyance. The problem is, of course, interwoven with many unanswered questions regarding the nature of the affective life ; for our purposes it is sufficient to note that the rejection of such conceptions has become a cardinal point for most varieties of behaviourism.

[1] *Behavior* (1914), p. 256 f.
[2] Thorndike and Herrick, " Watson's ' Behavior,' " *J. An. Beh.*, V, 1915.

The first definitions of behaviourism were necessarily in rather negative terms ; for example, in terms of the exclusion of parts of the subject matter of contemporary psychology. The movement began gradually, however, to develop a system of positive assumptions and to work these into a psychological system. Even in his earliest work, Watson emphasized the right of the behaviourist to think of "mental" processes as internal forms of behaviour, the relation of language to thought being especially stressed. We shall return to the point.

In the meantime, the conditioned response method was beginning to be widely applied in human psychology, with profound consequences for psychological theory,[1] and perhaps most of all for the theory of behaviourism. Lashley,[2] for example, demonstrated that the conditioned salivary reflex could be elicited in human beings through the sight of chocolate candy, a small cup against the parotid gland collecting quantities of saliva which varied with the nearness of the stimulus. New possibilities of the method were shown by Cason,[3] who found that the pupillary reflex can be conditioned by the simultaneous presentation of visual and auditory stimuli. A sound may in time produce those pupillary contractions which resulted originally from light.

An application of the conditioned response method to the problem of the nature of intelligence has been made by Mateer.[4] Utilizing a method developed by Krasnogorski,[5] she placed a chocolate drop in the mouth of a child when she bandaged his eyes. A record was made of the number of repetitions required to cause the child to open its mouth immediately upon the application of the bandage. A group of children from less than a year to seven years of age was studied, and to those from three to seven she gave standard intelligence tests. The number of repetitions necessary for conditioning was found to have a large negative correlation

---

[1] See the summary and bibliography in Cason, " The Conditioned Reflex or Conditioned Response as a Common Activity of Living Organisms," *Psychol. Bull.*, XXII, 1925.

[2] " The Human Salivary Reflex and Its Use in Psychology," *Psychol. Rev.*, xxiii, 1916.

[3] " The Conditioned Pupillary Reflex," *J. Exp. Psychol.*, V, 1922. See also his " The Conditioned Eyelid Reflex," *ibid*.

[4] *Child Behavior* (1918).

[5] *Ueber die Bildung der künstlichen Bedingungsreflexe bei Säuglingen* (1907).

T

with intelligence scores. Moreover, the children who learned most quickly to open the mouth when the signal was given were in general the ones who learned most quickly to cease doing so when the touches were no longer followed by chocolate. The experiment, while obviously crude, is highly significant both for the problem of the nature of the relation between intelligence and learning, and as an expression of the widespread belief that the speed of conditioning is an important element, if not, in fact, the chief element, in the organism's ability to adapt itself to new situations.[1]

Of course it was inevitable that profound changes in the definition of the learning process should follow from such studies, and that they should lead toward a restatement of the whole problem as to the mechanism by which connections between stimuli and responses are altered. Many years elapsed, however, before a group of behaviourists saw their way clear to utilize these simple doctrines in the construction of a systematic psychology which should reduce such time-honoured problems as instinct, perception, judgment, intelligence, and reasoning to these elementary forms of response. For one result of such intensive study of the conditioned response, and of the recognition of its importance for the theory of learning, has been the recent tendency among some American psychologists to believe that *all* learning is simply conditioning, and that the conditioned response is the true *unit* of learned behaviour.[2]

A few illustrations will serve to show how "learning through conditioning" may be substituted for the concept of the influence of satisfaction and annoyance as a determinant to action. If a rat is placed before two runways which contain, respectively, food and electric-shock apparatus, we may proceed to study objectively the factors which enable him, through trial-and-error, to choose the alley with the food. A circle, for example, may always appear above the door which leads to food, and a triangle above the other, the right and left placement of both food and shock being frequently reversed. Of course, he learns quickly if the circle and triangle are kept on their respective sides; but

[1] Experiments in conditioning, from the earth-worm to man, seem in general to indicate a significant relation between the speed of conditioning and the complexity of the nervous system.

[2] Watson, *Behaviorism* (1925), p. 157f. Smith and Guthrie, (*General Psychology in Terms of Behavior* 1921), are forerunners of this view.

if the stimuli are frequently reversed, the rat typically requires many dozen trials to learn to enter the " circle " alley consistently and without error, as the circle is shifted from side to side. Now, one may say, this is a case of simple conditioned response ; the approach reactions previously present in response to food have simply been " conditioned to " the circle. The circle acts as a substitute stimulus, just as the tuning-fork is a substitute stimulus for meat.

The same theory applies to a slightly more complicated performance manifest in the task of learning to escape from a maze. If the hungry animal is placed at the centre, and food outside, random running follows, in the course of which blind alleys and " correct " turns occur. Blind alleys are gradually eliminated, and " correct " turns more frequently made, because the latter lead to food ; each point in the course of the maze which does, in fact, lead to food becomes in time a substitute stimulus eliciting the approach-reaction. Afferent (" sensory ") impulses from the muscles are emphasized as conditioning stimuli.[1] In a group of animals which had learned the maze, Watson[2] had (years before his formulation of behaviourism) extirpated the eyes and essential mechanisms connected with hearing, smell, and other senses, and found that the maze could still be run ; he suggested that incoming neural impulses from the muscles were sufficient to guide the animal. Each turn at an opening within the maze served as stimulus for the next set of muscular contractions. From the standpoint of the theory under discussion, the movements had built up habits in which each muscular response served as a *substitute stimulus* for the next response.

Some difficulties in this explanation have appeared. In the case of learning complicated mazes, food may be reached so long after certain of the " correct " movements that it is difficult to see how conditioning could occur.[3] The rejoinder that the last steps in the maze are first learned through

---

[1] They had, of course, been emphasized before ; James's chapter on Habit is a classical instance.

[2] " Kinesthetic and Organic Sensations : Their Rôle in the Reactions of the White Rat to the Maze," *Psychol. Rev., Monogr. Suppl.*, VIII, 1907 (whole No. 33).

[3] The length of time which may elapse in successful conditioning, between substitute and original stimulus, must, of course, be established separately for each species and each situation.

conditioning to the food, and that the elimination of blind alleys occurs in regular *reverse* order through successive conditioning of muscular responses, is rendered dubious by the fact that experimental evidence shows no such orderly progression in the acquisition of the necessary habits.[1]

As we have seen, one of Watson's most important theoretical contributions has been the suggestion,[2] and as time elapsed, the insistence[3] that all the phenomena of " inner " life are in reality the functioning of mechanisms which are as objective, though not as observable, as gross muscular contractions. In particular, imagination and thought have been stated in terms of " implicit " muscular behaviour, especially the behaviour of the speech-organs and other mechanisms which symbolize lines of overt conduct. The study of language is therefore of paramount importance for the formulation of behaviourist theory.

A word is appropriate about the study of language during the nineteenth century. The relation of language to thought occupied many of the associationists.[4] In the second and third quarters of the century a number of philologists devoted themselves to the question of the origin of language,[5] and collected data to support the hypothesis that all languages must have started from simple roots, these roots building themselves into higher and higher organizations by the process of psychological association ; such words as " blackboard " and " nevertheless " were held to be paradigms for all late linguistic developments. On the other hand, some scholars showed with fair plausibility that many

---

[1] " No apparent relation exists between the serial position of a cul-de-sac with respect to the foodbox and the temporal order of elimination in the maze here employed . . . . . "——Warden, " Some Factors Determining the Order of Elimination of Cul-de-Sacs in the Maze," *J. Exp. Psychol.*, VI, 1923. See, however, Carr, " The Distribution and Elimination of Errors in the Maze," *J. An. Beh.*, VII, 1917.

[2] " Psychology as the Behaviorist Views it," *Psychol. Rev.*, XX, 1913.

[3] *Behaviorism* (1925).

[4] The problem engaged the close attention of Taine (*On Intelligence*, 1870), and has recently been attacked systematically by Ogden and Richards in *The Meaning of Meaning* (1923).

[5] A famous triad of explanations comprises : (1) the doctrine that words were originally copies of sounds,—the " bow-wow theory "; (2) the doctrine that they were originally interjections,—the " pooh-pooh theory " ; (3) the doctrine that " everything which is struck rings,"—the " ding-dong theory."

languages are rich in roots which are neither phonetically nor ideationally simple. Another branch of inquiry was the study of the phonetic changes which marked the divergence of linguistic stocks from a common origin. The brothers Grimm, for example, showed specific steps which had taken place in the differentiation of the Germanic tongues. The problem of the origin of language tended to fade as its complexities and difficulties were realized ; and empirical problems in phonetics tended to take its place. Phonetics became, in fact, an experimental science. A most important step was the invention of the Marey tambour[1], which made it possible to ascertain the time relations of the movements involved in speech. This was extensively used by Scripture[2] at about the turn of the century. In the same period, students of early childhood (notably Stern[3]) made observations upon individual development in the use of phonetic combinations. Naturally, the process by which language is acquired was soon subjected to intensive analysis. A clear statement of part of the problem was given by Holt.[4] He pointed out that words, acting as substitutes for situations, *evoke the same responses* which the situations themselves would elicit.[5] The " meaning " of a word, he held, is nothing but a conditioned response to that word. We can see this most plainly in the case of movements which have arisen in the history of the individual in relation to specific objects ; for example, in the act of reaching for things. If, for example, the child reaches toward a bottle, and the word " bottle " is repeated many times in connection with it, in the course of time saying the word " bottle " will produce in the child the reaching movement ; a conditioned response has been established. What the word " bottle " *means* is the behaviour in reference to the bottle. In other words, behaviourism has involved the abandonment of the associationist view that words arouse simply *ideas*. It is clear that we have shifted responses from the field of association to the domain of

[1] An air chamber which may be connected on one side (by means of rubber tubing) with various parts of the speech apparatus, and equipped on its other side with a rubber diaphragm, the movements of which control a marker upon a revolving drum.
[2] *The Elements of Experimental Phonetics* (1901).
[3] See p. 284.
[4] *The Freudian Wish* (1915).
[5] This obvious fact was, of course, not put forward as a new discovery, but the grasping of its implications for behaviourism was important.

muscular responses. This hypothesis goes so far, in fact, as to maintain that even those words that refer to purposes and attitudes function by the conditioned response mechanism ; purposes and attitudes are muscular behaviour which differs from overt activity only in respect to the amount of movement involved.[1] When a person, thinking through a problem, says to himself : " That forces me to halt in my thinking," the word " halt " acts as the overt command to halt would act.

It is necessary, of course, to distinguish between " passive language habits " (the response to words) and " active language habits " (the use of words). The interpretation of passive language habits in behaviour terms turned out, as we have seen, to be very simple. But active language was a larger problem. To this problem Watson addressed himself in a paper presented to the *International Congress of Philosophy and Psychology*[2] in 1920 ; his view was later set forth in the second edition (1924) of his *Psychology from the Standpoint of a Behaviorist*, and in *Behaviorism* (1925). Starting with the random babblings of the child, he asserted that any sounds that cause other persons to minister to the child's needs tend in the long run to be repeated more often than sounds which bring little or no result.[3] Consequently, the child develops not only a set of nursery words understood and used by the family, but, purely through such trial-and-error variations, sounds which, by approximating genuine words, bring quicker and better results. No mechanism of learning need be supposed other than those manifest in the rat's learning the maze, or the cat's learning to escape from the puzzle-box. The child learns to say " ta-ta," and later " doll," by the same mechanism. If the word " ta-ta " is used and is understood by others to mean doll, it serves the purpose ; the only thing necessary is that it should work. Whenever it fails to work, further trial-and-error occurs until " doll " is uttered.

In the view just stated, the *imitation* of words can only be explained by assuming an extraordinary amount of random

[1] See Hobbes, p. 17.
[2] In a symposium : " Is Thinking Merely the Action of Language Mechanisms ? " (Published *Brit. J. Psychol.*, XI, 1920.) Though Watson was not present, his paper was the subject of much discussion.
[3] This would, of course, be cited by Thorndike's followers as a case of the " law of effect." From the behaviourists' viewpoint we are dealing simply with the elimination of irrelevant responses (see p. 270).

activity which develops, step by step, a child's ability to duplicate what it hears or sees. Observation of the extra-ordinary degree of successful imitation present in the second year of life has suggested the need of an explanation which will not insist upon the laborious process just described, yet will avoid recourse to the defunct theory of the "instinct of imitation." F. H. Allport[1] has utilized for the purpose a doctrine developed by J. M. Baldwin[2] a quarter-century before, the " circular reflex."   Baldwin had asserted that the constant repetition of a movement might be due to the fact that each movement serves as a stimulus for its own repetition ; as, for instance, when a monkey was observed to slap a surface of water over and over again.   Allport has assumed that the child's random utterances stimulate its auditory area while its motor-speech centres are still active ; a connection is thus established which may lead to almost endless repetition of a sound.   Such a reaction having been established between the hearing of a sound and the uttering of it, it is easy to see how the utterance of a sound by another individual may cause, immediately, the child's repetition of it.   This view seems really a supplement to the Watsonian view, rather than a direct contradiction of it.

This shows the process by which the chief terms used in thinking, namely, words, are learned as separate units ; they are now integrated, in like manner with other forms of behaviour, into " higher units." The next step is to show how this overt language is replaced by internal language, that is, how we learn to talk to ourselves instead of talking aloud. Watson[3] is here again the chief contributor to the theory. He suggests that the child's vocalization is eliminated through social pressure, so that children, in talking to themselves, no longer talk aloud, but in a whisper. Only one modification is necessary to change ordinary speech to a whisper, namely, that the vocal chords should be relaxed instead of innervated. All the rest of the speech-mechanism works as before. Finally, whispering itself is eliminated, yet speech movements continue ; " implicit " language activity continues in the form of constant changes

[1] *Social Psychology* (1924).

[2] *Mental Development in the Child and the Race* (1895).

[3] *Psychology from the Standpoint of a Behaviorist*, 2nd ed. (1924), p. 343 f.

in tension among the various speech-mechanisms, which are duplicates of the movement involved in overt speech.

It will be recalled that several authors[1] had described thinking in terms of mental experimentation, and had shown the close similarity between thought and overt trial-and-error behaviour. Ruger had shown that a good deal of this trial-and-error activity exists in the thought processes involved in solving new and complicated problems. Now the trial-and-error mechanism, as described by Ruger, consisted, to a large extent, in the manipulation of ideas or attitudes. These processes lend themselves to construction in terms of language-mechanisms. Thinking consists, therefore, for the behaviourist, of speech-movements made on a very small scale, and substituted for overt acts.[2] Trial-and-error goes on in implicit language behaviour, each word or phrase in the thinking process serving as a substitute for some act. No longer do we find " ideas," but speech-movements, as the elements involved in thinking.

As trial-and-error occurs, some of these combinations lead to overt activities which have been conditioned to their respective verbal stimuli. Certain manual and verbal activities are conditioned to each other.[3] Behaviourism, therefore, has stated the thought processes in terms of language which, through the conditioned response, serves in place of similarly conditioned overt acts. To be sure, there must be forms of thinking which are not verbal, and these are stated by behaviourists in terms of gesture, of movements of the hands, feet, neck, trunk, and especially of the eyes.[4] The elaborate study of eye-movements, begun by Helmholtz, had been continued by many experimenters. The relation of these movements to the reading-process became a fertile field of inquiry early in the present century, and it was easy for the behaviourist to press such studies into his service by

[1] See p. 252.
[2] Bain, Ribot, and others had described speech-movements which occur in the process of thinking ; but the *identification* of such movements with the thinking process is the work of Watson.
[3] The point is elaborated in Watson's *Behaviorism* (1925).
[4] But behaviourists insist that speech-movements may rarely be wholly eliminated. Children seldom, if ever, succeed in completely eliminating the tongue and lip movements associated with the original printed words. The deaf and dumb use their fingers to think with : Watson has, in fact, reminded the incredulous that Laura Bridgman could be observed to talk in her sleep by means of her fingers.

suggesting that memory for verbal material, as well as for events observed, may be in part the repetition of eye-movements which have occurred before, though, to be sure, they are repeated in abbreviated form. Slight ("implicit") gestures and delicate eye-movements co-operate constantly with speech-movements in the complex processes of thought. Though the brain remains a connecting station, it is for the behaviourist no more intelligible to say that we think with the brain than that we walk with the spinal cord.[1]

In place of the classical doctrine of the association of ideas, behaviourism substitutes the conception of an ordered series of *motor* responses. The centre of gravity is moved, so to speak, from the cortex to the periphery. The facts pertaining to " mental set " or the " motives " which give direction to the thought process occasion no difficulty. Such mental sets are themselves, in part, a matter of verbal organization which plays its part in the total conditioning, while motives are intraorganic stimuli—" visceral tensions " or other disturbances which may give rise to verbal trial-and-error, just as they set going overt muscular trial-and-error, until some act puts an end to the tension.

As regards experimental evidence for the behaviouristic theory of the process of thinking, many investigations[2] have indeed shown a relation between the movements of the tongue and the thinking process, indicating that in some cases of silent thought the tongue actually traces the form of overt speech. Recent evidence seems to indicate, however, that the identity of form between " uttered " and " thought " syllables is at least very far from universal.[3] The rejoinder of the behaviourists lays stress on variations in muscular tonus too delicate to be observed, and on symbolic movements executed by other parts of the speech-mechanism, or indeed of the whole body.

No less important for behaviourism has been the consistent exclusion of the concept of " ideational " behaviour and of

---

[1] The associationists, from Hartley on, although writing of the " association of ideas," had with few exceptions assumed that the real basis for mental connections lies in brain connections. Behaviourism undertook to get rid not only of " mental " connections, but of emphasis upon the mechanisms of cortical connection.

[2] *E.g.*, Reed, " The Existence and Function of Inner Speech in Thought Processes," *J. Exp. Psychol.*, I, 1916.

[3] Thorson, " The Relation of Tongue-Movements to Internal Speech," *J. Exp. Psychol.*, VIII, 1925.

the claim that animals and men are capable of sudden "insight" into situations in terms other than those of previous learning and the operation of trial-and-error. An emphasis on the genetic method leads the behaviourist always to inquire regarding the organism's previous conditioning. Imitation itself is regarded not as the perception of the utility of duplicating an observed act, but as a type of behaviour which appears only as motor mechanisms have been practised, ineffective acts having been rejected and effective ones gradually selected. As the sparrow *gradually* learns to approximate the song of the canaries with which he is caged, but can, after such learning, copy a trill with sudden and dramatic success,[1] so all imitative conduct is based on the previous mastery of the necessary elements.

The popularity of behaviourism in the United States has been so great that a multitude of experiments, as well as a multitude of theories, are loosely termed "behaviouristic," although little indeed of the behaviourist system may be involved. Behaviourism has become in many quarters simply a name for mechanistic psychology,[2] or has been reduced to a mere *emphasis* upon objective, as opposed to subjective, data. The description of experience known only to the subject, as in dreams, is admitted even by Watson. Indeed, the proportions and significance of the movement would be greatly understated, were we to confine the term to a set of experiments or to the programme of 1914. Accurately or inaccurately, "behaviourism" means to many psychologists simply the biological approach to human personality, through which all its possibilities are to be examined and utilized. It promises that psychology shall one day make itself as objective as physical science, and that all its facts shall be verified in the manner of the physical experiment.

---

[1] Conradi, "Song and Call-notes of English Sparrows when Reared by Canaries," *Am. J. Psychol.*, XVI, 1905.

[2] "To me the essence of behaviourism is the belief that the study of man will reveal nothing except what is adequately describable in the concepts of mechanics and chemistry, and this far outweighs the question of the method by which the study is conducted."—Lashley, "The Behavioristic Interpretation of Consciousness," *Psychol. Rev.*, XXX, 1923. Such quotations might be multiplied indefinitely. For many the term "behaviourism" simply summarizes the whole trend towards "natural-science" psychology, and in particular, the trend away from psycho-physical dualism.

CHAPTER XVII

CHILD PSYCHOLOGY

" CHILD psychology " became a field for systematic research towards the close of the nineteenth century. But its development might well be traced from the Renaissance and the humanistic interest in children. One might note evidences in the sixteenth and seventeenth centuries that the child was coming into his rights as an individual, as something more than an incomplete man or woman. In the seventeenth century Comenius published a picture book *for children*.[1] A trend of considerable significance for the purpose of understanding the origin of child psychology was the educational movement (p. 50) associated with the names of Rousseau and Pestalozzi. Education began to mean the free development of the child's abilities. This was closely related to the apotheosis of all that was " natural," and to the doctrine of *laissez-faire*. Education was to be a means of enabling the child to attain his own latent selfhood and capacities. The first intensive study of the child came in this period, in the biographical observations of childish growth recorded by Tiedemann.[2] Though the educational contributions of Froebel and Herbart intervened, no marked advance in child psychology was made for over fifty years. A few works of importance were written about the middle of the nineteenth century. But it was not until experimental physiology and the evolutionary movement began to bring their forces to bear that child psychology came into its own. Darwin himself made a direct contribution through the publication of a series of observations entitled " A Biographical Sketch of an Infant."[3]   Taine[4] offered a similar sketch.

---

[1] *Mother Goose* was written a little later.
[2] *Beobachtungen über die Entwicklung der Seelenfähigkeiten bei Kindern* (1787). Pestalozzi had kept a three-weeks' record of the behaviour of his little son.
[3] *Mind*, II, 1877.
[4] *Rev. Philos.*, I, 1876.

There appeared in 1881 a much more systematic and important study by the German physiologist, Preyer, under the title *The Mind of the Child*. Preyer made careful observations upon the reflexes present at birth, or at an early age, and on the more and more elaborate forms of behaviour which appeared at successive stages. It was natural enough that his work should take account even of complex psychological phenomena and that it should be regarded as marking out a new field for the experimental psychologist. Just as experimental physiology had led earlier in the century to the experimental study of adult psychology, so in the present instance child psychology arose not from previous psychology but from investigations in its sister science.

Aside from his classical description of the reflex acts with which the child begins its life, perhaps the most engaging of Preyer's observations relates to imitation. He told of eliciting imitative movements in the child by his own frequent repetition of certain acts. For example, he reported that his infant son pouted on observing his father to do so. But we learn that this was only after many repetitions by the father ; the modern reader would be glad to know what repertory was exhibited during the father's previous poutings. The experiment is significant not for Preyer's conclusions, concerning which more recent evidence and interpretation continues to conflict, but in the fact that experimental study was actually under way.

Educational theory and practice were making rapid advances, and in connection with these, child psychology was greatly needed. In Spain, for example, a country in which psychology had made but little progress, a National Museum of Pedagogy was founded (at Madrid) in 1882, while significant work on pedagogy was appearing in the *Boletin de la Institucion Libre de Enseñanza* (1876). But a further stimulus was needed before child study could become an international concern. The spark which made the interest in child psychology kindle into a conflagration was the influence of Hall. The *Pedagogical Seminary*, founded by him in 1891, presented data which, in the spirit of Preyer, went far beyond the practical problems of education, to include child study for its own sake. The questionnaire method, though fraught with sources of error, made possible the rapid accumulation of material which awakened the hope of a systematic understanding of childish emotion, imagination, and thought. In 1893 there came together at the Chicago Exposition a group of persons interested in child study. Many of them were educators, whose chief concern with the psychology of the child lay in its educational implications. Their many aims had as yet been shaped into no clear purpose. But through their conference, and the inspiration which Hall imparted, they acquired a sense of unity and confidence which was destined to give child study and, above all, child psychology, a new impetus.

A movement of international importance directly followed. Two years later, Sully, founder of the new *British Association for Child Study*, published his widely popular *Studies of Childhood*. A similar organization for child study was shortly formed in Paris, and kindred organizations were established in several other cities of France. Binet's studies of the thought processes of his own children (p. 239) were carried out shortly thereafter, and in 1904 he began to devise those intelligence tests (p. 348) for " young children " from which such a vast quantity of research in the psychology of both children and adults has followed. In Germany the movement took more precisely an educational form, in close connection with the school system. Emphasis was placed upon class-room experimentation. One of the leaders was Meumann, whose use of mental tests in the schools[1] stimulated much subsequent research. The child-study movement rapidly spread to the Scandinavian countries, to Belgium and the Netherlands. In Italy the movement found its way already prepared by years of excellent medical and biological study of the child,[2] while in Switzerland, always eminent in educational contributions, the expressly psychological features of the movement were welcomed. In the United States attention was given especially to the study of the learning process and to the measurement of the various attainments of the school child (*e.g.*, spelling, reading, handwriting).

Studies of learning, of practice and fatigue, of the optimum

---

[1] *Zeitschr. f. exp. Pädagog.*, I, 1905. His *Haus- und Schularbeit* (1914) included pioneer studies in the influence of the class-room situation upon the child's capacity for study. See p. 298.

[2] Melzi, de Sanctis, and Ferrari were among the leading spirits in this movement, about the turn of the century. Marro's *La Pubertà* was published in 1897.

conditions for work, and, above all, of individual differences, transformed the nature of the relations between psychology and education. A comparison of Bain's *Education as a Science* (1878), on the one hand, with Claparède's *Experimental Pedagogy* (1905) and Thorndike's *Educational Psychology* (1913–14), shows at a glance the advent of a new discipline, an " educational psychology " the literature of which is too vast for any sort of summary here.

Now to return for a moment to the personal work of Hall. Unfortunately this was of far less value and importance than his work as a stimulus to others—though his volume, *Adolescence* (1904), was for many years a standard. It happened that a contribution through which his work became known was the " recapitulation theory." In the early years of Darwinism, Haeckel had pointed out that the human embryo passes through stages which resemble certain stages through which the race has passed ; such phenomena as the " gill-slits " of the embryo were the basis for Haeckel's " biogenetic law " (1866), the celebrated statement that " ontogeny repeats phylogeny."[1] Darwinian, and, more especially, Spencerian evolutionism had in the same period given rise to numerous theories as to the cultural evolution through which human societies have passed. The two principles were synthesized by Hall : the child passes through a series of stages similar to stages in the life of the group. The little child goes through a hunting period when he catches frogs ; a building period when he makes sand-houses at the seashore ; and so on. This served also as a theory of play ; the child's play is the prosecution of activities belonging to the cultural stage to which his own stage of development corresponds. There was a simple grandeur in all this which appealed to the imagination. The public seized upon the " recapitulation theory " with enthusiasm. The study of the child and the shaping of his life were to be illumined by history ; his progress from infancy to maturity was to be facilitated by offering him constant opportunities to express those impulses which belonged to each succeeding stage in an inevitable cycle. It was Hall's misfortune to be far better known as the sponsor of the recapitulation theory than as the contributor of any other working principle. The

---

[1] The theory has been attenuated by many modifications, but some instances of the principle continue to attract the attention of zoologists.

theory survived as a centre of psychological controversy for many years, and still exerts considerable influence in education. Based, as it was, on faulty anthropology, it could but mislead students of childhood, who have, in fact, failed to find any uniform pattern of stages in the child's interests, except in so far as the child's own physical and intellectual growth and his social surroundings impose them.

In the same years in which the recapitulation theory won its adherents, another theory of play was put forward by Groos.[1] This was in some ways similar to a theory offered by Spencer.[2] Spencer had explained play as an outlet for surplus energy. Groos found value in the notion of energy which could be directed to activities not biologically necessary at the moment. But he maintained that play is also a preparation for life activities ; play is the exercise of tendencies which are later on to be dominant in the struggle for existence. Play is, in fact, gentle rehearsal of those various activities which are to be the central interest of adult individuals. The impulses which are to be all-important for the adult are already present in some form in the young child or animal. This is stated in terms of Darwinian evolution. The offspring which practised these activities would naturally be able to carry them out more effectively, when older, than those which did not practise them. And those species which play would tend to survive in competition with those which do not ; those species are best adapted to their environment whose members get their instinctive equipment into serviceable form before the instincts are needed. This hypothesis, that play is the exercise of instincts prior to their full development, has won much favour.

But more important than any of these theoretical interpretations of childish activity, there began, under the inspiration of the work of Preyer and Hall, a series of careful studies of the development of individual children from birth onwards. What had been boldly suggested by Pestalozzi, Darwin, and others, what had been so appealingly described by Preyer, was now carried out in detail. The first of these careful records of the daily accomplishments of the newborn was that of Shinn[3] (1893), whose observations on the development

---

[1] *The Play of Animals* (1896) ; *The Play of Man* (1899).

[2] *Principles of Psychology*, II, Part IX, Chapter IX.

[3] " Notes on the Development of a Child," *Univ. of California Studies* 1893 ; some of the material was rewritten in popular form and became widely known under the title *The Biography of a Baby* (1900).

of the eye-hand co-ordination are of special interest. This work was immediately followed by that of K. C. Moore,[1] whose study, though following Shinn's method in many respects, contained much new material. She carried it through several years of childhood, thus obtaining a rich store of material on the acquisition of language.

A few years later Stern made further important studies of linguistic development.[2] The vocabulary studies reported by Stern have been followed within recent years by the work of Drever,[3] Descoeudres,[4] and others.[5] The study of language as an index to the thought of the child, undertaken by Stern, has recently received close examination by Piaget,[6] whose records of childish association and reasoning, and of the reveries of childhood, are not only full of absorbingly interesting material, but help greatly towards the classification and quantitative tabulation of childish interests and activities.

In the last decade of the nineteenth century there began also the systematic study of the maladjustments of childhood, for which the neurological and psychiatric studies of Italian " pædologists " had prepared the way. In 1896 Witmer founded in Philadelphia a " Psychological Clinic " for " problem children," *i.e.*, those maladjusted in their emotional life, or of defective intelligence, or otherwise handicapped in their relation to school and family. Medical and psychological studies were combined. As other clinics followed, and as psychiatric methods developed, attention has turned from the immediate physical results of diseases and faulty nutrition to the social and emotional effects of such handicaps, together with conflicts arising in home, school or play relationships. In the analysis of factors contributing to the child's difficulties in fitting into society, increasing use has been made of those testing methods which began with Binet's 1905 scale (p. 349). Such clinics have within recent years become a necessary adjunct to the life of all the larger

---

[1] " The Mental Development of a Child," *Psychol. Rev., Monogr. Suppl.,* I, 1896.

[2] *Ber. ü. d. I. Kong. exp. Psychol.,* 1904.

[3] *E.g.,* " The Vocabulary of a Free Kindergarten Child," *J. Exp. Ped.,* V, 1919.

[4] *Le développement de l'enfant de deux à sept ans* (1922).

[5] The study of the child's early phonetic repertory has been studied by Blanton, " The Behavior of the Human Infant During the First Thirty Days of Life," *Psychol. Rev.,* XXIV, 1917.

[6] *The Language and Thought of the Child* (1923).

American cities, serving the city school systems, the juvenile courts, and the social-service agencies.

The present century, especially in the period since the war, has shown an increasing tendency to abandon easy generalisations about the course of childish growth as a whole, and to insist more and more on the specialized study of specific problems. Not only has the "problem child" in recent years become such a speciality, but investigators devote themselves to the detailed study of specific problems in certain periods, such as the acquisition and elimination of loves and fears.[1] Just as Piaget has sought to find in the child's language a key to the mechanisms of motive and thought which in the adult are so bafflingly complex, so others[2] have explored the emotional behaviour of pre-school children. Another illustration of the same tendency to specialization is the study of children's drawings,[3] in order to determine just what the drawings express and what they mean to the child, and the stages through which the child attains to the conventional adult methods of representation. Other fields recently explored are : children's dreams, children's heroes, imaginary playmates, etc.[4]

Great historical importance attaches to the introduction of many new experimental methods in the study of newborn infants, by J. B. Watson and his collaborators[5] at the Phipps Clinic, Baltimore, beginning in 1917. Watson devoted himself to two problems : first, the repertory of acts found prior to all learning ; and second, the experimental study of the learning process. It is strange that from Preyer's work until 1917 child psychology had been studied for the most part through "observational" methods with no close control. Watson had an opportunity to study the behaviour of infants who remained continuously in the hospital, subject to a daily routine whose details could be almost fully known. He was able in many cases to observe children from birth up to or beyond their two-hundredth day.

First, as regards the experiments upon behaviour at birth

[1] M. C. Jones, "The Elimination of Children's Fears," *J. Exp. Psychol.*, VII, 1924.

[2] L. R. Marston, "Emotions of Young Children," *Univ. of Iowa Studies in Child Welfare*, III, 1925.

[3] Kerschensteiner's important work, *Die Entwicklung der zeichnerischen Begabung*, was published as early as 1905.

[4] See, for example, Kimmins, *Children's Dreams* (1920).

[5] The most important findings are presented in Watson's *Psychology from the Standpoint of a Behaviorist*, 2nd ed. (1924), Chapters 6 and 7.

U

and shortly thereafter. Watson repeated and confirmed Preyer's studies of many of the reflexes present at birth ; the list of reflexes reported by Preyer was, however, amplified. The demonstration of innate orientation of the eyeballs to light is of special interest. Studies were made on the use of the right and the left hand in early infancy ; an instrumental record of the activity of the two hands showed that most infants displayed no distinct preference.

As to the much more complicated problem of the instinctive and emotional make-up of newborn children, Watson undertook to investigate empirically that repertory of innate patterns to which so many speculative studies had given attention. He reported clear-cut reaction-patterns of three main types. These he entitled " fear," " rage," and " love " (the last being defined as roughly equivalent to Freud's term " sex "). The stimuli which produced fear were sudden loud sounds and loss of support ; fear was easily elicited by allowing the child to drop a short distance into the attendant's arms or by pulling at the blanket as he fell asleep. The reaction-pattern included sudden catching of the breath, followed by crying, and in the case of loss of support, clutching movements. In older children, falling to one side or crawling away were observed ; these were not demonstrated to be innate. Rage was elicited by hampering the child's movements. The holding of one arm against the side, or even the pressure of cotton pads about the head (in studies of eye-co-ordination) evoked it. The response consisted of crying, stiffening of the body, slashing or striking movements with the arms, drawing the legs up and down, and holding the breath. The stimuli to love or sex activity were found to consist of stroking or manipulation of the erogenous zones ; rocking, patting, etc. The responses included cooing and gurgling (and the sudden cessation of crying). Sometimes the arms were extended (this was believed by Watson to be the forerunner of the adult embrace). Smiling and laughing were frequent elements in the picture. These three patterns of response could be elicited at or shortly after birth. Watson ventures the hypothesis that there are no other complex reaction-patterns besides these three. (We shall return to the point in Chapter XX.)

Watson's second major contribution was the demonstration of the practicality of altering original nature by the conditioned-response method. He showed experimentally the conditioning of fear responses to stimuli which held no fear for the inexperienced child. He brought before his subjects, children between 100 and 325 days old, several common domestic animals. Not only was no fear evinced ; in many cases the children grasped at the rabbit's ears, at the cat's nose, etc. Then to some of the children animals were presented simultaneously with the loud striking of an iron bar, already found capable of eliciting the fear response. After a few such joint stimulations, the presentation of the animal alone was sufficient to evoke the fear response. Moreover, when a furry animal had thus become an object of fear, furry objects, such as a muff or a fur coat, directly aroused fear ; the response was " transferred " to a similar object.[1] Such conditioning, and the transfer of responses, Watson believes to be the basis for those complex forms of activity which are ordinarily called instincts. Instincts are in reality, he believes, a few primitive patterns with endless conditioned responses built upon them.

Within the last few years the experimental study of young children has gone on apace. These studies have ventured to classify not only innate acts and the time of their first appearance, but the age at which various habits are acquired and the steps through which such acquisition is made possible.[2] The tendency to specialization, already noted, has made possible the intensive study of motor and emotional habits in the first years of life.[3] The present decade is characterized not only by the multiplication of special studies, but by the foundation of numerous institutes intended to foster an integrated scientific attack on the problems of child development. In the meantime the conviction appears to be widespread that it is through such painstaking study of special factors in growth[4] and learning that an understanding of adult personality is to be achieved. Investigation, for example, into the processes by which the child learns, whether learning the alphabet or a standard of conduct, not only throws a flood of light on what he is at a given age,

[1] This sort of "transference" is, of course, the analogue of the traditional "association by similarity."

[2] E.g., M. C. Jones, "The Development of Early Behavior Patterns in Young Children," Ped. Sem., XXXIII, 1926.

[3] E.g., Woolley, "David, a Study of the Experience of a Nursery School in Training a Child adopted from an Institution," Child Welfare League of America, Case Studies, II, 1925.

[4] E.g., Gesell, The Mental Growth of the Pre-school Child (1925).

but shows more clearly the significance of these habits in the structure of the adult personality. The psychiatry of childhood[1] is of special importance here ; for the study of the child's maladjustments, and the processes by which these maladjustments arise, has begun to suggest very strongly that childhood experiences may literally predetermine normality or abnormality in the adult. The age at which various forms of activity appear, their interrelations in possible "types," their organization into an integrated personality, are all being studied by investigators in the field of child psychology.   Yet, important as these problems are for our understanding of the child as a child, they are even more significant for our interpretation of personality as a whole. For example, the "short sample" methods of observing behaviour,[2] which have been developed for use with children, are suggesting new ways of studying adults accurately in normal settings.   Experiments with this technique have demonstrated the possibility of obtaining reliable information on various aspects of personality by a series of detailed objective reports on behaviour during short intervals, usually two to five minutes in length.   Twenty or thirty such "short samples" of activity in the child's normal setting are found to show high reliability and to offer an exceedingly valuable supplement to the case-study.   The work of C. Bühler[3] has shown the possibility of bringing a wide range of significant problems in the formation of personality under experimental control ; differences in domination and submissiveness have been experimentally shown before the age of one year.   For the most part these broader problems of personality differences have not as yet been pursued by techniques of quantitative refinement apparent in studies of children's activity, laughter, and verbal expression.   Thomas and her collaborators[4] have made it clear in their attack on these aspects of behaviour that the beginnings of social response may be studied with the same accuracy that is customary in standard laboratory problems.

---

[1] E.g., Thom, *Habit Clinics for the Child of Pre-school Age* (1924).

[2] Goodenough, "Measuring behaviour traits by means of repeated short samples," *J. Juv. Res.*, XII, 1928 ; Olson, *The Measurement of Nervous Habits in Normal Children* (1929).

[3] *Kindheit und Jugend* (1928).

[4] *Some New Techniques for Studying Social Behaviour* (1929).

CHAPTER XVIII

SOCIAL PSYCHOLOGY AND THE PSYCHOLOGY OF RELIGION

It is evident that the State is a creation of Nature, and that man is by nature a political animal. And he who by nature, and not by mere accident, is without a State, is either above humanity or below it.— *Aristotle.*

THE development of "social psychology" as a distinct discipline began, like that of child psychology, rather suddenly in the 'nineties. We have little that is expressly psychological by way of background ; our background consists chiefly of those developments in anthropology and sociology which we briefly sketched above (p. 130 f.). But the reader will recall that a journal for "folk psychology" had been founded in Germany by Steinthal and Lazarus, in which characteristic differences between human groups were portrayed. Wundt appropriated folk-psychology as a province in which his own psychological principles were applied to data collected from the social sciences (p. 172). Since Wundt's work, this domain of folk-psychology, with special emphasis on the psychological interpretation of the life of primitive groups, has been left chiefly to anthropologists and sociologists.[1] A few whose training has been chiefly or largely psychological have indeed delved into these mines ; in particular, several British psychologists, following the lead of Rivers[2] and C. S. Myers,[3] have made a serious attempt to understand the psychology of primitive peoples in terms borrowed from established psychological principles.[4] But a much larger number of psychologists have been interested chiefly in the activities of more

[1] See, for example, the writings of Sumner and Marett.
[2] Rivers's "Observations on the Senses of the Todas" (*Rep. Brit. Ass. Adv. Sci.*, LXXIV, 1904) was followed by a series of studies in which ethnology and psychology are combined. See especially *The History of Melanesian Society* (1915).
[3] *E.g.*, "A Study of Rhythm in Primitive Music," *Brit. J. Psychol.*, I, 1905.
[4] See, *e.g.*, Bartlett, *Psychology and Primitive Culture* (1923).

advanced peoples, especially those of their own cultural heritage.

Though searching, of course, for psychological principles of universal validity, the attempt to give a psychological description of our own social life has been the chief feature of " social psychology." To be sure, in this field, too, more sociologists than psychologists have laboured ; but a development has occurred which has marked out a field now organically connected with the work of psychology as a separate science. The exploration of this field commenced with the attempt to show the laws by which groups[1] control the conduct of their members, and how individuals within the group act upon one another. As a separate discipline, social psychology began in the writings of Tarde,[2] Sighele,[3] and Le Bon.[4]

Sighele and Le Bon devoted their chief attention to crowd psychology, endeavouring to define the ways in which the behaviour of crowds differs from the behaviour of individuals acting alone. These contributions were largely influenced by the French psychiatric movement, as expressed in the work of Charcot and his successors. Emphasis was laid on pathological phenomena such as the extreme suggestibility of the hysteric. These scholars proceeded from the belief that crowds exhibit a universal and frequently a morbid lack of rationality, being swayed by their leaders' suggestions or by situations that arouse blind and unrestrained impulses. Instead of emphasizing the influence of one person upon another in the normal state, they paid special attention to the phenomena of hypnosis, which they conceived as a condition in which one person is subservient to the will and instruction of another. Much clinical material was available to show how the individual could be reduced to an automaton by virtue of suggestions imposed upon him.

Le Bon applied these concepts to historical material, with especially frequent references to the French Revolution.

---

[1] We cannot here discuss the long and heated controversy as to the existence of a social mind as distinct from individual minds. The controversy, important as it is for *social theory*, does not seem to have contributed to the development of principles for social psychology. (See, however, p. 133, footnote, and p. 307)

[2] *The Laws of Imitation* (1890).

[3] *La Coppia Criminale* (1893)

[4] *The Crowd* (1895).

Group suggestibility was the key to mass-movements, their inception, climax, and decline. A description was given of the general characteristics of crowds, with emphasis upon the fact that by virtue of their heterogeneous make-up they must be held together by ideas of a simple and fairly universal character. This meant that the ideas that govern the crowd put it on a lower intellectual and moral plane than would be set by its highest, or indeed, by its average, member. Le Bon succeeded in painting a brilliantly vivid picture of these crowds which in English we should tend to call mobs ; the picture of collective madness and primitiveness which he outlined has indeed become classical. Its most characteristic feature is the loss of the sense of individuality ; the feeling that one belongs to a group, and derives tremendous, in fact, insuperable, power from affiliation with vast numbers. From this follows the inhibition of whatever is purely individual by all that which the group has in common. The intelligence manifested by the group must be low, as low as that of the lowest member, if all are to understand the goal, and if the mob is to be held together. Under good leadership the mob may be capable of heroic achievement ; but it is all too common to find the crowd morally bankrupt. The part played by the hypnotist in individual psychiatric experience is here played either by the leader, or by the crowd as a whole, as each member responds to the rest. Despite these attempts to formulate laws, Le Bon's book is in general descriptive rather than analytical.

In Tarde's *The Laws of Imitation* a very different purpose is apparent. Tarde attempted a logical analysis of the forms of social interaction, proceeding to the formulation of a series of general and special laws.[1] Unfortunately " imitation," as a central principle to explain the influence of men upon their fellows, was not reduced to any minute analysis. In fact, Tarde's pages are full of material which seems to belong to suggestibility, as Liébeault had defined it, as well as of material describing such deliberate copying of the behaviour of others as displays a rational basis far removed from the automatisms of the hypnotized subject. But we are one step nearer to psychological *analysis* than we are with Le Bon ; a psychological mechanism is postulated by which the

[1] Bagehot had already emphasized the social importance of imitation (*Physics and Politics*, 1869).

group influences the individual, or by which individuals influence one another; and this mechanism is shown at work in a wide range of situations.

A few of Tarde's specific contributions will show the richness of his conception. One of Tarde's laws states that cities serve as models for imitation by outlying regions. Since it is in the cities that social changes are most rapidly effected, they provide a mechanism by means of which the imitation of one another, among country people, may be replaced by an imitation of those changes within the city that constitute the basis of " progress." Tarde's explanation of public opinion and of group decisions is illuminating. It is only when *small groups* of individuals have so modified one another's attitudes as to produce some kind of *unity*, that a basis is formed for understanding, within the social group *as a whole*. Larger and larger groups are formed which possess a relative unity. But wherever individuals and groups are in a state of complete suspense and indecision, there exists not only no basis for unity, but no basis for discussion. Conflict itself is a product of conformities already achieved within groups. In much the same vein is the explanation of invention as an accumulation of imitations. Tarde shows how a conquering nation serves as a pattern for a conquered nation, the latter copying from its military superiors. We find this in ancient India despite the caste system. But there are definite limits within which the principle can work ; in some respects the lower castes are not allowed to copy the higher castes. Another of his laws relates to the copying of the habits of a higher social stratum by a lower, whether the basis of stratification be rank, family, economic success, or what not. Tarde's distinction between custom-imitation and fashion-imitation is also valuable.

The first book to bear the title *Social Psychology* was that of Ross (1908). His system of thought is essentially a continuation of Tarde's work. Ross quotes extensively from Tarde, adding much material to corroborate his teachings. Perhaps the most interesting feature of Ross's work is the abundant reference to current events, such events as happened a month or a year before the time of his writing, and the application of the principles of suggestion and imitation to their explanation. Ross's work, however, contains a penetrating psychological analysis of the mob[1]: the constriction of bodily movements in a dense throng serves to inhibit those individual acts which tend to keep alive individual self-consciousness, so that the immersion of the self in the group is readily effected. Moreover, Tarde's term " imitation " is replaced by a more critical use of the concept of suggestion, special emphasis being placed on verbal and facial expression, rather than on the crude conception of the copying of the acts of others. This doctrine is one of many that spring from Ross's conception of social psychology as a science treating of the influence of the social group upon the individual. Despite Ross's concern with " psychic planes and currents," he frequently thinks in terms of the psychology of individuals in relation to their groups, rather than in terms of social aggregates.

A new epoch begins with McDougall's *Introduction to Social Psychology* (1908).[2] McDougall gives us here an analysis of human nature as a group of instinctive tendencies which he believes to be fundamental to social life. He looks upon the complexity of human nature as a group of distinct innate predispositions, which, though combined and in many ways modified so as to result in quite complicated patterns, continue in all human life to be the mainsprings to action. Each instinct manifests three phases : cognitive, affective, and conative. Man is so constituted that certain stimuli arouse in him first, perceptual patterns, then emotions, and finally strivings from which follow overt acts. This doctrine was in the first place an attack upon the hedonistic tradition which had governed much of British thought during the nineteenth century. McDougall's doctrine reflected Stout's emphasis on *conation*.[3] It was an attempt to show that human action is governed not by the rational search for

---

[1] Much material being drawn from Sidis's *Psychology of Suggestion* (1898). An ingenious attempt to formulate laws governing group suggestibility appears in Ross's " laws of crazes," *e.g.*, " the higher the craze, the sharper the reaction from it " ; " a dynamic society is more craze-ridden than one moving along the ruts of custom."

[2] He tells us explicitly (*The Group Mind*, 1920) that this earlier work was not meant to be a book on social psychology, but an *introduction*, an analysis of human motivation which would make social life intelligible. *The Group Mind* itself was offered as his own " social psychology." The earlier book is, however, of much greater historical importance.

[3] See p. 229.

pleasure and the avoidance of pain, but by primitive urges, such as had been named by Hobbes, Cabanis, Gall, Bain, James, and many others, but had been almost totally neglected by students of man's social life, such as the political economists.

McDougall's theory of instincts will receive attention in Chapter XX ; our concern here is with this radical restatement of the nature of social psychology. Social life is not an entity to be understood in its own descriptive and explanatory terms ; on the contrary, it is rooted in the inborn nature of *individual* human beings, whose interactions involve no laws beyond those of individual psychology. The emphasis on the individual was vastly greater than was that of Ross. Moreover, instead of taking human beings for granted, and dealing with them (as a physicist might) as gross lumps which bump against one another, McDougall presented, so to speak. a chemical analysis of the constituent parts of human nature which are acted upon by social situations.

But something remained to be done. It was not enough to define human impulses ; there must be a description of other mental processes by virtue of which human beings take cognizance of their fellows and respond to stimulation from them. Following, therefore, upon his analysis of instinct, McDougall entered upon a psychological explanation of suggestion, imitation, and sympathy. Suggestion involved the acceptance of a proposition " in the absence of logically adequate grounds." James[1], among others, had already advocated the doctrine of " ideo-motor action "— the notion that the idea of an act is a direct stimulus to the act itself.[2] McDougall also postulated that ideas lead to their fulfilment, provided they are not inhibited. The great suggestibility of a little child is, in fact, gradually reduced as the wealth of experience provides ideas which act as inhibitors ; adult suggestibility is dependent upon relative freedom from the intervention of such inhibitions.[3]

[1] *Principles of Psychology*, II, p. 522.
[2] Thorndike has succeeded in showing (*Educational Psychology*, I. 1913, p. 181f.) that ideas have such a capacity only when the idea and the act have been connected through previous learning. But for McDougall's purposes, *learned* ideo-motor acts meet all the needs of the theory.
[3] As the child grows, he also becomes less " submissive " ; suggestibility is partly dependent upon the attitude of " self-abasement " in which inhibiting ideas are less effective.

But the comparative stability of personality in the face of ever-varying social stimulation requires further explanation. McDougall showed in his chapter on " Volition " that a variety of mechanisms is built up which make each individual a social self. Defining a sentiment[1] as an " organized system of emotional tendencies centred about some object," he suggested that the development through social influences of the " self-regarding " sentiment makes possible the identification of the self with one among a conflicting group of impulses, giving individual life a certain coherence and consistency. Imitation McDougall believed to exist as an unlearned type of response ; the point, however, was not stressed, nor were any important conclusions drawn from it.

McDougall's emphasis on the individual seemed to simplify enormously the problem for social psychology ; and his doctrine of instinct, in particular, enjoyed remarkable popularity. It occurred to psychologists, sociologists, and economists that they could undercut thereby a large part of the difficulty which the complexity of their subject matter imposed. Enthusiasm for the book spread like wildfire.[2] Not only was it largely influential as a text-book, but its conception was copied and extended right and left by both social theorists and educators.[3] The instinct doctrine became the guiding concept for many to whom psychology had been an untrodden field.

In the same decade, another line of development was manifest in the writings of a group of social theorists who placed the centre of gravity for social psychology not in the instinctive life but in the consciousness of *self* and of relations with other selves. We may notice, for instance, in the closing years of the nineteenth century such volumes as Giddings's *Principles of Sociology*, with its emphasis on " consciousness of kind " as the fundamental factor in the integration of social groups. James's description of the development of the " social self "[4] was followed by J. M. Baldwin's elabora-

---

[1] The conception had been developed by Shand, who had begun to write on " Character and the Emotions " as early as 1896 (*Mind*, N S., V.).

[2] It ran through fourteen editions in the first thirteen years.

[3] *E.g.*, Trotter, " *The Instincts of the Herd in Peace and War* (1916) ; Veblen, *The Instinct of Workmanship* (1914) ; Tead, *Instincts in Industry* (1918).

[4] *Op. cit.*, I, p. 293.

tion of the stages in selfhood[1] which result from the interaction of the individual and his fellows; our selfhood is essentially social. The organic unity of self-consciousness and our knowledge of other selves was also emphasized by Cooley,[2] all of whose work may be regarded as a protest against the notion of a sharp antithesis between the individual and society. Cooley's work borrows much from the teachings of Dewey and American functional psychology. He makes individual human nature essentially a product of its social environment. Moreover, the social environment of each individual may be subdivided into a " primary " group and a " secondary " group. The primary group consists of all those persons with whom any given individual makes continued personal contact. This group, rather than society at large, is the basis of the social self, as well as of its most important ideas, preferences, and opinions. Even intelligence itself Cooley regards as conditioned to a certain extent upon the mental habits of one's primary group.

Other important contributions to social psychology were in the meantime coming from authors who have emphasized the influence of economic,[3] climatic,[4] and geographical[5] influences on the life of social groups. Social psychologists have been forced, frequently with reluctance, to recognize that the " laws " of social psychology are to an extraordinary degree set by such climatic and economic factors; that man reacts upon his physical environment while reacting to his fellows, and that really significant social psychology must be organically related to the materials of all the social sciences. An interesting approach appears, for example, in Veblen's *Theory of the Leisure Class* (1899), in which we are given an economic interpretation of a variety of social attitudes. Historically, groups free from the drudgery of labour have enjoyed a sort of prestige which is fundamental to their own mental outlook, the " complacency with which they may legitimately be contemplated by themselves and by others " (p. 34); the fundamental facts of priesthood, war, and later,

[1] *Mental Development in the Child and the Race* (1895; see especially 3rd edition, 1906); *The Individual and Society* (1911).
[2] *Human Nature and the Social Order* (1902); *Social Organization, A Study of the Larger Mind* (1909).
[3] *E.g.*, J. L. and B. Hammond, *The Town Labourer* (1917).
[4] *E.g.*, Huntington, *Civilization and Climate* (1915).
[5] *E.g.*, Teggart, *The Processes of History* (1918).

mercantilism are at the root of social differentiations which no purely psychological analysis could ever disclose. Similarly, Sumner's *Folkways* (1907) made economic factors all-important in the origin of customs, and of the entire range of social ideals upon which religion, ethics, and law depend. In general, we may contrast such " sociological " interpretations of society with those " biological " interpretations which lay chief stress upon the inherited nature of individuals.

Social psychology was also greatly enriched during the first decade of the century by new material relating to the psychological origin of ethical codes. In particular, Westermarck's *Origin and Development of the Moral Ideas* (1906-8) offered a vast array of data on the ethical systems of primitive and advanced cultures, centring in the conception that " right " and " wrong " acts are so classified because of human tendencies to approve or disapprove, while these tendencies in turn depend on the gratification or misery which an individual's acts bring to his fellows. When society recognizes the general helpfulness or harmfulness of various courses of action, these acts come in time to be codified as right or wrong, or indeed as legal or illegal. Ethical judgments had, of course, been placed on a purely psychological basis long before (Hobbes, for example, was one of many who had offered such interpretations), but Westermarck's mass of material gave such a psychological interpretation a foundation which at last compelled general acceptance.[1]

A serious attempt has been made, within the past few years, to bring together material from history, anthropology, geography, and economics, in direct relation to distinctly psychological principles, so as to formulate a social psychology in which the laws of individual behaviour are seen in relation to their complex cultural settings.[2] Znaniecki's *The Laws of Social Psychology* (1925), for example, proceeds from this point of view.

Recent years have witnessed also a rapidly growing

---

[1] Not, of course, that the exact nature of the psychological factors is universally accepted as Westermarck stated them.

[2] " Social Psychology must take into account not only these mechanisms—the how we think, feel and act—but must deal with the content of mind and act—with *what* we think, feel and act, as well."—K. Young, in Barnes *et al.*, *The History and Prospects of the Social Sciences* (1925), p. 201–2.

disinclination to use "instinct" as a fundamental concept for social behaviour. On the one hand, emphasis has been placed on the plasticity of human nature, and the necessity of giving closer attention to the influence of those early environmental factors, especially social, which give the individual his ideas, his attitudes, and his governing "habits"; on this point the views of Dewey and Cooley seem to be winning almost universal acceptance. Even when fundamental impulses are emphasized, as in the writings of Thomas[1] and Dunlap,[2] these are seen not as explanations of specific modes of conduct, but simply as raw materials which are only fashioned into social conduct through a great number of mechanisms of social control. McDougall himself, to whom the "instinct" vogue was so largely due, has repeatedly insisted that instincts may be almost indefinitely modified, both in respect to the stimuli arousing them and in respect to the acts to which they lead, their emotional core alone remaining clearly recognizable. Together with this widespread movement has come a renewed interest in the mechanism of personality itself, and (again reflecting the influence of Baldwin, Dewey, and Cooley) a desire to work out the principles by which the socialized "self" develops.

Probably the most striking event in contemporary social psychology is the introduction of experimental method. The pioneer work in this field may be divided into three heads. The first is the study of the influence of groups on individual behaviour. Early in the present century, attempts[3] were made to compare work done alone with work done in the presence of one or more companions; German educators in particular pursued the problem for the sake of defining the value of "home-work" as contrasted with "school-work" (p. 281). In 1914, Moede[4] began a series of vitally interesting experiments on the influence of social groups in accelerating or retarding the speed of individual activity, and in increasing or decreasing the vigour of muscular work. One of the most important of his findings related to the influence of rivalry in decreasing the speed of fast workers and increasing the

[1] Stated as early as 1917 : Jennings, Watson, Meyer, and Thomas, *Suggestions of Modern Science Concerning Education.*
[2] " Foundations of Social Psychology," *Psychol. Rev.*, XXX, 1923.
[3] *E.g.*, Mayer, *Arch. f. d. ges. Psychol.*, I, 1903 ; Schmidt, *Sammlung v. Abh. z. psychol. Pädagogie* I, 1904.
[4] *Zeitschr. f. pädag. Psychol.*, XV, 1914.

speed of slow workers. He measured also the influence of competition between groups ; membership on a team drew forth a greater expenditure of energy than had been elicited in solitary work or in competition with a single opponent.

F. H. Allport[1] has made a series of such studies on the influence of the group upon association, judgment, attention, etc. His results point to the influence of the group in accelerating the speed of work. A series of judgments as to the pleasantness or unpleasantness of odours was also made by subjects who in some cases worked alone and in others together. While working together, the extremes of pleasantness and unpleasantness were much less frequently reported ; this was interpreted as an aspect of the tendency of social groups to bring individual judgments more or less into conformity with the group level. Equally interesting is the experiment of H. T. Moore on " The Comparative Influence of Majority and Expert Opinion on Individual Judgments."[2] In matters of linguistic usage, ethics, and musical agreeableness, individual judgment was shown to be profoundly altered when the individual was informed of the majority opinions ; the influence of expert opinion was also striking.

A second field of inquiry to which much attention is being given is the measurement of personality traits, with special reference to traits which are important for social contacts. Such measurements, though occupying a large place in contemporary writings on social psychology, may be more adequately discussed in relation to the measurement of emotion in Chapter XXII.

A third field comprises the attempts to measure such phenomena as public opinion. Within the last few years studies have been made of such attitudes as " liberalism " and " conservatism." Typical of such work is Neumann's' survey of the attitudes of American high-school students on many national and international issues. A definite conviction of the superiority of American institutions over those of other nations was found to be accompanied by general

---

[1] *E.g.,* " The Influence of the Group upon Association and Thought," *J. Exp. Psychol.,* III, 1920.
[2] *Am. J. Psychol.,* XXXII, 1921.
[3] *A Study of International Attitudes of High School Students,* etc. (1926).

unwillingness to see American institutions imposed upon other nations, and by strong dislike of secret diplomacy. F. H. Allport and D. A. Hartman[1] have shown that variation from extreme conservative to extreme radical views permits of many gradations, the majority of subjects taking more or less a " middle ground." They found also that those whose opinions were decidedly atypical were more confident of their opinions than were those in the middle of the distribution ; and suggested that personality factors known to the psychiatrist under such captions as " compensation " are of deep significance. Allport's *Social Psychology* (1924), and his more recent publications, indicate nothing less than a determination to envisage the entire field of social psychology in terms familiar to the experimental psychologist and the psychiatrist, and capable ultimately of constituting an exact experimental science. The same conception, and a wealth of experimental data, are offered in the " collective reflexology " of Bekhterev.[2] His experiments on the differences between individuals thinking alone and individuals thinking co-operatively on a common task are of special interest. The territory shared by social psychology and political science has been successfully invaded by Rice,[3] who has shown the possibility of analysing statistically many of the phenomena of public opinion, such as the diffusion of political sentiment from one region to another, and the part played by commercial centres in facilitating such diffusion.

The closing years of the nineteenth century witnessed also the beginning of more systematic attempts to analyse empirically the psychological principles underlying religious experiences and practices.

The anthropological approach to religion in the hands of German and British students had already yielded promising results (see p. 130). Tylor's " animism " had proved an especially helpful concept, together with his emphasis upon dreams as experiences which cause primitive man to conceive the soul as an entity apart from the body.

In the 'nineties an extensive revision of Tylor's animism

[1] " The Measurement and Motivation of Atypical Opinion in a Certain Group," *Am. Pol. Sci. Rev.*, XIX, 1925.
[2] *E.g.*, *Zeitschr. f. ang. Psychol.*, XXIV, 1924.
[3] *Quantitative Methods in Politics* (1928).

was suggested by a work which did not pretend to be based on wide empirical observation, but on a single culture. Codrington[1] found among the Melanesians that instead of the personalizing tendency there exists the tendency to think of a vaguely defined power which belongs to gods, to spirits, or even to living men or objects with which they come in contact. The character of such power cannot be described in our language as either " personal " or " impersonal." This power—" mana "—may be helpful or harmful to humankind ; contact with it means so much for human welfare that ceremonials and taboos have arisen to make man's relations with it free from danger, or blest through its aid. It is a notion not unlike that which attends our own superstitious belief in charms or amulets ; " mana " is, however, almost a substance, and, though of vaguely spiritual origin, may directly impart fertility to a garden or deadliness to a weapon. We have here something quite different from strict animism. The religion of the Melanesians has been found to have an analogue in other cultures, and it may well be that no *sharp* distinction exists between animistic and mana-istic attitudes ; where thinking is so indefinite, the tendency to think of a stone as somehow personal is in some cases not far removed from thinking of it as filled with a dread power. The mana concept has made wide conquests, sometimes modifying the theory of animism and sometimes attaching itself to that theory.

But we must turn to another movement which began in the same decade. The intensive study of *individual religious experience* began with Stanley Hall's studies of childhood (see p. 280), in which he included a large quantity of material on the religious experiences of children. He made studies, for example, of the child's idea of God, his notions of right and wrong, the experience of change of heart or conversion. These studies were conducted largely by the questionnaire method, and necessarily failed to ascertain the exact nature of the environmental forces at work.

In the last few years of the century Starbuck brought together a celebrated collection of manuscripts contributed by a host of individuals who recounted the history of their

---

[1] *The Melanesians* (1891). The systematic interpretation and clarification of the concept is largely the work of Marett (*e.g.*, *The Threshold of Religion*, 1909).

X

own religious experiences.[1]   The experiences were especially full of the sense of sin, the necessity for conversion, the process of unification of the soul with God.   This collection of manuscripts constitutes, both in its extent and in the detail of its report, a much more serious contribution than Hall's ; in fact, it meant the first great inductive approach to religious experience.   Starbuck's chief use of the manuscripts[2] was in relation to the problem of religious conversion. He noted the great frequency of cases in which a struggle among discordant elements in personality had been resolved by means of sudden emphasis upon concepts and values which, through satisfying deep needs, gave the individual new unity and stability.   It was shown by Starbuck[3] that there is a " critical period " for the struggle of the self in its attempt to make its adjustment to the forces of the universe.   This " critical period " lies in the " teens " ; that is, in adolescence. A graph was worked out showing the relative frequency of conversion experiences at different ages.   They appear rarely before thirteen ; from year to year they become more frequent, the peak being attained at about sixteen ; thereafter they decline, so that very few occur after twenty.   Some purely social factors are to be considered, but there are important biological factors, especially the sexual and other emotional tensions and the abundant energy which plays its part in the widening of interests.   This " storm and stress " period in the life of the individual leads him toward forces which he believes to be ultimate ; and he seeks the resolution of his conflicts through an adjustment, the pattern of which is set by his environment.

This intensive study of the psychology of conversion formed a large part of the groundwork upon which James developed his lectures on *The Varieties of Religious Experience* (1902). James not only made extensive use of the manuscripts collected by Starbuck, but went through much historical material on religious experience, particularly records of the lives of great mystics and religious leaders.

---

[1] Many of the manuscripts were written with a personal directness and earnestness which reminds one of Richard Jeffries's *The Story of My Heart*. A large proportion of these experiences were so intense as to provoke the question whether they were indeed typical of everyday religion.

[2] *The Psychology of Religion* (1899).

[3] And shortly thereafter confirmed by Coe (*The Spiritual Life*, 1900).

He opened his discussion with a consideration of the relation of the morbid to the religious. He took serious account of the work of authors who had emphasized the frequency of mental abnormality among religious leaders ; but he insisted that the question of mental instability throws no light upon the *value* of experience—the existential approach to religion leaves entirely open the question of its significance.[1] George Fox's evident abnormality, as a problem in psychology, has nothing to teach us regarding the beauty and power of his message. The intense and dynamic, though ill-balanced person may be a genuine leader, and in a field where emotion is such a vital factor, disintegration may alternate with significant achievement. The achievement may be worth more than the cost of the neuropathic signs that come with it. There is, however, a deeper significance in this relation of religion to psychopathology. James was concerned to show that our whole system of values in regard to social experiences has been woefully narrow ; that if we are going to understand civilization at all, we must stop the uncritical use of the terms " normal " and " abnormal," and abandon the tendency to fling aside things that do not harmonize with smooth, easy-rolling, everyday experience. He kept recurring to this protest against the habit of making stability of mind the criterion of social worth.

James outlined two fundamental types of religious experience. The first is the religion of " healthy-mindedness," in which the world is taken as a joyful place to live in, with the conviction that all that appears evil is incidental or irrelevant in the face of fundamental goodness, summed up in the words : " God's in His heaven, all's right with the world." This religion of healthy-mindedness is one that does not understand why people should be pessimistic ; it is in accord with the widespread nineteenth-century movement of mental healing through belief in the *unreality of sickness*.[2] He

[1] He was frankly and deeply interested, for example, in the use of drugs in inducing mystical states ; the physical factors did not for him involve the exclusion of the claims of mysticism.

[2] James appears to have appraised the strength of the movement more justly than his contemporaries ; witness the extraordinary wealth in recent years of popular psychology which " radiates sunshine," and the conviction that health is to be had for the asking. The vogue of the New Nancy movement (p. 144, Coué) seems largely attributable to the same source. The urge for a " healthy-minded " denial of the existence of evil has, to be sure, spread far beyond the limits of religion

expressed little respect for this attitude, believing that it involved direct rejection of undeniably real and omnipresent misery and anguish. " Civilization is founded on the shambles " (p. 163). If we refuse to recognize this fact, we blind ourselves to deep and terrible realities.

In contrast with healthy-mindedness is the religion of the " sick soul." The personal narratives of disillusionment and despair which he quotes remind one of those insanities in which the individual feels that something is fundamentally wrong with the world itself, and finds it full of suffering and misery. This view, James urges, is more complete than that of the healthy-minded ; it faces the whole of life and finds a need for some kind of conquest of evil, or some reconciliation in which evil can, through a new way of life, be made to contribute to the good. Some see conflict first between various parts of the world they experience. They are unable to understand why the same universe creates both kindness and bitterness. But the struggle to understand the universe involves also the problem of the relation of the individual himself to the world. The individual finds himself striving towards the attainment of happiness, or the happiness of his fellows ; yet he commits acts which cause distress to himself or to those whom he loves. He finds himself in a tortured relation both with his world and with his own nature. Wherever the self conceives the powers controlling the universe in personal terms, the evil within one's individual nature is felt to be a violation of one's relation with the universe ; sin inflicts suffering upon God Himself. The conflict within the self must somehow be resolved. The soul feels itself torn into two parts, and must be integrated. It tries in vain to find satisfaction in " the senses." This leads to a crisis, and this crisis necessarily takes the form of a struggle involving the ejection of some parts of the personality from the realm of consciousness.[1] Suddenly a solution is

as such ; methods which in the nineteenth century were largely tinged with religious colouring have in recent years become a method of " strengthening one's will, " or making one's personality "magnetic" with a view to practical success.

[1] The concept of the subconscious had been so widely heralded by Carpenter, von Hartmann, Janet, F. W. H. Myers, and James's own earlier writings that the assumption that disturbing tendencies were forced into the subconscious was a matter of course, leading, in fact, to no significant adverse criticisms. Singularly enough, no reference was made to the Freudian psychology.

reached through which the individual identifies himself with what he feels to be good, abandoning his interest in all those dominating satisfactions which appear to be in conflict with his new purpose. Conversion represents a transformation of the self, in which petty aims are subordinated ; in other words, the subconscious powerfully assists conscious strivings toward the transformation. Conversion, therefore, is the unification of the self through absorption in one group of ideals which evoke such profound devotion that conflicting forces lose their potency.

The last third of *The Varieties of Religious Experience* is devoted to a study of mysticism. James regarded mysticism as that form of experience in which we come into contact with elements in the universe which we cannot grasp through sensory or intellectual processes ; as James puts it, a window into an invisible world, a way of seeing into realities which are ordinarily hidden. After describing several aspects of mystic experience—such as the fact that to the mystic it is ineffable, and that it takes on the character of complete and absolute reality—he comes to two generalizations as to the content of these states. First, mystic experiences are regularly optimistic, not in the care-free manner of the healthy-minded, but through the *conquest* of despair ; they reveal the universe as ultimately good. Secondly, they give a picture of harmony ; they represent the world as *unified*. To be sure, James goes on in characteristic fashion to give exceptions, describing the mysticism of despair and conflict. But this typical optimism and sense of harmony are for him crucial in determining both the claims of mysticism to validity and the significance of mysticism for the world of values. These aspects of mysticism serve to show that, notwithstanding the multitude of religious backgrounds from which mysticism arises, mystics do nevertheless seize upon something which is more than the product of time and place. Moreover, they achieve for the individual a sense of grasping the meaning of the whole universe, and hence an authority which is absolute. James went the whole way in maintaining that the mystic experience is a genuine, valid way of getting into touch with aspects of the world that one cannot apprehend through reason. But though the authority of the experience is absolute for the individual, and though full sympathy may be extended to those who live with such a faith, James regards such experiences, by virtue of their very ineffability, as authoritative only for those to whom they directly come.

James's *Varieties*, partly because of his immense prestige, and partly through the earnestness, sympathy, and literary brilliance of the presentation, served to widen enormously the circle of readers within that new field which Starbuck had outlined. It aroused intense interest among students of religion, and served for years as the basis of discussion in religious psychology. Psychologists, educators, and biographers worked over James's material in the conviction that the phenomena of religion had at last become a subdivision of psychological science.

During the first decade of the present century the emphasis upon the individual began nevertheless to give way to a fuller recognition of the social aspects of religion, especially the part played by religion in the expression of social values. An important figure in this shift of emphasis was King. " The social group may be said to furnish the matrix from which are differentiated all permanent notions of value, and these are primarily conscious attitudes aroused in connection with activities which mediate problems more or less important for the perpetuation of the social body."[1] Similarly, in Ames's *Psychology of Religious Experience* (1910) the social rather than the individual aspects of religious life were emphasized. With Ames, religion is the sense of the " highest social values." But religion is defined in the terms of the functional psychology, with emphasis on genetic and comparative material. Religion consists of beliefs, practices, and regulations which make possible the attainment of certain social values ; it is, therefore, largely ethical. Ames discusses, for example, the changing conception of God which occurred generation after generation among the Jews, relating it to economic factors and to the diffusion of culture. The tribal god had been, in this and in other cultures, Ames believes, a personalized representation of that on which the tribe subsisted ; the transition from a bull-god to an anthropomorphic deity was effected through a widening of the values which the group hoped to obtain through worship. Later, the anthropomorphic God became even the God of all humanity, or the

---

[1] *The Development of Religion* (1910), p. 84.

Spirit of the Universe. Ames's material is essentially psychological, although the data are drawn from anthropology and history.[1] He was the first to utilize on a large scale such anthropological material in the formulation of psychological principles which would prove of general validity.[2] Magic, custom, and taboo were treated in the same spirit. Especially suggestive was his use of the conception (though not the name) of the conditioned response as the basis for the origin of magic and taboo. " Among the Malays, those who work in the mines are required to wear special clothing and speak a particular language, as those who first worked in them. Success in securing the ore is apparently as dependent upon the use of the ancient coat and speech as upon skill and labor."[3] Ames insisted that the nineteenth-century explanation of such customs through the " association of ideas " was both cumbersome and inaccurate.[4] Habits are in large measure established, he believed, through a simple, almost a mechanical, attachment of responses, by analogy, to new situations.

Emphasis upon the essentially social nature of religion has, however, been carried much further by Durkheim,[5] who on the basis of a study of Australian religion concludes that individual experience offers no adequate clue to the understanding of religious phenomena. Religion is a special form of emotional and valuational experience which *groups*, in the interests of collective ceremonial, instil ; he postulated, in fact, a *collective* religious consciousness. Lévy-Bruhl[6] has been influenced in this direction, though his chief contribution is probably his emphasis upon the " pre-logical," mystical thinking of primitive peoples.

[1] The work of other scholars had, of course, already clarified the historical situation ; Ames's contribution lay precisely in subjecting historical material to a systematic psychological analysis.

[2] Systematic inductive studies of our own contemporary religious life (such as are attempted in journals of religion) have not as yet yielded psychological *principles* comparable in clarity with those contributed by the anthropologists. Field studies such as F. M. Davenport's *Primitive Traits in Religious Revivals* (1905) are, of course, valuable, but most of the phenomena of contemporary European and American religious psychology have been very inadequately studied.

[3] Summarized by Ames from W. W. Skeat's *Malay Magic*, p. 253 f.

[4] The brilliant theories of Frazer (*The Golden Bough*, 1890 and later) cling to explanations of religious behaviour in terms of " association by contiguity " and " association by similarity."

[5] *The Elementary Forms of the Religious Life* (1912).

[6] *E.g.*, *Primitive Mentality* (1923).

Ames's highly suggestive list of concepts from individual psychology, in the interpretation of group religious phenomena, was followed in a few years by several works which sought to bring together, and to show in their mutual relations, biographical material on individual religious experience and anthropological data on religious practices. Leuba, who had already attracted attention as a student of individual religious life,[1] offered such a synthesis in *A Psychological Study of Religion* (1912). The content of the mystic experience is given, he held, by suggestion, just as the content of the hypnotic experience is suggested either by others or by the subject himself.[2] Another contribution of Leuba is a statistical study of the *Belief in God and Immortality* (1916) prevailing in American society. His conclusions, based on extensive questionnaire material, are to the effect that, in general, students in the last two years of college believe in a personal God[3] and in immortality to a lesser extent than those who are doing their first two years' work ; while professors in universities have less belief in God and immortality than students have. Leuba relates his data to an extensive study of the history of these beliefs, and presents his questionnaire material as part of the evidence for his view that the prevalence of these beliefs is declining. The work is especially interesting because of its attempt to subject religious phenomena to quantitative treatment, as well as because of its use of historical material in its relation to material capable of immediate empirical analysis.

Coe[4] devotes much energy to dispelling the conception of religion as an independent group of functions. Religion arises in " social immediacy " rather than in reason, and belief in superhuman persons involves no special mystery. The child's belief in God arises exactly as does his belief in human

[1] Through his *Studies in the Psychology of Religious Phenomena* (1896) and other contributions.

[2] Special attention was given to mysticism, which was extensively described in terms of the physiological background and the evidence for a thoroughgoing naturalistic explanation of the phenomena. The view is more fully stated and defended in his *Psychology of Religious Mysticism* (1925).

[3] The term " personal God " was defined, in different questionnaires, in two slightly different ways. The second, apparently preferable, definition is indicated in the words " I believe in a God to whom one may pray in the expectation of receiving an answer. By answer I mean more than the subjective psychological effect of prayer."

[4] *Psychology of Religion* (1916).

beings he has never seen. Coe adheres to Leuba's view that religious experience is conditioned by the social group. The content of mystical experience is conditioned by the expectation of the individual ; that is, it results from suggestion. He lays emphasis also upon physical disorders which produce a state favourable to mysticism, and concludes that religious mysticism has no unique quality which differentiates it from aberrant emotionalism found elsewhere ; and he questions James's contention as to the value of such states, noting in fact the frequency with which they fail to produce anything of consequence in the way of socially constructive endeavour. Having laid the setting for religion in group life, and in the interaction of persons rather than in the experience of " individual men in their solitude " (as had James), it is easy for Coe to complete that integration of anthropological with contemporary " personal " material which had been so urgently demanded. It is only in the hands of Coe that the mana concept has been fully utilized in connection with material from psychology proper. The mana concept is related to mystical attitudes induced by the group ; the semi-personal character of mana is related to social immediacy itself. Another doctrine drawn from contemporary psychology is that of the " attitude " as developed by the American " functional " school. Attitudes, as motor adjustments, play a large part in giving meaning to events which primitive man cannot clearly understand ; and the mana concept is explicable in terms of emotional attitudes induced by group contact with mysterious powers whose influence is fraught with social consequences.

Another recent study which has drawn its materials from a wealth of historical and anthropological sources, with equal interest in individual and group religion, is the work of Pratt.[1] The book is particularly rich in materials indicating the co-operation, and at times the conflict, between tradition and mysticism ; and the values of mysticism are found to depend not so much on their general origin as on their specific forms and content.

Finally, despite the huge difficulties involved, Girgensohn[2] and his pupils have undertaken an *experimental* analysis of religious consciousness, with special emphasis on its affective character.

[1] *The Religious Consciousness* (1920).
[2] *E.g., Ber. ü.d. VIII. Kong. f. exp. Psychol.*, 1924.

CHAPTER XIX

PSYCHOANALYSIS

Well-educated physicians, at any rate, say that we should pay close attention to dreams . . . . The most skilful interpreter of dreams is he who can discern resemblances . . . . As the picture in the water, so the dream can be similarly distorted.—*Aristotle*.

WE must now retrace our steps to the decade of the 'eighties; for we have to discuss a vast development which must be surveyed as a unit. Indeed, the life of the founder and presiding genius of psychoanalysis has meant the continuous evolution of doctrines which are best understood in their biographic setting.

Sigmund Freud, a young Viennese physician, was occupying himself in the late 'seventies with such orthodox medical investigations as the embryology of the nervous system. He made contact with an older man, Breuer, who was engaged in the study of hysteria and kindred complaints. Hysteria was, at that time, treated by many physicians according to the methods which had been so ably demonstrated by Charcot; the use of hypnotic suggestion was of paramount importance. Freud became acquainted with the use of hypnosis as a technique for the removal of such hysterical symptoms as functional paralysis, anæsthesia, and amnesia.

In 1880, there came to the attention of Breuer a case of hysteria the study of which aroused questions in Freud's mind, the solution of which contained the kernel of a new system of treatment, and indeed a new system of psychology. A prominent symptom of the patient, a girl of twenty-one, was a violent repugnance to the act of drinking from a glass of water.[1] There was no evident reason, nothing in her background which she could report, to throw light on this strange aversion. The case was handled through hypnotic suggestion. While in a deep sleep-like state and under the

[1] This was but one symptom in a complicated case. See Freud's account in his Clark University lecture, " The Origin and Development of Psychoanalysis " (1909), *Am. J. Psychol.*, XXI, 1910.

influence of suggestion, she was led to a recollection of the event from which her difficulty had arisen. It was the fact that she had seen a pet dog drink from a glass, an incident which disgusted her so violently that she feared she would display her disgust in the presence of the dog's owner. She inhibited or " suppressed " her disgust, and the total experience was forced out of consciousness, so that until the time of the hypnotic treatment she had been unable to analyse the trouble. This case brought into brilliant light the possibility that an experience, though ejected from consciousness, might continue to play an important part in conduct.

Shortly thereafter Freud went to study with Charcot at Paris. Charcot had a clear-cut theory of hysteria, according to which the hysterical crisis and the hypnotic trance constituted the same alteration of personality ; much, therefore, of the clinical material which Freud witnessed was so presented as to suggest that hypnotic treatment bore an intimate and necessary relation to the understanding of hysteria. He had great admiration for Charcot, and was willing for years to proceed in accordance with the master's method. But Charcot made a singular remark one day that left an indelible impression on Freud's mind. A pupil had asked the master why a particular set of symptoms appeared in a particular case ; and Charcot replied, with animation, that such cases always had a sexual basis. And he repeated with emphasis, " Always, always, always ! " " Yes, but if he knows this," said Freud to himself, " why does he never say so ? " Freud states that Breuer, and the gynecologist Chrobak, had made remarks expressing the same belief in the importance of sexuality for nervous disorder ; and that when reminded of these remarks, they denied making them.[1]

Freud returned to his practice in Vienna and collaborated further with Breuer.[2] The use of hypnosis continued for several years to be a part of their method. They found indeed that they could by this means detect conflicting forces which had been present in personality, and had been forgotten through suppression. They could lead back, by suggestion,

---

[1] " History of the Psychoanalytic Movement," *Psychoanalytic Rev.* III, 1916, p. 406 f. In many of Freud's early publications, cases were presented in expurgated form.

[2] Freud also studied with Bernheim at Nancy, and was much impressed with the latter's studies of post-hypnotic amnesia.

to the recovery of these factors. They found that some
apparent cures could be effected in this way, in the sense
that the symptoms could be dissipated. But they discovered
a serious difficulty arising in the use of the hypnotic method.
At first the symptoms would disappear, but a little later
other symptoms would show themselves. A paralysis might
be dissipated, but six months later an anæsthesia or amnesia
might appear. Hysteria could not be permanently cured
through hypnotic methods. Instead of getting at the core
of the trouble, they merely dispelled its manifestations.

Breuer and Freud hit upon the device of allowing their
patients, while in a normal waking state, to talk freely about
anything that entered their minds, permitting their associations to lead back gradually to the sources of the difficulty.
This led the patients in some cases to become emotionally
absorbed in the physician (" transference "), a fact which
Breuer felt necessitated abandonment of the method.
Freud's insistence on continuing the " talking-out method,"
together with his growing conviction that sexuality was of
the most vital importance for hysteria, led to a parting of
the ways between Freud and Breuer. The two men maintained mutual respect, but it was impossible for them to
remain in close association because of their opinions on these
points.

Freud proceeded to develop this new method. He told
the patient simply to attempt an honest narrative of his free
associations ; the origin of his symptoms would gradually
become clear. To be sure, this necessitated the consecutive
overcoming of " resistances," at points where the patient
said that he could not think of anything more, or that he was
thinking of something ugly which he hated to mention. At
these points there seemed to be not so much a genuine failure
of memory, through time, as an effect of the same mechanism
which had been involved in the suppression, namely, a
resistance against the free expression of a particular emotive
tendency. Freud learned by experience that resistances
were vitally important, and that it was at these very points
that something illuminating could, through the patient's
perseverance in the task, be disclosed. Resistances were
especially evident where associations of a sexual nature
appeared. The " psychoanalytic " method was this use of
free association ; with this method, psychoanalysis as such

began.   Through the patient's gradual recall of the emotional
episodes which had precipitated the conflict, and, in
particular, through the free recognition and release[1] of
pent-up emotion, the struggle could sometimes be terminated
and the patient's mental health restored.   More adequate
co-operation was secured than was possible through hypnosis,
for instead of dealing with a passive subject (and all hypnotic
subjects who merely follow the suggestion of the hypnotizer
are passive), he had the patient's active assistance towards
revealing the deeply submerged tendencies in personality.[2]

At this period (the last decade of the century) Freud had
not succeeded very far in relating specific types of symptoms
to specific types of emotional conflict ; nor had he any clear
notion as to the period in life at which such psychopathic
dispositions were at first formed.   There was no reason to
suppose that they necessarily involved anything more remote
than emotional experiences such as were apparent in cases
like that of the girl unable to drink from a glass of water.   He
was not as yet concerned to show an earlier origin, some
predisposing cause, for such manifestations in the life of the
patient.   But the cure of a symptom was sometimes followed
by new symptoms, and it became necessary to penetrate
deeper, *i.e.*, to go farther and farther back into the patient's
personal history.   Adult experience seemed to call for
emphasis upon the importance of childhood conflicts as basic
for adult maladjustment.

Freud did, moreover, encounter many psychoneuroses in
children.   A boy, for example, was afflicted by a strange
compulsion ; before he could go to sleep he had to arrange a
row of chairs beside his bed, pile pillows upon them, and turn
his face towards the wall.[3]   The study of the case showed that
he had been the victim of a sexual assault which had so
terrified him that ever afterwards a barricade must be placed
between the bed and the open room, and his face averted.

---

[1] *Abreaktion*, a part of the " cathartic method " already developed by
Breuer and Freud in conjunction with hypnotic technique.
[2] Such spatial and mechanical metaphors are prominent throughout
the history of psychoanalysis.   James, in discussing closely similar
material, said " in the end we fall back on the hackneyed symbolism
of a mechanical equilibrium " (*Varieties of Religious Experience*,
p. 197).   The metaphors were surely helpful at first; but with time their
value has been more and more seriously challenged.
[3] *Collected Papers* (1924), I, " Further Remarks on the Defence
Neuro-Psychoses " (*Neurolog. Zentralbl.*, 1896).

Thus the symptoms were *symbols* of the conflict. A great variety of such symbolic symptoms were presented in Freud's essays.

A clear divergence is apparent between Freud's interpretation of symptoms and the interpretation offered by Janet.[1] Janet had indeed emphasized the reality of aspects of personality which were so dissociated as to be no longer capable of control by the conscious self ; but with Freud emphasis was laid especially upon the *dynamics* of such dissociation. The same ultimate forces that are working in consciousness seemed to him to be working outside of consciousness. For Freud such unconscious impulses were capable of statement neither in purely physiological terms nor in terms of " impersonal " mental events ; they were personal in the same sense that our introspective consciousness is personal. It was, he believed, only by conflict that any element or impulse could be kept outside of personal *awareness*. But just as conflict was the explanation of dissociation, so it was held to be the clue to the particular *form* which the dissociation took, and, consequently, to the nature of the symptoms. The symptoms were, in a broad sense, symbols of the suppressed tendencies, symbols to be understood through examination of the course of the disease. Janet had himself thought that symptoms arose from " subconscious ideas," and that amnesia involved the narrowing of the field of consciousness, but had left the dynamics of the process untouched. For Freud this conception was eminently unsatisfactory[2] ; in a host of such cases, such as that of the governess, the symptom seemed clearly a symbol of a *conflict*.

During the 'nineties Freud also discovered that he could sometimes use another starting point for free association more fruitfully than the materials of everyday thought. He shifted his attention to the patient's dreams. Dreams had hitherto been studied in a rather haphazard fashion, though considerable attention had been given to the influence of physical stimuli,[3] especially to the position of the limbs.[4]

[1] *The Mental State of Hystericals* (1892).
[2] For Janet himself it was only a provisional, and not in any sense an explanatory, formulation.
[3] *E.g.*, Maury, *Le sommeil et les rêves* (3rd ed., 1865). See also *Annales med. psychol.*, 1854.
[4] Vold, *Expériences sur les rêves et en particulier ceux d'origine musculaire et optique* (1896).

Quite aside from its therapeutic significance, Freud's use of dreams was significant as part of the widespread movement to bring within the field of psychology materials lying outside that domain of clearly conscious and observable processes which had been generally recognized as its legitimate subject matter. Freud's work on *The Interpretation of Dreams* was finally published in 1900. Dreams he regarded as the expression of wishes. They are a means by which elements in personality which have been kept out of consciousness during everyday waking life can, through symbolism, express themselves with relative freedom from interference. Suppressed strivings find a way to express themselves. To say that dreams spring from the unconscious is not the same as to say that they spring from items which have *lapsed* from memory; on the contrary, the dream is a dynamic expression of forces which, though suppressed, are *struggling* to regain a place in consciousness. The dream seemed to be a beautiful illustration of the mechanism by which submerged or suppressed elements in personality, elements in conflict with the everyday " self," arc manifested. The everyday self is a group of tendencies which have been strengthened by social, especially ethical, indoctrination, tendencies which are a part of our accepted social life, necessary in the making of a living and the building up of a reputation. We live in a society which is intolerant of certain of our instinctive tendencies; among these. fear and sex tendencies are prominent, but fear tendencies are suppressed to a very much smaller degree than those of sex. Sexual tendencies are more or less constantly with us, and are therefore subject to far more rigorous suppression. Freud made much of the significance of dreams as symbolic representations of sex wishes.

Now there must be some factor in waking life which is not present in the dream, to explain why the dream takes on a form easily distinguished from the wish-fulfilments which appear in day-dreaming. It had long been known that people of orderly habits not infrequently dream of participating in burglaries, murders, and the like. Men of irreproachable character may curse like troopers in their sleep. It seemed to Freud that something in the waking life must act as a constant damper on latent tendencies, which show themselves in the dream. But even in the dream there was evidence of restraint, and to this restraint he gave the name of " the censorship." Now, censorship during sleep is very much less effective than suppression during waking hours, and so allows forbidden tendencies some degree of freedom. Nevertheless, it continues in sleep to prevent the *direct* and unambiguous expression of suppressed materials, forcing them to take on a disguise. This disguise or symbolism is analogous to the symbolism already noticed in the case of the psychoneurotic symptoms. But how is the dream symbolism to be interpreted ?

Many dreams, especially those of children, seem to be *direct* wish-fulfilments. They are like day-dreams. They deal with *unsuppressed* wishes, and picture the fulfilment of such wishes. A child who had eagerly wished to climb a certain mountain dreamt that he climbed it. Another child had been boating, and was bitterly disappointed when she came to the shore ; in her dream that night she went boating again, and the trip was longer.[1] We find, Freud believes, relatively few such dreams in adults. Some common types are, however, apparent, notably " comfort " dreams : a drowsy man wishes on a cold winter's morning that he could keep his appointments without getting up, he falls asleep again and in a dream keeps the appointments. But the majority of adult dreams are not so simple ; the key to them is the interpretation of symbols.

As he analysed more and more dreams, Freud arrived at the conviction that there are, despite their infinite variety, certain striking uniformities in their contents, much greater in number than we should expect to find by chance. The dream of being in public, clad only in night-clothes, kept reappearing. Dreams of flying and of being pursued were very frequent. Freud felt himself forced to the hypothesis that certain stock symbols are to be found in the dreams of all sorts of people, symbols which regularly and with very few exceptions mean the same thing wherever they appear. Many of these symbols bore an evident resemblance to the thing symbolized ; this was especially emphasized in the case of sexual symbols. The interpretation of many symbols was, however, very difficult, necessitating a detailed analysis of their origin. Symbols may, he observed, be handed on

---

[1] These cases appear in Freud's *General Introduction to Psychoanalysis* (Hall trans., 1920), p. 102.

from generation to generation (the serpent has been used as a symbol of the healing art from pre-Homeric times to the present) ; symbols used by the social group may be accepted by the individual.

But symbolism is not the only mechanism by which suppressed tendencies may appear in altered form in the dream. The elements of the dream may be not a direct but a condensed or inverted narrative of a sequence of events unconsciously wished. The " manifest dream " is a distorted representation of the " latent dream." And whereas the latent dream is a *wish*, the manifest dream appears as an *event ;* the indicative mood appears, so to speak, in place of the optative. During the dream the censorship is sufficiently lax to permit the latent dream (*i.e.*, wishes struggling for fulfilment) to find expression in such a way as to escape recognition by the self. The dream, like the neurotic symptom, is a compromise between the suppressed and the suppressing tendencies. The nature of such struggle and compromise is shown in the nightmare, which becomes more and more terrifying until the dreamer wakes up. The disguise covering the suppressed tendencies becomes too thin, and the self, terrified lest the suppressed wishes break forth into clear consciousness, takes full control of the situation. Freud did not dismiss the evidence which shows that nightmares, as well as many other dreams, may arise from such simple physical causes as indigestion ; but he regarded such explanations merely as legitimate comments on some of the materials of the manifest dream, not as an explanation of the fact of dreaming, nor of the character of the dream. Similarly, he was not concerned to deny that many elements in dreams are recollections of recent waking events, but he insisted that the particular materials chosen for the manifest dream appeared because of their effectiveness for the purpose of the latent dream.

Two illustrations will show Freud's use of these hypotheses. A woman dreamt that she attended the funeral of a small nephew. She was very fond of the boy, and did not understand why she should have dreamt of his death. Analysis showed that some time earlier she had attended the funeral of another nephew, and had met on this occasion a young physician with whom she was in love. The dream was a simple way of saying she wished that the physician

Y

would return. The manifest dream revealed but little of the latent dream. The symbolism was fairly simple. Another illustration[1] in which the interpretation is much less simple is more characteristic of the mass of published dream analyses. A young woman who had been married for several years dreamt that she went to the theatre with her husband. On arrival at the theatre they found the house only half filled. Her husband told her of a young woman and her bridegroom who had wished to come, but had been unable. She thought this " no misfortune " for them. In point of fact, she (the dreamer) had recently bought theatre tickets in advance, paying a surcharge for them, only to find that one side of the orchestra was almost empty, and her mind kept running upon the theme " too hasty." The meaning of the dream as given by Freud was that painful associations surrounded the incident of buying tickets *too early*, because this was symbolic of her own unconscious protest against too early a marriage.

Such interpretations have been, in general, difficult to support by convincing evidence. Freud and his pupils have emphasized the fact that the interpretations are frequently accepted by the patient, and play a part in the process of self-understanding which helps towards cure. But since the influence of suggestion cannot be excluded, both arguments have failed of convincingness. Freudian dream-psychology has therefore been subject, among his followers, to all sorts of revisions, and has been one of the aspects of his system selected for especially vigorous attack by psychologists who have demanded experimental confirmation of his major tenets. The method of free association, with or without the use of dream material, did unravel the skein of many a tangled personality ; but the question remained open whether this was chiefly due to Freud's interpretation of symbols or simply to his emphasis on the importance of conflict and suppression—an emphasis which, aside from all theories of symbolism, led the patient to struggle towards a rediscovery of the forgotten episodes underlying his troubles.

But in this intensive dream-study the psychoanalytic method has been kept in constant use, and in the course of it many new problems have been raised. Practically all

[1] *General Introduction to Psychoanalysis*, p. 98. The case is here much abbreviated.

varieties of psychoanalysis have emphasized dream-material. But it is to be remembered that both the psychoanalytic method and its application to dream-material were worked out by Freud before psychoanalysis became a school or a movement. Freud worked, in fact, alone, until about the beginning of the new century.[1]

In 1902, a group of medical students in Vienna began to join with him in a seminar for the study of psychoanalysis. Psychoanalysis became, in a few years, a " movement " of wide proportions. In this period Freud published a book applying his working concepts to new materials, *The Psychopathology of Everyday Life* (1904). The thesis of the book was very simple in comparison with his dream-psychology. Not only in neurotic symptoms, he held, but in the everyday acts of normal persons, there is constant evidence that any tendency which is forced out of consciousness continues to struggle for expression, and, though failing to appear in consciousness, influences thought and action. The most casual slips of tongue or pen, the forgetting of familiar names, and all sorts of oddities and blunders which interfere with our deliberate purposes, reflect a real though unacknowledged motive. At a time of rather strained relations, a man's wife gave him a book which she thought might interest him ; the book was promptly lost and his efforts to find it were vain. Later she exerted herself to care for her husband's mother in a serious illness. Returning home one day with enthusiasm for her devotion, he immediately found the book. The original losing of the book was a symbolic expression of the fact that he had lost his affection for his wife. He had forgotten the book because it was a token of her. Similarly, through regaining his affection for her, the obstacle to recalling the whereabouts of the book was removed.

In the same period Freud published his contribution to the theory of wit.[2] In this he emphasized the rôle of wit in suddenly liberating suppressed impulses, "letting the cat out of the bag." The practical joke is funny in so far as there is genuine antagonism against the victim ; jokes upon

---

[1] His observations were frequently published several years after they had been made ; the indifference of the public gave him a leisure which he felt saved him from the pressure later exerted upon him as the leader of a school. (" History of the Psychoanalytic Movement," *Psychoanalytic Rev.*, III, 1916, p. 418.)

[2] *Wit and its Relation to the Unconscious* (1905).

pompous or self-righteous persons or upon " hated rivals " are funny, while jokes against the helpless are merely brutal. Humorous stories, moreover, can be classified in respect to the type of emotion released. One group of stories resembles the practical joke ; persons or institutions towards which a forced deference is maintained may be seen stripped of their dignity. Another group gives release to sex-suppressions. Another group comprises puns, the explanation of which shows beautifully the ambition of the Freudian teaching to become no mere commentary on emotional life, but a genuine system of psychology. The pun is funny because it frees our minds from a particular kind of constraint, namely, that constraint which logical thought and the forms of grammar impose upon us. We are forced to use the same old words with the same old meanings year in and year out.[1] Through using words in an unaccustomed sense, the punster and his hearers are released from the strain of being logical. Anything that allows the sudden release of pent-up energies gives a sudden, in fact an explosive, satisfaction.

Wit is, however, merely one of many ways in which the mind constantly seeks freedom from restraint. Early in life the child learns the stern necessity of thinking for practical purposes, the " reality motive."[2] He continues, however, the simple and satisfying habit of letting his thoughts roam at times where they will. The struggle against accepting a painful reality may show itself in a tendency to interpret our own conduct and motives as we should wish them to be. The process of finding " good reasons " for acts of which we are covertly ashamed has been given by Jones the name of " rationalization."[3] If the behaviour of others suggests that they entertain an unfavourable attitude toward us, we resort to " defence-mechanisms "[4]; we strive to put ourselves in a favourable light or to convince ourselves that their approval means nothing to us.

During the last twenty years have come thick and fast a series of contributions regarding the theory of sexuality and of the ego, constituting the later Freudian period of

---

[1] Unless we use them as Humpty Dumpty did.
[2] See, e.g., Beyond the Pleasure Principle (1920).
[3] " Rationalization in Everyday Life," J. Abn. Psychol., III, 1908-9.
[4] Similar, of course, to the defence of the neurotic against his suppressed impulses ; the idea of defence has been emphasized throughout the history of psychoanalysis.

psychoanalysis. They may be said to be the essence of contemporary psychoanalysis, as distinguished from the invention and extension of the psychoanalytic method itself, which was the chief achievement of the earlier period. In the early period Freud was in general content to find most of the causes of the neuroses in the emotional conflicts of adult life. He had, however, as we noted above, observed psychoneuroses whose origin lay in childhood. Further study of such material constantly drove him further back into individual history, even to the point of attaching paramount importance to the sexual life of early infancy. The earlier viewpoint was represented, for example, by tracing a symptom, a slip of speech, etc., back to some suppression in adult life. In Freud's subsequent work, suppression has been regarded not simply as the result of the conflict of present forces, but as the most recent manifestation of a history of emotional conflict which goes back to an origin in the sexual maladjustments of the little child. An early elaboration of much of this system of thought was presented in *Three Contributions to the Theory of Sex* (1905). The extension of the doctrine has appeared in a number of articles and treatises which have not as yet been presented as an organized whole.

Most of this material was obtained from the study of adults, especially neurotic adults, whose memories were carried back by the psychoanalytic method to earlier and earlier stages in their development. A symptom in an adult might appear to go back to an adolescent conflict ; this might be found to lead to painful memories of an episode in the eighth year ; and these, in turn, might in time be found to involve memories from earlier childhood. Confirmation of some of the hypotheses obtained have, however, been sought through the psychoanalysis of children,[1] with results which are regarded by Freud as a verification of much that had been gleaned from adult memories.

From such analytic material, as well as from many scattered observations as to the ways of infants and children, Freud roughly outlined certain stages in individual sexual growth.[2] In early infancy there appears a wealth of response to which the term " sexuality " may be applied. It had long been suspected, for example, that such habits as thumb-

---

[1] See, *e.g.*, *Analysis of the Phobia of a Five-year-old Boy* (1909).
[2] See, *e.g.*, *General Introduction to Psychoanalysis*, p. 277 f.

sucking have something to do with sexuality. Freud found,
however, nothing in the infant which could be characterized
as a specific sex-impulse ; on the contrary, sexual manifestations were so extraordinarily " polymorphous " that it
seemed wiser to use the term " sexuality " to mean the whole
bundle of dispositions which are connected with the love-life,
whether associated with the organs of sex or not. Even the
" perversions " of adult life, e.g., sadism, are simply continuations of infantile responses which have never been repressed.
And even the dominating and submissive tendencies are
regarded as aspects of sexuality. The child discovers the
topography of his body, and therewith a group of satisfactions.
This leads to the fixation of a habit in which the child's
affections are directed to his own body instead of towards
another individual. This stage is designated " auto-
eroticism."[1]

Now the rather diffuse sexuality of early infancy undergoes
a series of repressions and modifications. The person most
intimately associated with the infant's sex feelings, as well
as with the satisfaction of his hunger, is of course the mother.
In the course of time, Freud believes, the little boy learns
that the father is not only a competitor for the mother's
affection, but may, and frequently does, interfere in the
child's close intimacy with the mother. Both of the parents,
and society in general as well, make it plain to the boy that
he may not have undisputed possession of his mother ; and
the father is, in fact, not only the competitor but the stern
incarnation of discipline. Love for the mother, Freud contends, must be in some way suppressed, while the father,
though still the object of affection, is at the same time hated.
To this mechanism Freud gave the name " Œdipus complex,"[2]
" complex " being a general term[3] for a constellation of affect-
ively toned ideas which have been suppressed. To a somewhat similar mechanism in the girl, the name " Electra "[4]
complex was given. Both the psychoanalytic evidence and
the reasoning based upon it are so complicated that our brief

[1] Freud calls this " the happy term invented by Havelock Ellis."
This is but one of many contributions for which Ellis's work has been
welcomed by psychoanalysts. (See Ellis, " Auto-Erotism : a Psychological Study," *Alienist and Neurologist*, XIX, 1898).
[2] Because Œdipus killed his father and married his mother.
[3] A term now obsolescent.
[4] On account of Electra's hatred of her mother.

summary must be especially inadequate at this point. It is, however, important to remember that the above picture may be profoundly modified by the child's tendency to " identify " himself with either parent.

But the child's love-energy, or " libido," may come in time to be attached to his whole body ; and this " narcistic " (or " narcissistic ") stage is characterized by self-absorption and vanity, one's mental as well as physical attributes becoming objects of affection. The social situation ultimately forces the child to find another love-object. He chooses individuals like himself, that is, those of his own sex. This " homosexual " stage, in which children show strong attachment chiefly to playmates of their own sex, gives place at last to devotion to the opposite sex ; and this passage to the "heterosexual" stage synchronizes with the rapid physical changes of early adolescence.

From the character of these stages it is evident that the sexual impulse is regarded as of extremely vague and indefinite character, which knows no set forms of behaviour. Only when the individual has passed through various stages can his affections undergo fixation of a stable and normal type. But the emotional attachments formed in each stage are not completely obliterated during progress to the next, and herein much of the distress of adult life resides. Whenever adjustment at a given stage fails, one tends to " regress " to a previous stage which brought satisfaction. The rejected lover turns to his old friends. Such flight away from an adult level of adjustment plays an important part in that escape from reality which characterizes many insanities ; regressions of many forms are prominent symptoms of several common mental disorders. But most of all, the attachments of infancy persist. Not only does the young man often seek a wife resembling his mother ; a filial attitude is evident as a component in adult love. The word "infantilism" is one of the major indices to the Freudian psychology.

But regression is only one of *many* mechanisms through which a conflict may be resolved. "Sublimation" is the discovery of a substitute object for the libido, some channel of expression which, by its close association with the one sought, will give partial satisfaction. The arts and sciences give vicarious satisfaction ; civilization itself is in large part the creature of energies which have been diverted from a sexual outlet. Both Freud and his followers have been much interested in the problem of demonstrating, in the work of creative artists, the presence of materials reflecting the unconscious sexual fantasies of the artist.[1] A similar process is evident in fetishism, in which a man becomes attached, for example, to the slipper of the loved one ; this peculiar fixation may remain even when the love for its wearer is suppressed.

But why should man build up elaborate systems of restraint ? Why should he not do as he pleases ? Why be bound by social restrictions, habits, conventions ? Because, after all, it is easiest, Freud thinks, for mankind to live under such restraints. From the Freudian point of view, humanity is in conflict with itself, has tendencies which make for discord ; and a struggle, in some form or other, is inevitable. The tendencies lumped together under the name of sexuality are apt to come into conflict with our relations with our fellows. Sex-tendencies are kept in subjection by a group of socially recognized " ego " tendencies, through which the individual struggles for self-maintenance and a place in society. The ego-tendencies, supported by society, constitute the agency of restraint. As we have seen, Freud believes that when energy is restrained it continues to struggle for a way out. It is a cardinal point in Freud's system that when energies are inhibited, they continue active in one guise or another. Now man, wherever he is found, has much the same emotional make-up and much the same restraints. The effect of man's conflict is to produce more or less similar culture the world over. Not only marriage and the family, but myth and folk-lore, religion and ceremonial, science,[2] language, music, pictorial and plastic art, and other cultural phenomena are full of materials for psychoanalytic study.

The first to offer a psychoanalytic interpretation of anthropological data was Abraham,[3] but Freud welcomed this extension of method, and contributed substantially to it.

[1] Freud, *Leonardo da Vinci* (1910).
[2] The curiosity motive implicit in science is regarded by Freud as emanating largely from childish curiosity regarding sex.
[3] *Traum und Mythus* (1908).

His comparison[1] of the " ambivalence " of the sacred and unclean with similarly ambivalent attitudes encountered among neurotics (and others), has provoked much discussion. His comments, however suggestive, do not appear to have won general assent from the only group qualified to judge of them, namely, the anthropologists.[2]

Now we come to Freud's interpretation of some of the phenomena which had throughout his career been the central problem for direct study, the neuroses.[3] Nearly all of these he has continued to attribute to sexual conflict ; but the decades have brought an increasing emphasis on the sexual struggles of childhood. Adult maladjustments occur because the way has been prepared by earlier emotional shocks. The *anxiety neurosis*,[4] which Freud has emphasized, is attributed to the arousal of intense sexual feeling followed by sudden repression. The Freudian interpretation of *obsessions* may be represented by an illustrative case.[5] A woman came to Freud suffering from a distressing obsession, an idea which she knew to be foolish, but which nevertheless she could not dispel. She felt that her husband was disloyal to her. The woman had recently seen a young and attractive officer with whom she had become infatuated. Being unwilling to acknowledge the fact, she had " projected " it to her husband. Such a process is somewhat similar to the act of " rationalization," by which we explain our conduct in such terms as to free us from the sense of guilt. In contrast with obsessions, *compulsions* are overt *acts* through which an affect, or rather the defence against it, constantly symbolizes itself ; many patients, like Lady Macbeth, wash their hands in an effort to wash away the sense of guilt. But the

---

[1] *Totem and Taboo* (first published in *Imago*, I-II, 1912-3).

[2] But a direct field-work application of psychoanalytic principles has recently been made by Malinowski in the study of the Trobriand Islanders, much of whose culture does seem to be illuminated by the application of the concepts of suppression and symbolism (*e.g.*, " Psychoanalysis and Anthropology," *Psyche*, IV, 1923-4).

[3] Though these are attributed to a psychophysical " trauma " or shock, no dualism of mind and body being assumed, some neuroses are traced to physiological disturbances, while others are stated in psychogenic terms. Early emphasis on the single dramatic trauma has been replaced by emphasis on the whole life-history.

[4] Described by Freud as early as 1894. See his *Collected Papers*, I, " The Justification for Detaching from Neurasthenia a Particular Syndrome, the Anxiety-Neurosis " (*Neurolog. Zentralbl.*, 1895).

[5] *General Introduction to Psychoanalysis*, p. 213 f.

line of separation between obsessions and compulsions is not always clear.[1]

Phobias present a somewhat similar mechanism. Objects excite a fear for which the patient has no explanation. Some phobias are not sharply distinguished from compulsions ; the fear of dirt (misophobia), for example, may provoke excessive hand-washing. The fear masks a desire which the patient is afraid to recognize. Whereas most phobias reported by Freud appear to be of sexual origin (by a mechanism somewhat similar to that of the nightmare as mentioned above), a case cited by Rivers[2] indicates a method of extending some of the Freudian concepts to other cases. An officer who showed good self-control under fire suffered from a strange terror on entering a dug-out. His personal history revealed recurrent fear of small rooms. The study of dreams made possible his recall of a violent fright at the age of four, when a dog in a dark passage-way had frightened him. Fear had been suppressed; but any small enclosure like the passage could at any time touch it off. The reference to suppression and the belief that suppression is the major cause for the persistence of the difficulty, distinguish such explanations sharply from the simple " conditioned response " explanations of Bekhterev[3] and others.

In " conversion hysteria " the suppressed affect is " converted " into a specific symptom, such as a paralysis, contracture, anæsthesia, or amnesia. The unconscious protest, for example, against seeing what is painful may lead to a functional blindness. Freud, Rivers, and others applied such conceptions to the study of the war-neuroses, believing that a paralysed arm, for example, was a compromise between fear and the attempt to suppress it.[4] The conversion hysteria of civil life, Freud believes, is regularly due to such compromise formations arising from sexual suppressions.

Though absolute insistence upon the patient's co-operation with the analyst, and upon his effort to face directly those painful episodes whose suppression has wrought such havoc, has been a constant feature of Freudian therapeutic method,

---

[1] The " counting mania " may arise when counting has been found to be an effectual mechanism of escape from a painful idea.

[2] *Instinct and the Unconscious* (1920), p. 170.

[3] *La psychologie objective* (1913).

[4] See Rivers, *op. cit.*

the technique of psychoanalysis has undergone numerous changes. Most important is the increasing insistence upon the functional significance of " transference,"[1] the process by which the patient transfers to the physician the love which, through suppression or distortion has failed of a free outlet. Having gained the patient's affection and full co-operation, the analyst is able, in completing his task, to give the patient such self-understanding that he or she may be freed from the transference and regain wholesome affection for a previous love-object or freely bestow it upon a new one. Transference is therefore essential to any Freudian analysis. Many other changes of emphasis and new points of technique have been outlined by Freud's pupils, Ferenczi and Rank.[2]

Along with these changes in technique, the most important development in Freudian theory in recent years is the formulation of a systematic doctrine regarding the structure of personality. The primordial impersonal cravings of the organism, governed by the pleasure principle, come into conflict with stern reality, so that the Ego (das Ich) is formed out of the Id (das Es). Later the Id subdivides further as a result of complicated interactions, including " identification " with each parent, and the Super-ego is formed, the disciplinary force which underlies conscience. Other aspects of Freudian theory which have been more and more emphasized are the castration complex resulting from fear of parental violence and the narcissistic love of the Ego for itself ; inferiority feelings arise from a " narcissistic wound." But here the architectonics of Freud's system have become so intricate as to defy any brief and simple exposition.[3]

Our brief sketch of the evolution of Freudian psychology presents a strange contrast with the development of that experimental psychology which has chiefly concerned us. Freud's work has outlined an approach to psychology radically different from that of any psychological system

---

[1] See chapter on " Transference " in Freud's *General Introduction to Psychoanalysis*.

[2] *The Development of Psychoanalysis* (1925).

[3] The development of Freud's thought may be traced in the following four books : *Beyond the Pleasure Principle* (1920) ; *Group Psychology and Analysis of the Ego* (1921) ; *The Ego and the Id* (1923) ; *Inhibition, Symptom, and Anxiety* (1927).

either ancient or modern. For, despite the constant recourse to theory, the system differs fundamentally from earlier speculative systems, in that it has arisen from and has constantly returned into the practical problems of personalities struggling for an adjustment to the world.

Among the Freudians of the first importance is a little group of disciples, already mentioned, who gathered with Freud early in the century for discussion. The number of his followers in Vienna and other Central European cities increased until the need for co-operation was expressed in a number of " congresses," where psychoanalytic methods and discoveries were discussed at length.

Among those who, as early as 1910, had achieved distinction as exponents of the Freudian position, were Abraham of Berlin and Brill of New York. It is but natural, however, that leadership of the school should remain in and near Vienna ; and notwithstanding the prominent position accorded to Ernest Jones[1] (at Toronto and London), the evolution of the school has been largely guided by Freud himself, aided by Ferenczi, Rank and others. A few typical contributions of these men may be noted. Ferenczi has written upon the " Stages in the Development of the Sense of Reality "[2]; Brill upon the psychology of the " only child."[3] Rank has laid great stress upon the " birth trauma,"[4] the shock undergone by the infant upon first meeting the adversities of extra-uterine existence.

But we must turn to the work of another " school." In 1904 there appeared a highly important experimental and theoretical study by Jung and Riklin, *Studies in Word-association*, the first substantial contribution of the " Zürich School." This work not only marked the advent into psychoanalysis of a method developed by experimental psychology (the word-association test), but introduced into psychiatric practice a system of thought in many ways strikingly similar to classical associationism. All mental life was conceived

---

[1] As editor of the *International Journal of Psychoanalysis*, 1920.
[2] In his " *Sex in Psychoanalysis* " (1916).
[3] " The Only or Favorite Child in Adult Life," in his volume *Psychoanalysis* (3rd ed., 1922).
[4] *Das Trauma der Geburt und seine Bedeutung für die Psychoanalyse* (1924).

as a tissue of associations ; every emotional pattern, every attitude, was to be construed as a network which the association-test must help to analyse.

A large part of the work was a simple inductive study, such as Wundt might have carried out ; the variation of association time with age, sex, and education was analysed, and associations were classified under captions closely similar to those of Trautscholdt (see p. 170f.) Here and in later association studies Jung has contributed much which experimental psychologists have been glad to accept. Typical of the possibilities of his method is the work of Fürst[1], who showed that " association type " (the distribution of associations under the various classification headings) displays striking family resemblances. But these quantitative uses interested the experimenters much less than the possibilities of the association-test as an instrument for the qualitative analysis of the emotional life of individuals. They gave close attention to responses which were exceptionally slow or exceptionally quick ; instances in which a response word was given over and over again ; or where the stimulus word was repeated by the subject ; or where he blushed, coughed, stammered, or gave other indications of emotional disturbance. Such " complex-indicators," or clues to concealed emotional conflict, were used in conjunction with the study of those word responses which directly betrayed emotion. But despite their great interest in the new method, Jung and his group did not regard the association method as a *substitute* for the psychoanalytic method of Freud, the subject's narrative of his spontaneous associations. Moreover, the new technique was welcomed by Freud as a supplement to the existing methods, and the relation of the two schools was at first quite amicable.

But Jung's system of thought diverged more and more from Freud's during the years immediately following, and this, together with personal differences, brought about a cleavage which makes it necessary to regard the Zürich school as a distinct entity. A cardinal point of difference lay in the theory of the " libido." For Jung, Freud's emphasis upon sexuality is unwarranted. The mainspring to human strivings is rather an undifferentiated life-energy which may

[1] See Jung, " The Association Method," *Am. J. Psychol.*, XXI, 1910.

pour itself into limitless channels.[1]   The unconscious, moreover, is not simply a repository for the suppressed experiences
of the individual.   It is a mass of symbolic material which
represents not only the cravings of the individual, but much
which has been handed down from ancestral experience.
Symbolism itself is not an evidence of suppression ; the
primitive nature of the unconscious directly involves the
tendency to think in symbols.   " Analytical psychology " in
Jung's hands has come to mean something very far from
Freud's concerns.   A Freudian psychoanalysis seeks to
enable the patient to understand his own plight and to
re-integrate his shattered personality ; or, in non-pathological
cases, simply to understand the genesis of his own fixations,
ambitions, fears, and aversions.   But with Jung the problem
is vastly more complicated.   Mythology and folk-lore,
history, religion, and the arts, must ever be gleaned anew
for " changes and symbols of the libido " which may throw
light on the patient's fantasies.   Such fantasies, which for
Freud had arisen from a relatively simple tendency to use
one's imagination for the direct satisfaction it yielded, rather
than for the attainment of practical purposes, became, for
Jung, the very centre of the life of the libido.   And, since
the individual's potentialities express themselves in myriad
forms, a psychoanalysis is never " finished " ; the task of the
analyst is to present constantly widening vistas of self-
realization.   This whole construction naturally seemed to the
Freudians to be as imaginative and unverifiable as their own
system had appeared to orthodox psychology.

The various manifestations of the libido did, however,
suggest to Jung a fundamental classification of personality
types.[2]   In some individuals emotion is directed outward,
toward the objective world.   The " extraverts " strive to
manipulate their environment.   The " introverts," on the
other hand, turn their energies within, toward the world of

---

[1] The importance of sexuality, however, is fully admitted.   " . . . we
see the desire, the libido, in the most diverse applications and forms.
We see the libido in the stage of childhood almost wholly occupied in the
instinct of nutrition . . . . With the development of the body there are
successively opened new spheres of application for the libido.   The
last sphere of application, and surpassing all the others in its functional
significance is sexuality."   Jung, *Psychology of the Unconscious* (1912),
p. 148.

[2] See, *e.g.*, *Collected Papers on Analytical Psychology* (1916), Chapter XI.

imagination ; among them arise poets and artists, those who live in the things of the spirit. Both extraversion and intro-version may, however, be manifested in many forms, and psychologists who have utilized the conception have tended to regard both types as merely extremes on a distribution-curve.[1] Introversion may easily lead to the habit of living entirely in the world of dreams, in such a fashion as to bring about an unsocial personality. The extreme form of such morbid self-absorption may be a clinical entity such as Kraepelin had delineated under the name *dementia præcox*[2] (see p. 171). Jung has more recently described introversion in terms which suggest much less of the pathological. He makes the point that, after all, the world of inner life is just as " real " as the objective world ; there is nothing invidious about the distinction.[3] Another great psychiatrist of Zürich, Bleuler, co-operated in the extension of this theory, giving this entity the name of *schizophrenia*,[4] to express the " splitting of personality " by which some of the subject's energies are dissevered from the rest. By emphasizing, however, internal toxic factors which arise during such maladjustments and play a part in the patient's intellectual deterioration, he removed the mental disorder from the confines of a purely " analytic " domain ; and Jung himself had at times stressed the toxic factors.

Jung's psychology, notwithstanding such references to mental disease, is centred in the normal rather than the abnormal. Just as Freud's doctrines, whatever their signi-ficance for normal life, have emanated largely from the study of sick personalities, so Jung's have in large part been based upon literary material. Jung's greater willingness to depart from psychiatric findings has helped to engender that bitter-ness which Freud epitomized through referring to the days in which Jung was " still content to be a mere psychoanalyst —and did not yet want to be a prophet."[5]

---

[1] " All studies seem to be agreed that we have not two distinct groups, but a normal curve with the majority of persons ambivert."— G. B. Watson, " Character Tests of 1926," *Vocational Guidance Magazine*, V, 1927.

[2] Jung's *The Psychology of Dementia Præcox* appeared in 1907.

[3] *Psychological Types* (1921). To use F. L. Wells's metaphor, " in the machinery of life, the extravert is a cog, while the introvert is a crank."

[4] See his *Theory of Schizophrenic Negativism* (1912).

[5] *General Introduction to Psychoanalysis*, p. 232.

Another important deviation from Freud's doctrine, again constituting a defection from the ranks of his followers, is the school founded at Vienna by Adler. Adler's earliest contributions had to do with the sense of inferiority which arises from some organic defect or inadequacy.[1] The unconscious strivings to offset this defect by "compensation" were held to be vitally important for the understanding of both normal and neurotic constitutions.[2] Some of Adler's doctrines regarding the ego were accepted by the Freudians[4] as a helpful but not a major contribution ; the younger man, plainly stating that he would not remain " in Freud's shadow " all his life, founded a separate school. The doctrine of the " inferiority complex " was elaborated, and the mechanism of compensation was illustrated from many fields of social life. Mental as well as physical inadequacies were recognized as starting points for the development of the " masculine protest " against a sense of insufficiency, while extensive study was made of instances of compensation in which the patient not only tends to correct but to *over-correct* his disability. It was not enough for the semi-invalid Roosevelt to become well ; he must ride at the head of his " Rough Riders." Emphasis has recently been placed upon the details of the social surroundings which shape the child's formulation of a " style of life " ; his ordinal position in the family is of special importance.[3] But mere " determinism " is a futile concept, Adler's " individual psychology " regards life as a struggle towards a goal.[4]

Though difficulties of perspective make an interpretation of present movements quite hazardous, an attempt must now be made to trace the spread of psychoanalytic doctrine, and to indicate briefly some of the points of its greatest influence upon psychology.

The dissemination of psychoanalysis through the German-speaking countries has gone on steadily since the opening years of the century. Though many great clinicians have looked upon it askance, its major tenets have at least become

[1] *Study of Organ Inferiority and its Psychical Compensations* (1907).
[2] *The Neurotic Constitution* (1912).
[3] *Practice and Theory of Individual Psychology* (1924).
[4] *Understanding Human Nature* (1927).

familiar to medical men. Upon the *psychology* of Germany, Austria, and Switzerland, however, it has exerted relatively little influence.

Neither upon the psychology nor upon the psychiatry of other Continental countries has its influence been comparable with that exerted in Great Britain and in the United States. A factor largely responsible for its introduction into American psychiatry was the activity of Brill, in translating several of Freud's works[1] ; while the lectures by both Freud and Jung at Clark University in 1909, in response to Hall's invitation, were of capital importance. In Great Britain, after 1914, the study of " war shock " brought about a very rapid and widespread dissemination of Freudian principles into psychiatry, and, especially through the work of Rivers,[2] into psychology ; the interpretation of such conditions in organic terms proved so unsuccessful as to make the study of motive and conflict an apparent necessity.

There were, however, already at work, in British and American psychiatry, forces with which psychoanalysis became easily assimilated. The work of Meyer and Hoch, for example, had never been a mere reflection of Freudian influence, yet their writings expressed a functional conception of mental disorder, in which the influence of organic disease was not comparable in importance with the psychogenic factors. Meyer's emphasis upon " faulty mental habits " and Hoch's suggestion that *dementia præcox* is most apt to arise in a " shut-in " personality, are not simply instances of the adoption of Freudian method in psychiatry ; they are, rather, the expression of a trend towards personality-study which had been moving forward under the influence both of the psychoanalysts and of Kraepelin, Janet, Morton Prince, and countless other students of psychopathology. Not only is it difficult, in recent American and British psychiatry, to tell just how much should be designated psychoanalytic ; it is exceedingly hard to define to what extent the influence of Freud and his followers outlined new problems and concepts, and to what extent they merely added form and colour to an existing tendency towards the study of conflict, dissociation, and other dynamic factors in personality-disturbance.

[1] The translation of *The Interpretation of Dreams*, appearing in 1913, attracted a considerable amount of attention.
[2] See, *e.g.*, *Instinct and the Unconscious* (1920).

z

And although there appears to be a tendency for the adherents of rival therapeutic schools to emphasize sharply the lines of cleavage established by their Continental leaders, much eclecticism nevertheless prevails, both in the combination of doctrines taken from Freud, Jung, Adler, and other related schools, and in the admixture of these with the more "orthodox" teachings of Kraepelin and "clinical psychiatry."

Psychology itself has been much more reluctant to admit the doctrines of psychoanalysis, though this reluctance appears greater in America than in Britain. And its spread among "clinical" psychologists has greatly outstripped its advance in the psychology of classroom and laboratory. The greater prevalence of experimental psychology in America, and the tendency of British students to entertain considerably less confidence as to the possibilities of experimental method in relation to the most complicated problems of personality, seem to be directly related to the somewhat more cordial reception which psychoanalysis has enjoyed in Britain. The opinion of Rivers[1] that Freud had contributed more to the understanding of personality than had experimental psychology, the presentation of Freud's work as the "new psychology" in J. A. Thomson's *Outline of Science* (1922), and the recent appearance in Great Britain of many educational texts written from a psychoanalytic approach, cannot easily be duplicated from recent American history.

The chief grounds of objection have been, first, the concept of the unconscious, and the quasi-animistic language which speaks of "libido," "censorship," and the "ego"; secondly, the emphasis upon sex and especially upon infantile sexuality, which is distinctive of Freud's approach; and thirdly, the impossibility of experimental or statistical control of complicated factors unearthed by the intricate and arduous process of psychoanalysis. The "unhappy divisions" existing among practitioners have contributed to such distrust. But while so much uncertainty and open hostility attach to these doctrines, and indeed in many quarters to the whole movement, terms like "rationalization," "compensation," "defence-mechanism," and "projection," are rapidly becoming current. Not only such

[1] Expressed in an informal address at the *New School for Social Research*, New York City, 1919.

specific concepts, but the habit of thinking in terms of a struggling personality divided against itself, unaware of many of its own motives, and seeking through devious channels satisfactions which it cannot or will not clearly define, has become a prominent feature in that general transition from structural to functional problems which has already engaged our attention.

CHAPTER XX

INSTINCT

" You are right," he replied ; " every desire in itself has to do with its natural object in its simply abstract form, but the accessories of the desire determine the quality of the object."—*Plato*.

ГHE present century has brought many changes in regard to the interpretation of those forms of behaviour which in the nineteenth century were rather vaguely described as " instinctive." Perhaps the leading characteristic of the prevalent conception of instinct was the idea of a perfect adaptive mechanism which made possible the effective execution of a complex act prior to all experience and without knowledge of the end which it served. In accordance with the conception of man as a rational creature, a notion which has been kept alive especially by idealism and by the Scottish school, a contrast was frequently drawn between the instinctive behaviour of the brute and the reasoned conduct of man. Darwin (*Descent of Man*, 1871) had challenged this sharp distinction, and James urged that man actually had more instincts than any other mammal.[1]

The anecdotal and speculative literature on instinct during the late nineteenth and early twentieth centuries was very voluminous. A guiding principle in this discussion was Lloyd Morgan's version of the " law of parsimony," to the effect that " in no case may we interpret an action as the outcome of the exercise of a higher psychical faculty, if it can be interpreted as the outcome of the exercise of one which stands lower in the psychological scale."[2] For psychology this meant that instinct was to be invoked, rather than intelligence, wherever both explanations of the activities of animals seemed legitimate. It is a double-edged sword which has turned against Lloyd Morgan's views in recent years, for instinct has proved to be one of the most complex of all

[1] *Principles of Psychology* (1890), II, p. 403.
[2] *Introduction to Comparative Psychology* (1894), p. 53.

psychological conceptions ; the clarification of its meaning has been a chief task of recent experimental and theoretical analysis.

The late nineteenth century, however, witnessed a great advance in the physico-chemical explanation of life and behaviour, and it became common to interpret not only animal but human conduct in the simplest possible mechanistic terms. The concept of the " tropism " (as in the work of Loeb) was especially fruitful ; there appeared to be no sharp distinction between the turning of a plant to the light and the swarming of lowly organisms from a darker to a lighter region. Furthermore, it was easy to see that much of the activity of very lowly forms was curiously similar to the positive and negative reaction-tendencies—the eating, fleeing, and attacking behaviour—of higher forms.[1] It became easy to think of both human and animal instincts as merely more complex forms of such primitive physico-chemical responses. On the other hand, Jennings (*Behavior of the Lower Organisms*, 1906) presented a mass of data which showed that even the protozoa possess reaction-patterns of some degree of complexity.

In this same period the movement towards a functional psychology was destined to give to instinct a position of the greatest importance. McDougall, profoundly influenced by Stout, was the chief figure. In 1908 the conception of instinct was redefined and given a position of all-embracing importance in the interpretation of conduct by McDougall's[2] doctrine of the relation of instinct to emotion, and his interpretation of nearly all behaviour as the expression of innate impulses. As primary instincts he listed flight, repulsion, curiosity, pugnacity, self-abasement, self-assertion, and parental instinct. To these a group of less well-defined instincts, including gregariousness and the sex-impulse, was added.[3] McDougall's list was short in comparison with that of James ; many of the more complex activities described by James were regarded by McDougall as compounds of two or more instincts, or as learned behaviour. But McDougall's list, historically important though it was, was of less significance than his analysis of the *nature* of instinct. Each instinct,

[1] *E.g.*, Loeb, *Der Heliotropismus der Tiere* (1890).
[2] *An Introduction to Social Psychology* (1908).
[3] Later editions have included alterations in the list.

he held, comprises three parts, cognitive, affective, and conative.   Men (and many animals) are by nature equipped with
a disposition by virtue of which the perception of certain
stimuli leads to definite and characteristic emotions, and these,
in turn, to definite strivings from which motor behaviour
follows.   The first and third aspects of this complex response
are susceptible to much modification.   (McDougall expressly
rejected the hypothesis that the association of ideas was the
clue to all modification of behaviour, and laid emphasis upon
a pattern which appears to be simply that of the conditioned
response.)   But the central emotional phase of the instinct
remains the clue upon which its detection must always depend.
Every instinct must contain an emotion as its core, and every
emotion is the central affective portion of an instinct.   This
simplification of the baffling problem of the relation of
instinct to emotion attracted much attention[1] and won many
adherents.   The hypothesis was in fact systematically
perfect ;   however much its accuracy might be doubted,
its clarity was directly compelling.   Perhaps the most
important of the many influences exerted by McDougall's
book was the attainment of the purpose (expressed in the
Preface) of replacing the still current psychological hedonism
by the doctrine of an impulsive ("hormic") basis for
conduct.

   Thorndike's *Original Nature of Man*[2] (1913) presented a
very much longer list of instincts.   Rejecting McDougall's
selection of the emotion as the central and always distinguishable core of the instinct, he urged the desirability of
classifying instinctive acts in terms of the types of
unlearned overt behaviour manifested ;   thus there were
several *kinds* of " fear " behaviour.   Further, many complex
activities regarded by McDougall as arising from the modification of his primary instincts were regarded by Thorndike as
independent ("kindliness," for example, which McDougall
regarded as an expression of "tender emotion," was for
Thorndike a distinct inherited impulse).   McDougall's and
Thorndike's catalogues of instincts enjoyed wide popularity,
both as keys to the interpretation of human motives and as
tools in educational practice.

   [1] See, for example, the symposium on " Instinct and Intelligence,"
Brit. J. Psychol., III, 1909-10.
   [2] Volume I of his revised *Educational Psychology*.

Woodworth (*Dynamic Psychology*, 1918), while accepting the reality of human instincts, argued that they were not the sole, nor even the main, "springs of human conduct." His list of instincts borrowed much from previous discussions, but he gave expression to the belief that, in addition to the definite instincts, there exist certain innate capacities whose pattern is less definitely fixed by nature ; here appear, for example, innate mathematical and musical ability. Such innate capacities might prove a simpler explanation for the mathematician's absorption in his work than the assumption that some disguised instinct is symbolized in the manipulation of numbers. Even when an activity is clearly pursued in the interests of some instinct, as when a man makes money to assuage his hunger, the "mechanism" may, in some cases, become a "drive," and continue as such even after the instinct is satisfied. Almost any means to an end may, under the right conditions, itself become a "drive."

In 1919, Dunlap[1] called in question the whole instinct doctrine as it had been developed by McDougall, Thorndike, Woodworth, and others, pointing out that the conduct of human beings is actually so extraordinarily complex that the concept of the pure or isolated instinct is of no real value. Upon this there followed within a few years a rapid succession of "anti-instinct" writings.[2]

This attack on the instinct doctrine has taken many forms, of which only a few can be considered here. Views somewhat similar to Dunlap's have been developed by Kantor.[3] His "organismic psychology" pictures each response as the behaviour of the organism as a whole, in which the attempt to isolate instincts is futile. Kantor, like Watson, makes the interpenetration of innate and learned factors the basis for all complex forms of activity ; but he goes farther than Watson, refusing to utilize even those elementary instinctive patterns which Watson had been content to describe as isolated units. Watsonian behaviourism, to be sure, had already insisted that behaviour is to be seen as a totality ;

[1] "Are There Any Instincts ? " *J. Abn. Psychol.*, XIV, 1919–20.
[2] Bernard's *Instinct* (1924), lists over three hundred books and articles on the topic, many of which are expressions of the controversy which began in 1919.
[3] "A Functional Interpretation of Human Instincts," *Psychol. Rev.*, XXVII, 1920; "The Problem of Instinct and its Relation to Social Psychology," *J. Abn. Psychol. and Soc. Psychol.*, XVIII, 1923–4.

the writings of Kantor have more fully expounded the implications of such a view.

Watson's *Psychology from the Standpoint of a Behaviorist* (1919) introduced into *human* psychology a conception similar to that already offered in his *Behavior: an Introduction to Comparative Psychology* (1914), namely, that the term instinct should be used to denote " a combination of congenital responses unfolding serially under appropriate stimulation . . . a series of concatenated reflexes."[1] The view defended in the *Psychology from the Standpoint of a Behaviorist,* his first systematic discussion of human psychology, was, however, more radical ; he dispensed altogether with the great majority of human instincts postulated by previous writers. He listed under the caption of " instinct " a number of reflexes found in early childhood, such as the series of reflexes connected with hunger, and as " emotions " (implicit, mainly visceral, pattern-responses) three reactions appearing immediately after birth : fear, rage, and love.   In a survey of James's and Thorndike's lists of human instincts he repudiated the claim that such complex activities as " hunting " and " gregariousness," etc., are innate. He insisted on the significance of consolidation between innate and habitual factors in the production of compounds easily mistaken for instincts.

The most sweeping attack on the instinct concept was that of Kuo.[2] Not contenting himself with the demolition of human instincts, and emphasizing especially the data from animal psychology, he insisted that there are no complex innate patterns whatever. Kuo urged that the only clear-cut mechanism to be found beyond that of the simple reflex is an internal adjustment, to which he gave the name " behaviour-set." The behaviour-set lowers the threshold for certain stimuli and raises it for others. If we consider the animal as a bundle of reflex-arcs, some are facilitated, others inhibited by the behaviour-set of the moment. But the behaviour-set is itself a learned (that is, a conditioned) adjustment. The separate reflexes, varying with the behaviour-set, are integrated through trial-and-error ; but the behaviour-set itself varies with the animal's experience.

[1] P. 106 of *Behavior.*
[2] " Giving Up Instincts in Psychology," *J. Philos.*, XVIII, 1921 ; " How Are Our Instincts Acquired ? " *Psychol. Rev.*, XXIX, 1922.

Some postural attitudes, for example, are effective in food-getting or fighting ; the conditioning process operates not only upon the eating or struggling reflexes, but upon the postures which play so large a part in the animal's adjustment. Nothing, therefore, is left of instinct.[1]

F. H. Allport,[2] emphasizing the data from Watson's experiments, reduces most of the socially significant human activities to habits based upon six " prepotent reflexes." The stimuli which may elicit these become, through conditioning, very numerous, and the forms of response undergo a parallel " efferent modification." In view of his emphasis upon intraorganic stimuli, attention has several times been called to similarities between his own system and that of McDougall. An examination, however, of Allport's treatment of such important social phenomena as crowds, public opinion, etc., shows these to be attributed to very primitive reflex tendencies, such as the " sensitive-zone reflexes " aroused in tickling, together with primitive tendencies to struggle, withdraw, and the like. Even such patterns as fear, rage, and sex conduct are treated not as complex pattern instincts but (following Watson) as learned behaviour based upon very simple and primitive infantile reflexes.

While such attacks upon the instinct doctrine have gathered headway among psychologists, the sociologists and economists have not been loath to speed the parting guest ; Ogburn[3] and Bernard[4], among others, have brought together an extensive collection of material to indicate that social behaviour is more intelligibly conceived in terms of a social pattern carried on by tradition than in terms of patterns inherited by the individual.

Strangely enough, few of the many authors who have taken

---

[1] McDougall, in replying to these various attacks, has made it clear that he is willing to concede much as regards the modifiability of instinct, but that his chief interest is in the emotional core of the patterns, and in the " purposive striving " which distinguishes instinct from a mechanical process. In this teleological conception he has had the support of several British and American psychologists, notably Tolman (*e.g.* " Instinct and Purpose," *Psychol. Rev.*, XXVII, 1920) ; though the forms of teleology are diverse and the frankly " animistic " conception of purpose is distinctively McDougall's own. See " The Use and Abuse of Instinct in Social Psychology," *J. Abn. and Soc. Psychol.*, XVI. 1921-2.
[2] *Social Psychology* (1924), Chapter III.
[3] *Social Change* (1923).
[4] *Instinct* (1924) ; *An Introduction to Social Psychology* (1926)

part in the discussion have availed themselves of the experimental data on animal behaviour which have been accumu-
lating during the present century.   The emphasis upon such
data has recently served to clarify much which the data from
human psychology could not directly disclose.   The studies
of Allport, Woodworth, Watson, Lashley, and others, have
called attention to materials pertinent to the controversy,
while the last few years have yielded new experimental
results.

The Peckhams' book, *Wasps, Social and Solitary*, had
shown as early as 1905 that some supposedly fixed patterns
of response, for example, the behaviour of some species of
wasps which sting a caterpillar so as to paralyse it, was not
actually so efficient and invariable as had been assumed.
A few years later Craig,[1] studying the sexual behaviour of
male doves reared in isolation, found that the pattern of
sexual response appeared in the young male dove without
any education whatever, but that the pattern could be elicited
by the one living object with which the isolated birds had
contact, namely, the experimenter's hand.[2]   Clearly, the
problem of complex inherited reaction-patterns had to be
distinguished from the problem of the stimuli which arouse
them.   The same comment applies to much subsequent
work, *e.g.*, to the demonstration by Yerkes and Bloomfield[3]
of the fact that young kittens did in some cases kill and eat
mice, without undergoing instruction in the art ; the range
of stimuli upon which kittens might pounce was not determined.   A systematic study of the rôle of instinct in sex-
behaviour is that of C. P. Stone.[4]   Using the male albino rat,
he found several distinct kinds of activities that he could
classify as sexual.   Some of these activities were very efficient
when the male was first brought near the female, but some of
them were very inefficient at first and required practice.
Stone's work tends to discredit, on the one hand, the " lump "
treatment of instinct, so to speak, as this had come down from
McDougall, the tendency to regard the instinct as a single

[1] " Male Doves Reared in Isolation," *J. An. Beh.*, IV, 1914.
[2] Whitman (*Orthogenic Evolution in Pigeons*, III, 1919) has found that
male ring-doves reared among carrier-pigeons will not mate with females
of their own species, but with carriers.
[3] " Do Kittens Instinctively Kill Mice ? " *Psychol. Bull.*, VII, 1910.
[4] " The Congenital Sexual Behavior of the Young Male Albino Rat,"
J. Comp. Psychol., II, 1922.

entity. The results are, on the other hand, explicitly stated by Stone to be incompatible with such anti-instinct views as had been offered by Kuo. That there are complex inherited patterns in the rat which operate efficiently the first time seems clear.

Nevertheless much light has been thrown on the problem by the concept of the threshold, emphasized by Kuo, but current in psychology especially since the work of Sherrington.[1] The study of hunger is illustrative. Cannon[2] had shown that the physical basis of hunger-pangs lies in the contraction of unstriped muscles of the stomach. Watson,[3] in his study of infants, had found that the sucking reflex could be much more easily elicited when the child was hungry than immediately after feeding. Putting the two facts together, it seemed possible to think of the "hunger instinct" in terms of the raising and lowering of reflex thresholds in consequence of variations in an intraorganic state. Woodworth[4] had suggested in 1921 that instinct could be regarded as a "drive" which facilitated some action-systems and inhibited others. The work of C. R. Moore,[5] Stone[6], and others has made it clear that the threshold for sexual behaviour is lowered by the internal secretions of sex ; the arousal of the reflex patterns of sexual activity depends, in fact, upon these internal chemical factors. Lashley summarizes the evidence concisely : " We are forced to the conclusion that it [the chemical factor] acts in some way to lower the resistance of definite reflex pathways so as to integrate or make excitable the reflex mechanisms of the sexual reactions."[7] Much of the outline of the controversy became blurred through this introduction of the concept of the threshold,

---

[1] *The Integrative Action of the Nervous System* (1906).

[2] *The Mechanical Factors of Digestion* (1911).

[3] *Psychology from the Standpoint of a Behaviorist.* 2nd ed. (1924), pp. 259-60.

[4] *Psychology, A Study of Mental Life* (1921), Chapter VI.

[5] " On the Physiological Properties of the Gonads as Controllers of Somatic and Psychical Characteristics," I, The Rat, *J. Exp. Zool.*, XXVIII, 1919.

[6] " Experimental Studies of Two Important Factors Underlying Masculine Sexual Behaviour : the Nervous System and the Internal Secretion of the Testis," *J. Exp. Psychol.*, VI, 1923 ; " Further Study of Sensory Functions in the Activation of Sexual Behaviour in the Young Male Albino Rat," *J. Comp. Psychol.*, III, 1923.

[7] " Contributions of Freudism to Psychology : III, Physiological Analysis of the Libido," *Psychol. Rev.*, XXXI, 1924, pp. 196-7.

the fact becoming evident that the disagreement between the friends and the enemies of instinct was in large part terminological. The tendency is apparent in recent work to think in terms of action systems which are more freely aroused in some situations than in others, the distinctive difference between reflex and instinct (if the latter term be admitted) lying in an intraorganic condition. This intraorganic factor, though corresponding to Kuo's " behaviour set," appears to be, at least in many cases, innate[1] ; but the possibility of very early, perhaps even pre-natal, conditioning, must of course be kept in mind.

F. H. Allport[2] and others of the anti-instinct group have emphasized the impossibility of proving the innate nature of complex human responses except when these appear at birth or immediately thereafter ; and in the absence of proof that such behaviour as " collecting," " curiosity," and " gregariousness " are innate, they have contended that environment offers a more probable explanation. One *possibility*, however, they regard as still open for the instinct-defenders ; namely, that such instincts, though not present at birth, " mature " later[3] ; just as the infant's teeth, though absent at birth, can scarcely be explained as " learned." They have, consequently, devoted their attention to the *elimination* of this " maturation " hypothesis. Allport makes good use, for example, of work published as early as 1913 by Shepard and Breed.[4] These experimenters placed chicks, as soon as hatched, in small boxes in which it was not possible for them to peck ; another group of chicks was allowed to peck for food as soon as they emerged from the shell. The first group was divided into a number of sub-groups, liberated from the boxes at various intervals after hatching. Daily records were kept of the progress of all these groups in reaching adult proficiency in pecking. The data showed that all groups improved rapidly with practice, but that those liberated late started with as poor a score as those which pecked on the first day of their lives. This Allport offers as evidence that no specific maturation was present, in terms of

---

[1] See Carlson, *The Control of Hunger in Health and Disease* (1916), for evidence that hunger contractions occur before birth.

[2] *Social Psychology* (1924).

[3] See, *e.g.*, James, *Principles of Psychology* II, p. 398.

[4] " Maturation and Use in the Development of an Instinct," *J. An. Beh.*, III, 1913.

definite sensori-motor connections which had ripened in the first few days. The data of Shepard and Breed, however, indicated that those liberated late very rapidly overtook their fellows, so that, at ten days of age, all groups were approximately equal. Allport interpreted this as the result of a *general* neuro-muscular growth rather than of *specific* maturation at some point in the nervous system.

But the facts do not appear to be so simple ; some good instances of specific maturation have been reported. Tilney and Casamajor[1], for example, using many litters of kittens, discovered extraordinary uniformity in the sudden appearance of such complex patterns as the animal's ability to raise itself on its hind quarters and some escape-reactions : and histological study showed that a great variety of such suddenly-appearing patterns depended directly upon the maturation of specific neural pathways, in consequence of the development of the myelin sheath within the necessary tracts. Even if all the facts were clear in the case of other species, it is doubtful whether psychology is yet in a position to determine the status of the maturation problem for human beings. A few cases of maturation in human beings appear to exist (the disappearance of the infantile Babinski reflex is known to be due to myelinization of the pyramidal tract), but such simple reactions throw no clear light on the nature of more complex patterns.

There exists, of course, a great mass of experimental evidence on the instinct problem collected by zoologists, of which psychologists have taken very little account. In fact, the disregard of the existing factual material pertinent to the problem has been an essential part of the rapid change of opinion, governed to such a large degree by controversialism and the desire to impose a stark simplicity upon the varieties of human and animal conduct. Much more analytical study appears needed to determine just what reaction-patterns are present in each species at birth, to what extent and in what ways these are governed by intraorganic conditions, in what ways they are modified, and to what extent maturation, interwoven with the learning process, may play its part. Students of animal behaviour have in recent years begun to provide us with just such materials. The work of Stone, mentioned

[1] " Myelinogeny as Applied to the Study of Behavior," *Arch. of Neurol. and Psychiatry*, XII, 1924.

above, illustrates the tendency of the controversy over *instinct in general* to give place to the genetic study of the intricacies of *specific* behaviour patterns. J. B. Watson's study of infant behaviour and the many recent studies of behaviour patterns as they undergo alteration early in life[1] have in the same way made possible a more systematic inductive study of human instincts.

[1] M. C. Jones, " The Development of Early Behaviour Patterns in Young Children," *Ped. Sem.*, XXXIII, 1926.

CHAPTER XXI

THE MEASUREMENT OF INTELLIGENCE

Reason, however, in the sense of intelligence, is not found equally in all animals, nor in all men.—*Aristotle.*

No movement is more characteristic of contemporary psychology than the endeavour to devise adequate means of measuring human abilities. Theories of intelligence and the practical attempt at measurement have been interwoven to a degree necessitating their joint treatment. As the work has progressed, however, quantitative data have accumulated faster than they have been assimilated, and our *emphasis*, if we are to give a fair picture of the development, must be upon the technical rather than upon the theoretical advances.

Ebbinghaus's measurement of learning and memory led immediately to Jacobs's study of the "memory span" (see p. 192), while in the same period tests of simple sensory and motor functions became popular. As early as 1890 Cattell[1] outlined some of the problems of "mental testing." In 1894 he and Farrand[2] gave a number of tests to college freshmen and seniors, measuring reaction-time, free and controlled association, and other simple mental and physical functions.

In 1897 Ebbinghaus[3] offered both a theory of intelligence and a technique by which intellectual capacity was to be measured. Intelligence, he suggested, is the ability to combine or integrate. His "completion tests" consisted of sentences containing gaps to be filled in by the subject. The paradigm "who dragged whom around the walls of what?" or rather, as it would have appeared in Ebbinghaus's scheme, "——— dragged ——— around the walls of ———," illustrates the method. Such tests lent themselves to the study of information as in the case just

---

[1] " Mental Tests and Measurements," *Mind*, XV, 1890.
[2] Cattell and Farrand, " Physical and Mental Measurements of the Students of Columbia University," *Psychol. Rev.*, III, 1896.
[3] *Zeitschr. f. Psychol.*, XIII, 1897.

stated, or of an original activity of the subject, as in the sentence, "the bitter ———— swept into the unheated ————, and the shuddering ———— no longer barked but whined." Ebbinghaus was chiefly concerned with the ability to integrate the items presented with other items necessary to complete a pattern, that is, with *intelligence* as he understood it, rather than information. The method has proved susceptible of numerous uses. Not only sentences but pictures may be thus mutilated and restored ; in fact, the ability to fill in gaps has been measured in a great many forms, both verbal and non-verbal. Although Ebbinghaus's theory of intelligence has not won general acceptance, his tests have done so, and have in fact been found to correlate highly with other measures of general ability.

The use of tests of simple sensori-motor and associative functions was continued, especially in the United States. Kirkpatrick,[1] working with a large number of subjects, compared such mental-test scores with achievement as shown in other ways, for example, with school work. In 1903 Kelly[2] and in 1906 Norsworthy[3] compared, by means of such tests, normal and defective children. The results indicated that the feeble-minded tended to do distinctly less well than the normal, but that there was a fairly even transition from the lowest to the highest scores. In Norsworthy's language, the feeble-minded were not a " species " ; the more intelligent of the feeble-minded could not be sharply distinguished from the least intelligent of the normal.

During the 'nineties Binet had occupied himself with attempts to devise suitable measures of intelligence. In 1904, the year after Binet's publication of his experimental study of thought processes (p. 239), the Minister of Public instruction appointed Binet as a member of a commission on special classes in the schools. When children were failing in the school work for their age, it was important to differentiate between the mentally deficient and the indifferent or lazy. In collaboration with Simon, Binet undertook the task of devising tests suited to the immediate practical task

---

[1] " Individual Tests of School Children," *Psychol. Rev.*, VII, 1900.
[2] " Psychophysical Tests of Normal and Abnormal Children," *Psychol. Rev.*, X.
[3] " The Psychology of Mentally Deficient Children," *Arch. of Psychol.*, No. I.

of detecting and measuring mental defect. They offered in 1905 a set of tests arranged from the simplest to the most difficult, but without further standardization.[1] Among these were tests requiring the naming of designated objects, the comparison of lengths of lines, the repetition of digits, the completion of sentences, and the comprehension of questions.[2] In 1908 this scale was revised,[3] practical experience having shown that some of the tests were harder and others easier than was at first supposed. Another very important change was introduced. The tests were arranged according to the age levels, experimentally determined, at which the average child performed them successfully, from three to twelve years inclusive. A child's " mental age " was the level which he attained on this scale ; the child of six might be able to pass the tests for age seven or eight, or only those for age four or five. This scale was translated and adapted for American use by Goddard[4] in 1910. In the following year Healy and G. Fernald published a set of tests which at once became widely known.[5]

Binet offered another revision of his scale in 1911, the year of his death.[6] His steady progress in the devising of tests was accompanied by much indecision and many changes of opinion regarding the essential characteristics of intelligence. Among the many definitions of intelligence which he suggested at one time or another, probably the most characteristic of his trend of thought is one in which not a *single* capacity but a combination of *three* different capacities was emphasized. Intelligence, he suggested, is the ability to understand directions, to maintain a mental set, and to apply " auto-criticism " (the correction of one's own errors).

The problems of intelligence-testing began to attract much attention in Germany, where Meumann had already conducted pioneer investigations. Stern[7] made an important contribution to method by suggesting a change in the calculation of test scores. Binet had been content to measure sub-

[1] *Année Psychol.*, XI, 1905 (several articles).

[2] De Sanctis published a short scale of mental tests in the year following, *Annal. di Neurologia*, XXIV, 1906.

[3] *Année Psychol.*, XIV, 1908.

[4] " A Measuring Scale for Intelligence," *The Training School*, VI, 1910.

[5] " Tests for Practical Mental Classification," *Psychol. Monogr.*, XIII, 1910–11.

[6] *Année Psychol.*, XVII, 1911.

[7] *The Psychological Methods of Testing Intelligence* (1912).
AA

normality by subtracting mental age from chronological age. Stern urged that the absolute retardation in years was of less importance than the relative retardation ; and suggested the use of the Intelligence Quotient (I Q), obtained by dividing the mental age by the chronological age. He showed, moreover, that this quotient is fairly constant, from year to year, for most children.

Another important step in technique was Terman's[1] revision of the Binet Scale. His " Stanford Revision " of 1916 was based upon work with about one thousand subjects, and standardized in the form of tests for age-levels from three years to eighteen (the sixteen-year-old tests were devised for adults, while the eighteen-year-old tests were for " superior " adults). Many of Binet's tests were placed at higher or lower age-levels than those at which Binet had placed them, and new tests were added. Each age-level was represented by a battery of tests, each test being assigned a certain number of month-credits. It was possible, therefore, to reckon the subject's Intelligence Quotient or " IQ," as Stern had suggested, in terms of the ratio of mental age to chronological age. A child attaining a score of 120 months, but only 100 months old, would have an " IQ " of 1·20. This intelligence quotient was found by Terman, as by Stern, to be fairly constant from year to year.[2]

Another revision, the Yerkes-Bridges Point Scale,[3] had in the meantime been published, making use of a series of tests of gradually increasing difficulty, the authors believing that the concept of mental age was of very doubtful value. Terman's scale has nevertheless been by far the most popular of scales for individual testing, and the concept of mental age continues to be employed in a great many other intelligence tests.[4] Kuhlmann's[5] revision of the Binet scale, including

---

[1] *The Measurement of Intelligence* (1916).

[2] *The Intelligence of School Children* (1919). Marked variation in I Q has, however, been reported by Woolley, " The Validity of Standards of Mental Measurement in Young Childhood," *School and Society*, XXI, 1925, and by others.

[3] Yerkes, Bridges, and Hardwick, *A Point Scale for Measuring Mental Ability* (1915). These tests allowed fractional credits instead of scoring the response to each test simply as right or wrong.

[4] A very similar revision of the Binet-Simon scale is the work of Herring, *Herring Revision of the Binet-Simon Tests, and Verbal and Abstract Elements in Intelligence Examinations* (1924).

[5] *A Handbook of Mental Tests* (1922).

tests below the three-year level, has more recently come into use. Its emphasis on language factors is less than that of the Stanford scale. One other revision must be noted, the elaborate and systematic work of Burt,[1] adapted especially for use in Great Britain.[2]

The necessity for " performance tests " for those suffering from linguistic (or sensory) handicaps had already been met by the Seguin, Witmer, and Healy form-boards. Holes of various sizes were, for example, to be filled by appropriate blocks. The *standardization* of performance tests and the construction of scales for mental age occurred very shortly after Terman's work. The Pintner-Paterson[3] scale makes use of such materials as a Healy test consisting of dissected pictures which are to be reconstructed, and many similar tests in which the recognition of spatial relations is emphasized. A great many performance tests and a considerable number of performance " scales " are now in use. The results from such performance tests, however, have made it clear that the ability to manipulate things is scarcely the same as the ability to manipulate words (or other symbols). Whereas it is generally agreed that any two batteries of intelligence tests ought to correlate with one another at least as high as + ·70, batteries of performance tests have usually been found to correlate less than + ·50 with the ordinary intelligence tests.

Notwithstanding the very large number of children examined in schools and clinics by the Stanford test, immediately upon its publication, it was not civil but military experience which made clear the fact that such an extensive testing programme called, in many cases, for " group tests " rather than "individual tests." In 1917 psychologists devised for use in the United States Army a group scale " Alpha " for literate English-speaking recruits, and a group scale " Beta " for illiterates and non-English-speaking recruits.[4] The Alpha comprised a " following directions " test, arithmetic and information tests, and much other verbal material ; the " Beta," though of a paper-and-pencil

---

[1] *Mental and Scholastic Tests* (1921).

[2] Some differences between British and American test usage, as in the case of coinage, are inevitable. Burt's revision, however, is not a mere adaptation of any American scale.

[3] *A Scale of Performance Tests* (1917).

[4] *Memoirs of the National Academy of Sciences*, XV, 1921.

variety, emphasized the subject's ability to grasp spatial and other non-verbal relations which could be visually represented. Shortly thereafter, the use of group tests in surveys of the public schools became frequent, and many tests for different age-levels were prepared. The educational uses of intelligence tests[1] in the United States are reflected in hundreds of titles in psychological and educational journals, and cannot even be summarized here. Among the most important of such uses are first, the classification of pupils in accordance with their intelligence, in order that pupils widely separated in mental age may not be forced into the same group, and second, the examination of the probable cause for poor scholarship so that (as the French authorities wished) laziness may be distinguished from dullness. In general, group tests are more frequently used for classification, and individual tests for the analysis of maladjustment. The devising of satisfactory tests for the higher levels of intelligence has necessarily proved difficult, but has attained a degree of success sufficient to cause many American colleges to utilize such tests for the classification of applicants for admission and for other administrative purposes.[2]

The testing movement has engaged less attention in Great Britain and on the Continent than in the United States. But a number of investigators, notably Meumann and Stern, Bobertag[3] and Jaederholm,[4] have contributed materially to the advancement of testing methods in education and in industry, while Stern's[5] theory of intelligence has exerted a special influence. Intelligence, he urged, is "general mental adaptability to new problems and conditions of life." The difficulty of separating innate from acquired abilities, already evident in the work of Cattell, Ebbinghaus, and Binet, was directly faced. Tests of intelligence were regarded as valid in so far as the tasks imposed were genuinely new. Some degree of similarity must, of course, exist between the new tasks and some established habit, but intelligence is precisely the ability to utilize old responses in relatively new situations. James had written, " Geniuses are, by common consent, considered to

---

[1] And of many "educational" and "achievement" tests.
[2] See, for example, Wood. *Measurement in Higher Education* (1923).
[3] *E.g., Zeitschr. f. angewandte Psychol.*, V, 1911.
[4] *E.g., Zeitschr. f. angewandte Psychol.*, XI, 1916.
[5] *The Psychological Methods of Testing Intelligence* (1912).

differ from ordinary minds by an unusual development of association by similarity."[1] Stern's definition makes use both of this conception of recognizing similarities and of the notion of adaptation or adjustment.

The development of the technique of testing, especially for practical purposes, has been so rapid in the United States that relatively little attention has been given to the analysis of the nature of intelligence. Terman[2] has emphasized the ability to think conceptually. Thorndike has emphasized the relative independence of each specific function, and the conception that intelligence is not " homogeneous "[3] : intelligence might be regarded as the sum-total of many distinct functions. Such a *multi-factor* theory is in sharp contrast to those *uni-factor* theories (*e.g.*, that of Ebbinghaus) which regard intelligence as a single function. The fact that the various tests of abilities do not correlate perfectly with one another has seemed to present serious difficulties for any uni-factor theory, while the fact that most tests of abilities do present *some* positive correlation with one another has offered similar difficulties for the " multi-factor " theories.

Various compromises have been urged. The great advance of testing technique and, in particular, of statistical method in connection with it, has brought into great prominence a theory offered by Spearman[4] as early as 1904. It is necessary, Spearman believes, to take account in every human ability of two factors, one general and one specific. General ability, or " G," plays some part in nearly every human activity. In some activities, such as science, philosophy, and executive tasks, success depends largely upon this general factor. In other functions, such as skill in many of the arts and crafts, the importance of general ability is much less marked, success depending on much more specific aptitudes. Each individual possesses many such

---

[1] *Principles of Psychology*, II, p. 348.
[2] In symposium noted on p. 354.
[3] See, *e.g.*, *Educational Psychology*, III (1914). There is, of course, a close relation between the theory of intelligence and the theory of the transfer of training (see p. 254). Thorndike, for example, would regard any two intellectual functions as entirely distinct except in so far as they possess *identical elements*.
[4] " General Intelligence Objectively Determined and Measured," *Am. J. Psychol.*, XV, 1904. See also " The Theory of Two Factors," *Psychol. Rev.*, XXI, 1914, and *The Abilities of Man*, etc. (1927).

specific abilities, each one of which may, like "G," be measured. Every activity, in fact, calls into play at least one special ability or " S," while nearly all demand also the use of " G." Tasks in which " G " is relatively important may be said to involve " G " in greater " saturation " than those in which it plays a minor part. " G " can never be *directly* measured, but through the study of correlations many functions involving " G " may be compared in such fashion as to make its *indirect* measurement possible.

Thomson[1], on the other hand, has urged against this theory the fact that even " chance " combinations, such as those obtained by throwing dice, reveal a " general " factor, while Spearman has replied[2] that this factor lies not in the dice, but in the manner in which the results were grouped by the experimenter. Notwithstanding the great statistical complexity of the evidence and the unwillingness of most psychologists to reach a final conclusion at present, the theory has provided a clear and valuable hypothesis for research.

Many modifications of Spearman's theory have been suggested. For example, Woodrow[3] postulates between general ability and each of the special abilities, a level of abilities less general than the one and less specific than the other. Between arithmetical ability and general intelligence there may lie, for example, an all-round mathematical ability. Mathematical ability, verbal ability, etc., may be designated " group factors " ; Kelley,[4] Garrett, and others have, with greatly improved technique, offered evidence for the reality of independent group factors of this sort.

An international symposium[5] on the nature of intelligence in 1921 yielded many new theories, but none which have won general assent. In some quarters the attempt to define intelligence is regarded as premature, the investigators contenting themselves with the opinion nicely phrased by Thorndike that " intelligence is the thing that psychologists

---

[1] " General versus Group Factors in Mental Activities," *Psychol. Rev.*, XXVII, 1920.

[2] " Recent Contributions to the ' Theory of Two Factors,' " *Brit J. Psychol.*, XIII, 1922-23.

[3] *Brightness and Dullness in Children* (1919), Chapter XI.

[4] *Crossroads in the Mind of Man* (1928).

[5] " Intelligence and Its Measurement," *J. Ed. Psychol.*, XII, 1921.

test when they test intelligence."[1]   This is, of course, not a *finale*, but merely an *interlude;* new theories of intelligence continually appear.

Though most of the evidence on the nature of intelligence appears to be of statistical character, experimental methods do not seem entirely inapplicable.   Woodrow has shown, for example, in normal and feeble-minded children, that intelligence-test scores are closely related to the ability to learn.[2] It may well be that a closer liaison between intelligence-testing on the one hand and the experimental psychology of learning on the other hand are already in the process of giving a more satisfactory answer to the problem of intelligence.

The psychologist's preoccupation with measurements of intelligence has been accompanied in recent years by an intensive study of the inheritance of intellectual endowment. Research on the inheritance of mental traits has very naturally seen its most rapid development in relation to intellectual inheritance, rather than in relation to those aspects of personality which have yielded more slowly to quantitative attack. Perhaps ninety per cent. of all the work done in the field of mental inheritance has concerned itself with intelligence.

As early as 1869 Galton had undertaken to show in his *Hereditary Genius* that superior intelligence is inherited. His method, the study of lines of descent and of collateral branches, a procedure known as the pedigree method, was adopted in 1877 by Dugdale, who (though himself an environmentalist) showed in *The Jukes* the continuance of mental deficiency within the family stock for several generations.[3] Many investigations of mental deficiency by the pedigree method have followed, of which perhaps the best known is Goddard's *The Kallikak Family* (1912).   In the early years

---

[1] In an informal address (unpublished).   Thorndike's recent work emphasizes four major " intellectual " functions ; the sum of abilities in these functions correlates highly with scores on standard intelligence tests.   See his *Measurement of Intelligence* (1926).

[2] " Practice and Transference in Normal and Feeble-minded Children," *J. Ed. Psychol.*, VIII, 1917.   See also the more detailed experimental and theoretical analysis of learning contributed by Pyle in his *Nature and Development of Learning Capacity* (1925).

[3] In 1916, the work was brought up to date by Estabrook, in *The Jukes in 1915.*

of the century another pedigree study, in which heredity and environment were directly compared, was presented in Woods's article, " Mental and Moral Heredity in Royalty."[1] He consulted such historical and biographical material as is available in relation to royal families, with a view to determining to what extent various levels of ability are traceable to heredity. (The study of royal families has a decided advantage, since historical data make possible the tracing of the line through many centuries.) He offered evidence to show that the wide variations in ability are not attributable to education.

The pedigree method has inevitably been subject to some suspicion, because of the inaccuracy of the historical and questionnaire methods upon which it perforce relies. Many other traits have, however, been suggestively studied in the same way, and within recent years the use of questionnaires has been supplanted to some extent by more direct case studies of the living individuals concerned. Such a combination of case method with pedigree method, in the study of children of unusual ability, is found in the recent work of Terman[2] and his collaborators.

But the status of the whole problem of mental inheritance was greatly affected by the rediscovery,[3] about 1900, of Mendel's laws of inheritance. Mendel[4] had discovered, a little past the middle of the nineteenth century, a series of fundamental laws of heredity. First, in studying familiar plants, such as the sweet pea, he found that individuals of unlike colour yielded hybrid offspring resembling one parent much more than the other. The colour of one parent was " dominant." Now, when such hybrids were mated, twenty-five per cent. of their offspring reverted to the colour which had disappeared in the first hybrid generation ; they displayed the " recessive " trait which had characterized one grandparent. Seventy-five per cent. showed the " dominant " character. It was evident that the " skipping of generations " need no longer remain a mystery. It was important to distinguish between " body-plasm " and " germ-plasm," and to look in the latter for the elements which, in ever-

---

[1] *Popular Science Monthly*, LXI, 1902 ; LXII, 1903. (Also in book form.)

[2] *Genetic Studies of Genius*, I (1925).

[3] Independently by De Vries, Correns, and Tschermak.

[4] *Versuche über Pflanzenhybriden* (1865-9).

varying combinations, give rise to the diversities of body-structure. Germinal elements, though recessive for a while, may, when uniting with other recessive elements, cause the reappearance of a body character. This view seemed to imply that a large number of changes which occur from generation to generation can be explained not by the influence of changes occurring in the body, but by the reshifting of elements in the germ-cells. In the 'eighties and 'nineties Weismann[1] showed clearly that the germ-cells preserve a continuity of their own ; that each germ-cell can be traced back in its lineage to other germ-cells, and that germ-cells are rather remarkably free from influence from the vicissitudes of the body which has enclosed them. He showed experimentally that it is possible to injure body-structure without affecting the germ-cells. This conception has necessarily been of profound import for all studies of heredity ; its significance for psychology has been seen in the rigid exclusion of explanations of mental life in terms of " ancestral experience " and " ancestral habits." To be sure, psychologists had been wary (even in the heyday of Lamarck) of assuming the inheritance of acquired characters, but they became doubly so after Weismann's work. Changes from generation to generation were now explained solely in terms of variations within the germ-cells themselves. Later De Vries[2] pointed out that the germ-cell might undergo *mutation*, and that a new species might arise as the result of such germinal changes. This made it possible to think of changes in species not so much in terms of slight variations, such as Darwin had emphasized, as in terms of large and permanent alterations in the germinal constitution.

With this work of Weismann and De Vries, and with the rediscovery of the Mendelian principles, an attempt was made to apply these Mendelian concepts to the phenomena of human heredity. The publications of the *Eugenics Record Office*[3] have combined a thorough-going Mendelism with the use of the pedigree method. Davenport[4] has urged, for example, that both mental deficiency and certain defects in self-control are true Mendelian traits. The complexity of the mental

---

[1] *E.g.*, *The Germ Plasm* (1893).
[2] *Die Mutationstheorie* (1900).
[3] At Cold Spring Harbor, New York.
[4] *The Hill Folk* (1912) ; *The Feebly Inhibited* (1915).

traits whose hereditary principles are sought, and the difficulty of accurately gauging environmental influences, have prevented most of these contributions from attracting wide attention.

A very large mass of material has, however, been collected by Goddard[1] on the subject of the inheritance of mental deficiency, with results which have aroused much discussion. Goddard first studied the inmates of the Training School at Vineland, New Jersey, and then proceeded to investigate their parents, grandparents, brothers and sisters, uncles and aunts, etc. He collected his data through the efforts of case-workers who visited the homes and neighbourhoods from which the inmates came. They gathered data regarding the mentality, the activities, and the economic and social position of each near relative. In a great many cases fairly definite proof of feeble-mindedness was found even when the data were obtained at second hand. Some of the relatives were universally reported to be " half-witted " ; of others it was learned that they were not only respected but maintaining themselves in callings requiring considerable intelligence. Where evidence was consistent, the case was reported in the form of " normal " or " feeble-minded " ; when inconsistent, it was classified as " undetermined." Granting the many sources of error in such information, the data obtained show such a large proportion of unclassified cases as to suggest that considerable caution was used. The data on normals and defectives were in definite and precise terms for tabulation.

Goddard's more than 1,700 cases were then scrutinized with respect to the Mendelian formula ; early inspection of the figures suggested the hypothesis that primary feeble-mindedness (that is, mental defect not due to accident or illness) is a Mendelian trait recessive to normal intelligence ; thus feeble-mindedness would appear only when germinal taint enters from both the paternal and maternal lines. He then undertook to verify the hypothesis, by determining whether it was possible to " predict " the status of the children of the mating of two individuals whose family trees had been studied. When both parents are feeble-minded (excluding, of course, cases due to accident and disease), *all* the children should by hypothesis be feeble-minded. The

---

[1] *Feeble-mindedness: Its Causes and Consequences* (1914).

status of 482 such children was ascertained; of these, 476 were feeble-minded. Another group of cases includes those where one parent was feeble-minded and the other, though normal, presumably carried a recessive germinal taint ; where F represents feeble-minded, and N normal, such a mating would be indicated FF-NF. The theoretical expectation from 371 cases would be $185\frac{1}{2}$ normal and the same number feeble-minded ; actually, the numbers were 178 and 193 respectively. (The evidence for the NF constitution of any parent depends, of course, on the parent's own ancestry and the collateral branches. If one of his parents is classified as normal, and the other as congenitally feeble-minded, or if some of his brothers are feeble-minded, he should, if himself normal, be classified as NF. Goddard's hypothesis was applied to the whole mass of data, not merely to one generation, with a view to determining whether the working hypothesis accorded with the figures obtained.) Next came the offspring of NN and FF parents—one parent being of sound stock, so far as known, on both sides, the other parent being congenitally feeble-minded. Here, if the hypothesis is correct, all children should be of NF constitution, " normality " being a dominant trait. The findings are in accord with the hypothesis ; no one of 34 such children was feeble-minded. The combination NF with NF would give one feeble-minded child to three normal children ; the findings were 39 out of 146. Again, with NN parentage on one side and NF on the other, the prediction would be that there would be no FF offspring whatever, with which prediction the data perfectly agree.

It is frequently said that accurate data can never be obtained by the case-study methods employed here and elsewhere in surveys of mental deficiency. But the result of confusion and error in quantitative procedure is regularly to produce chaos and indefiniteness ; it is not apt to produce definite results consistent with a clear hypothesis. Still, the major objection to Goddard's findings has arisen from considerations relating to the " normal distribution " of intelligence—the fact, already noted, that the feeble-minded do not constitute a separate " species," but are simply those individuals whose intelligence lies below an arbitrarily selected point on a distribution curve. All that we know about heredity forces us to think of intelligence as depending

not on one, but on many hereditary factors ("genes");
and, consequently, to think of mental defect as an expression
not of one specific germinal defect but of a much more complex genetic composite.   Actually, Goddard gave consideration to this "multi-factor" interpretation.   And it does not
really appear to contradict his findings; we know, for
example, that, although human *stature* depends on *many*
"genes," nevertheless, a certain type of dwarfism is a Mendelian trait.   One gene may be so important in the picture that
no combination of other genes can atone for its absence.
At best, this is but speculation; the constitution of intelligence itself and of mental defect in particular is still far from
clear.   Goddard's exclusion of border-line and doubtful
cases made it possible to treat normal and feeble-minded as
opposed *types;* a much more complex technique would
be required to apply his conception to a large unselected
human group.

A similar Mendelian interpretation of two common mental
disorders, dementia præcox and the manic-depressive psycho-
sis, has been offered by Rosanoff and Orr.[1]   More recently
Myerson[2] has presented much material to discredit not only
the Mendelian interpretation of mental disorders, but even
the assertion that they are, in large part, traceable to heredity.
The work of geneticists has tended to make clear the wealth
and complexity of factors operative in the heredity of higher
forms, with the natural result that psychologists are not
inclined to look for the classical Mendelian ratios.   In the
meantime, psychiatry constantly contributes masses of data
on the environmental factors which appear to condition mental
disease, constantly revealing cases where—no matter how
important heredity may be—the impact of precipitating
factors must be reckoned of large importance.[3]

But with the refinement of intelligence tests, and with the
increasing recognition of the importance of *statistical
methods*, a more satisfactory approach to the problem of the
inheritance of intelligence has been offered.   With the

---

[1] " A Study of Heredity in Insanity in the Light of the Mendelian
Theory," *Am. J. Insan.*, LXVIII, 1911.   See also Rosanoff, " Dissim-
ilar Heredity in Mental Disease," *Am. J. Insan.*, LXX, 1913–4.
[2] *The Inheritance of Mental Diseases* (1925).
[3] Obscure physical factors have, of course, been given weight also.
A great many investigations have been published which, for example,
seek to establish a physico-chemical basis for dementia præcox.

recognition of the high probability that intelligence is a " multi-factor " trait, the meaning of correlation studies has been more clearly grasped ; such studies constitute our only adequate instrument for the determination of the behaviour of many genetic factors within family stocks. Pearson[1] showed as early as 1904 that brothers and sisters resemble one another in a variety of mental traits, to an extent closely comparable with results already obtained for admittedly hereditary physical traits. Whereas correlations between siblings in such traits as stature and cephalic index are about $+\cdot 50$, the resemblance in mental traits as reported by Pearson is nearly as large. The measurement of the latter traits was, however, based on ratings by acquaintances, especially upon teachers' estimates.[2]

Thorndike[3] made a statistical study of heredity based on direct measurement of individual abilities. He studied fifty pairs of twins, ranging in age from nine to fourteen years, in six mental functions, such as cancellation, addition, opposites, etc. He found that whereas the correlations between siblings (for these six mental functions) were in the neighbourhood of $+\cdot 30$, the correlations between twins were consistently upwards of $+\cdot 60$. This strongly suggested that the factor of heredity was of major importance. The difference between sibling and twin correlations is so large as to remind us of the difference between such correlations in the case of traits known to be hereditary. In reply to the natural contention that twins are subject to unusually similar environmental influences, Thorndike separated his group into " younger twins " and " older twins." He found no more resemblance between twins twelve to fourteen years of age than in those nine to eleven years of age, in spite of the fact that they had been subject on the average to three years more of environmental influence.

As Galton himself had recognized a generation before, this emphasis on twins is crucial in the approach to the problem of mental heredity. It may be said categorically

---

[1] " On the Laws of Inheritance in Man," *Biometrika*, III, Part ii.

[2] H. E. Jones, using Army Alpha, has reported rather high parent-child resemblances, *e.g.*, father-son, $r=.52$; mother-son, $r=.54$ (*Natl. Soc. for the Study of Education, Yearbook*, 1928).

[3] "Measurements of Twins," *Arch. of Phil., Psychol., and Sci. Meth.*, No. I, 1905.

that the germinal resemblance of twins is *in general* greater than that of siblings ; but early methods lumped together those most alike and those whose resemblances was less marked. The advance of biology in recent years has opened for the psychologist the problem of "identical twins." A recent study utilizing this distinction is Merriman's "The Intellectual Resemblance of Twins."[1] Merriman has shown that the correlations of twins in intelligence are not only much higher than the correlations found among ordinary siblings, but that the like-sex pairs must be sharply separated from the unlike-sex pairs.[2] Using the Stanford-Binet scale, he found that the correlation between unlike-sex pairs (38 cases) was +·504, a figure uncannily close to the +·50 expected by theory for fraternal resemblance in an inherited trait. But the correlation of intelligence in like-sex pairs of twins (67 cases) ran much higher, +·867 (the figure rising to +·908 in a group studied by the Beta test).

With the recognition, however, that variability in intelligence is the result of the combined effects of heredity and environment, special attention has been given to the study of cases in which the relative importance of the two can be directly estimated, *e.g.*, studies of foster children in which the change in IQ after exposure to a changed environment has been measured. The method of Freeman and his collaborators[3] differs from that of Burks,[4] yet the results agree in showing that environmental influences must be carefully weighed before the full value of an IQ can be judged.

Despite its difficulties, the quantitative analysis of individual abilities has made genuine progress, and we must now consider the way in which " the psychology of individual differences " has been able to make an approach toward the quantitative comparison of persons classified according to age, sex, race, and occupation.

First let us consider the variations of ability with age. In 1908 Binet established his " mental age " scale, which gave a

---

[1] *Psychol. Monogr.*, XXXIII, 1924.

[2] Identical twins (*i.e.*, those from the same ovum), are always of the same sex ; non-identical pairs may be of the same or of opposite sex.

[3] Freeman, Holzinger, and Mitchell, *Natl. Soc. for the Study of Education, Yearbook*, 1928.

[4] *Ibid.*

cross-section of certain abilities found in children at age-levels from three to twelve years. In the "Stanford Revision" Terman added tests for the period from twelve to sixteen years and made sixteen the level of "intellectual maturity." The assumption that the intelligence of most individuals does not progress beyond the sixteen-year level was based upon data from High School students and adult individuals. This assumption was crystallized in the standardization of the sixteen-year-old tests as tests for adults.[1] But data obtained in the United States Army[2] in 1917–18 strongly suggested that this sixteen-year level was too high. Several hundred soldiers took both the Stanford-Binet test and the Alpha test, making it possible to equate the scores on the two tests. Knowing what Stanford score corresponded to each Alpha score, it was possible to conclude from the vastly more extensive testing work in the Army that the average mental age of the white draft was somewhat under fourteen years. This did not, of course, indicate how much variability may exist in the age of attaining one's intellectual maturity ; it meant simply that the average intelligence of a fair sample of white male adults proved to be equal to the average intelligence of school children between thirteen and fourteen years of age. In 1919 Doll[3] undertook a study of over five hundred children from 9·5 to 15·5 years of age, from whose test scores he concluded that "*on the average*, or for 50 per cent. of presumably unselected cases, intelligence growth is practically complete at 13 years." This level was generally accepted for some time.[4]

On account of selective factors operative in the school population beyond fourteen, it proved difficult to gather satisfactory data on the variations in the exact form of the maturity curve in the neighbourhood of fourteen. Considerable change of opinion has occurred in recent years

---

[1] The eighteen-year-old tests, or tests for the "superior adult," were defensible either on the hypothesis that *some* individuals gain in intelligence beyond sixteen, or on the supposition that the unusually bright person may obtain a score which, because it does not fall within the scale, necessitates a higher standard (which for convenience takes the form of a higher age level).

[2] *Memoirs of the National Academy of Sciences*, XV, 1921 ; Brigham, *A Study of American Intelligence* (1923).

[3] "The Average Mental Age of Adults," *J. Appl. Psychol.*, III, 1919.

[4] Much discussion ensued as regards the educational and political implications of such alarming unintelligence.

as a result of the data of Thorndike,[1] Thurstone,[2] and others, indicating that measurable intelligence continues to increase even to eighteen years or beyond. Conclusions as to the average limit of intellectual growth, and especially as to individual differences, are not as yet clear.

To many behaviourists the discussion has been futile and irritating ; with their emphasis upon habit, they incline to the belief that intelligence-test scores may with proper training continue to rise indefinitely. To this the majority of students of in elligence-testing incline to reply that the test materials measure not stimulus-response patterns already acquired, but the ability to utilize such patterns in somewhat new contexts ; the ability to adjust oneself may, in fact, have an absolute limit.

The Army Alpha data threw some light also on the course of intellectual ability through the individual life-span. A sample of the Army population was classified according to age, from less than twenty to above fifty years. The data show a consistent decrease in intelligence throughout this span, the drop being slight from twenty to thirty, but somewhat accelerated thereafter. This drop is at least in part explicable by reference to selective factors. Men under twenty-one were mainly volunteers, and included reserve officers in training. The selective draft may have acted unevenly upon the span from twenty-one to thirty, while those above thirty were in large part "regular army men," among whom, through re-enlistment or return to civil life, many selective forces operate. On the other hand, those psychologists who emphasize learned rather than innate factors in test-performance naturally note that among older men there may be a decrease of *interest* in such verbal materials as comprise the bulk of the Alpha test, and of the ability to deal with them.

A much more direct and valuable attack upon the problem of the life-cycle of intelligence is that of Foster and Taylor.[3] They used many hundreds of subjects, for the purpose of a comparison of those above fifty years of age with those less

---

[1] *E.g.*, " On the Improvement in Intelligence Scores from Fourteen to Eighteen," *J. Ed. Psychol.*, XIV, 1923.

[2] " A Method of Scaling Psychological and Educational Tests," *J Ed. Psychol*, XVI, 1925.

[3] " The Applicability of Mental Tests to Persons over Fifty Years of Age," *J. Appl. Psychol.*, IV, 1920.

than thirty years of age.   Some members of each group were normal individuals, while some of each group were patients suffering from various mental disorders.   It was found that the average intelligence of the older groups was definitely below that of the younger groups, in respect to the performance on the tests used, but that the difference between old and young was much greater in some functions than in others.

While the literature on " sex differences " in intelligence and special abilities is voluminous, the extent of such differences appears in most investigations to be very slight, if indeed any difference whatever exists.   Binet's standards were constructed for age-levels irrespective of sex, and the work of Terman and many others has justified this procedure. The point has been made that the somewhat earlier adolescence of girls would lead us to expect some superiority of girls over boys in the neighbourhood of ten to twelve years of age, this disadvantage disappearing when both sexes have attained mid-adolescence ; but even this temporary difference is of small significance.   Many tests for adults, notably the Alpha, have indicated a slight superiority in the average score of men, but the fact that the information-items have usually been drawn largely from masculine pursuits appears to explain the findings.

The data of Wissler[1] and others suggested, early in the testing movement, that, despite the equality of averages, significant sex differences might exist in the field of variability. This has been widely challenged, and more recent work appears to indicate little if any sex difference.[2]   With reference to special abilities and disabilities, however, some fairly large and significant differences have been reported.   Early work with rating-scales and numerous studies of excellence in school subjects indicated some sex differences in interest and capacity, such as are reflected by feminine superiority in spelling and geography, masculine superiority in history and mathematics.   Thorndike, reviewing the data available in 1914, stated that the most striking of established sex differences lay in the fact that " only 15 per cent. of men are as much more interested in persons than in things as the median

---

[1] " The Correlation of Mental and Physical Traits," *Psychol. Rev.*, *Monogr. Suppl.*, III, 1899–1901 (whole No. 16).

[2] See L. S. Hollingworth, " Comparison of the Sexes in Mental Traits," *Psychol. Bull.*, XV, 1918.

BB

woman is."[1]   Nearly all the sex differences discussed by
him are so slight that thirty-five per cent. or more of one sex
surpass the median of the other.   With respect to results
from experimental methods, a number of students have
reported superior memory in girls and women, superior
ingenuity in boys and men.   One of the most striking of sex
differences has been demonstrated by E. K. Strong.[2]   A series
of advertisements was presented to each subject ; later these
were mixed with others which had not been seen, and the
subject was required to indicate which ones had been included
in the earlier presentation.   The men were greatly superior.
Strong then cut a number of advertisements into small pieces.
He presented these mixed with similar small pieces, again
using the recognition method.   Here the score of the women
greatly surpassed that of the men.[3]   This seems to indicate
that in this particular type of situation women excel in the
tendency to notice, and consequently to recall, details.
Even where any of the above, or, in fact, any reported sex
differences are of great magnitude, it has as yet proved impossible
to determine to what extent sex differences are biological
rather than cultural ; such determinations must apparently
wait upon a more adequate psychology of early childhood.

    The same comment holds, of course, for the numerous comparisons
of the sexes in suggestibility, of which the work of
Warner Brown[4] is the most thorough and elaborate.   Using
many methods, and materials taken from several sense-modalities,
he succeeded in keeping all his data in quantitative
form.   Illustrative of his procedure is the presentation to the
subject of a graded series of weights, each weight heavier
than the last, followed without interruption by a series in
which all weights were equal.   Suggestibility was indicated
by the tendency (already studied by Binet) to continue, for
many or few trials, the act of judging each new weight to be
heavier than the last.   The average suggestibility of women
was found to be somewhat greater than the average suggest-

---

[1] *Educational Psychology*, III, p. 201.   Thorndike's calculation is
based on the data of Heymans and Wiersma (see p. 381).
[2] " An Interesting Sex Difference," *Ped. Sem.*, XXII, 1915.
[3] Though published before the introduction of current measures of
statistical reliability, the differences are so huge as to appear to justify
Strong's conclusions.
[4] " Individual and Sex Differences in Suggestibility," *Univ. Calif.
Pub. in Psychol.*, II, 1916.

ibility of men, though much overlapping was present. The different tests of suggestibility, however, while giving positive correlation with one another, presented such low correlations as to force the experimenter to conclude that suggestibility is not a unit trait, but a disposition varying greatly with the situation confronted.

There seems reason to believe that special abilities and disabilities are, like intelligence, " normally distributed," being merely ends of the distribution curve.[1] The absence of striking sex differences in most special abilities and disabilities is, therefore, closely related to the fact of the absence of intellectual differences. One form of special disability, however, appears to constitute a marked exception, namely, the incidence of mental disorder. Using Kraepelin's classification, dementia præcox and paranoia seem to be somewhat commoner among men, manic-depressive psychoses commoner among women. If these disorders are indeed but exaggerations of tendencies implicit in the normal, it would appear that at one end of the distribution curve a socially significant difference may be found. But neither these data nor those indicating a higher prevalence of some psychoneuroses among women have been shown to be biological rather than environmental.

The study of race differences in intelligence has engaged the attention of many psychologists, especially in the United States. Studies indicating no clear differences between the sensory acuity of primitive peoples and that of advanced peoples were reported very early in the present century.[2] The first systematic experimental comparison of the intellectual capacities of races was that of Woodworth[3] at the St. Louis Exposition in 1904. The Seguin form-board was found useful in studying the " performance-test " ability of racial groups from all over the globe. Woodworth's conclusions were that in general the average abilities of the different races differed but little, while overlapping was large ; the only exception was the case of the negritos, whose abilities averaged distinctly less than that of other races.

---

[1] See L. S. Hollingworth, *Special Talents and Defects* (1923), p. 45.
[2] See Rivers, " Observations on the Senses of the Todas," *Brit. J. Psychol.*, I, 1904-5. Rivers's summary, " pure sense acuity is much the same in all races," is based on earlier work together with his own, and has not been overthrown by subsequent research.
[3] " Racial Differences in Mental Traits," *Science, N. S.*, XXXI, 1910.

The study of negro intelligence in the United States has received much attention. Beginning about 1910, attention was drawn by several students to the widespread retardation of negroes in the schools. Several studies of negro children and adults were made with intelligence-tests shortly thereafter. An early application of testing method was that of Ferguson.[1] Using four familiar tests of mental ability (of which he regarded the completion-test and the analogies-test[2] as the most satisfactory), he found large and consistent intellectual inferiority in the average attainment of several hundreds of negro children as compared with a large group of white children. Perhaps the most interesting result of Ferguson's work was the discovery that full-blooded negroes were on the average less intelligent than mulattoes, and even that mulattoes were less intelligent than quadroons ; the amount of white blood appeared to be correlated with intelligence. Ferguson's conclusions as to the relation of negro intelligence to white intelligence were amply confirmed by the study of negro recruits in 1917–18. Negroes averaged about three years lower than whites in mental age on the Alpha ; and while their performance on the Beta (non-verbal) test greatly surpassed their Alpha scores, it still fell far short of the white average.

Meanwhile, with the advent of the Stanford Revision of the Binet Scale, a series of studies of negro intelligence by this method began to appear.[3] The results have indicated with fair consistency that negro children and adults average somewhere in the general neighbourhood of ten points in intelligence quotient below the whites. The difficulties of properly evaluating environmental factors, which are especially acute in view of the inferior home of the negro, have been emphasized by Arlitt[4] and others ; and no matter how widespread the conviction that the negro is innately inferior, it is at least difficult in the face of such obstacles to establish the point clearly.

Of great importance in this connection and as a check upon

---

[1] "The Psychology of the Negro," *Arch. of Psychol.*, No. XXXVI, 1916.
[2] Such as : Man is to woman as boy is to——.
[3] Even prior to the Stanford Revision appeared A. C. Strong's article "Three Hundred Fifty White and Colored Children Measured by the Binet-Simon Measuring Scale of Intelligence," *Ped. Sem.*, XX, 1913.
[4] "On the Need for Caution in Establishing Race Norms," *J. Appl. Psychol.*, V. 1921.

all earlier studies is the recent work of Peterson.[1] He has undertaken to eliminate not only the verbal handicap which has been thought responsible for some of the reported race differences, but, in addition, the speed factor which may well play a large part in differentiating races. In the " disc-transfer " method, for example, negro and white children of various ages were allowed to manipulate discs to form a pre-determined pattern, their movements being governed by the rules of a game similar to " The Fox and the Goose and the Bag of Meal," but more complex. White children were found to work more rapidly, but when accuracy of perform-ance irrespective of speed was measured, white superiority was so slight as to be statistically unreliable. From this and other tests of conceptual thinking, he regards the distinction between speed and accuracy as all-important. Speed is at least conceivably a cultural product. Recent years have added a number of careful studies pointing more and more clearly to the importance of educational factors, and leading to a widespread tendency to reconsider the whole question of negro intelligence.[2]

The intelligence of a number of American Indian tribes has been tested.[3] Garth,[4] and Hunter and Sommermier[5] found among them not only intelligence distinctly below the white, but intelligence scores varying with the amount of white blood. The intelligence of full-blooded Indians appeared, however, to be above that of full-blooded negroes. Klineberg,[6] using a battery of performance tests, found, however, that a group of over a hundred Yakima Indian children presented *qualitative* differences from a white group, which appeared more significant than gross quantita-

---

[1] " The Comparative Abilities of White and Negro Children," *Comp. Psychol. Monogr.*, I, 1922–3 (serial No. 5). Peterson, Lanier, and Walker, " Comparisons of White and Negro Children in Certain Ingenuity and Speed Tests," *J. Comp. Psychol.*, V, 1925.

[2] See, for example, the point of view outlined by Garth in *Race Psychology* (1931).

[3] First by Rowe, " Five Hundred Forty-Seven White and Two Hundred Sixty-Eight Indian Children Tested by the Binet-Simon Tests," *Ped. Sem.*, XXI, 1914.

[4] *E.g.*, " The Results of Some Tests on Full and Mixed Blood Indians," *J. Appl. Psychol.*, V, 1921.

[5] " The Relation of Degree of Indian Blood to Score on the Otis Intelligence Test," *Psychol. Bull.*, XVIII, 1921.

[6] *J. Abn. Psychol. and Soc. Psychol.*, XXII, 1927-8.

tive differences. The Indian children at all age-levels worked more slowly than the whites, but made fewer errors.

This reminds one not only of Peterson's work with the negro, but of the writings of Boas[1] and many other anthropologists who believe that racial differences in intelligence consist not in significant differences in intellectual endowment, but in the types of activity emphasized by different cultures. To what extent the findings of Garth, Klineberg, and other students of the American Indian are of biological origin has not been determined.

Yeung,[2] Murdock,[3] Darsie,[4] and others have recently published studies of the intelligence of Mongolian groups, from which it appears clear that children who speak Chinese or Japanese at home tend to be inferior to whites in tests involving the use of English, but that on non-language tests significant differences between yellow and white disappear. The recent activity of Chinese and Japanese students in administering standard verbal tests in the schools of their own countries is now contributing material which should shortly give a much more satisfactory answer to the question of intellectual differences between major races.

The Army Alpha and Beta tests are still our chief source of information regarding the intelligence of subdivisions of the white race, although several more recent studies have obtained concordant results. On the army tests, both verbal and non-verbal, immigrants from the British Isles and from Canada gave scores closely comparable to those of American-born whites ; German and Scandinavian immigrants averaged slightly lower, while Italians, Poles, and Russians tended to make distinctly lower scores. In the absence of satisfactory data on these groups, when tested in their own countries, opinion is divided between three interpretations. These results may be significant of genuine racial differences ; they may be due to the " sampling " which all immigration involves ; they may be due to varying degrees of difficulty in meeting the test situation in America. Though there

[1] *The Mind of Primitive Man* (1911).
[2] "The Intelligence of Chinese Children in San Francisco and Vicinity," *J. Appl. Psychol.*, V, 1921.
[3] " A Study of Differences found between Races in Intellect and in Morality," *School and Society*, XXII, 1925.
[4] " Mental Capacity of American-born Japanese Children," *Comp. Psychol., Monogr.* III, 1925–26 (serial No. 15).

appears to be a drift toward the third interpretation in very recent publications, the opinions seem to claim adherents in the order just stated.

Many of the difficulties found in the study of race differences occur also in the study of occupational differences. Here, again, the Army data mark the beginnings of serious study of the problem, and here, also, subsequent studies have confirmed the results. A definite " intellectual hierarchy " was discovered, corresponding closely to an " occupational hierarchy " popularly recognized. The intelligence of (Taussig's) five major " non-competitive groups " —(a) professional, (b) semi-professional and higher business, (c) skilled, (d) semi-skilled, and (e) unskilled, follows in the order named, though with so much overlapping that many individuals in a given group attained not only to the median of the group above but even to that of the second group above. A more detailed analysis makes possible a similar comparison of specific occupational groups, e.g., carpenters with teamsters.

A fairly close relation has appeared between economic status and intelligence. Burt,[1] English,[2] and others[3] have shown that children classified according to the social status of their parents form a similar hierarchy, though again with considerable overlapping. The whole problem of the relation of inheritance to intelligence besets us here ; to what extent superior home environment may produce superior wits is still far from a measurable quantity.[4]

The study of occupational differences in intelligence is fraught with implications which have profoundly affected three major social problems, in a manner so definite as to constitute three subdivisions of contemporary " applied psychology." Vocational guidance, which took shape as a distinct social movement about 1910, through the efforts of British, German, and American educators, has perforce taken account of the fact that each occupation demands a certain

[1] " Experimental Tests of General Intelligence," *Brit. J. Psychol.* 1909-10.

[2] " An Experimental Study of the Mental Capacities of School Children Correlated with Social Status," *Psychol. Monogr.*, XXIII, 1917.

[3] *E.g.*, Pressey and Ralston, " The Relation of the General Intelligence of School Children to the Occupation of Their Fathers," *J. Appl. Psychol.*, III, 1919.

[4] Here the question of " constancy of the I Q " under different environments is especially pressing (see p. 350).

minimum standard of intelligence. The vocational guide has within recent years come to take it for granted that an intelligence test must be administered and that the applicant should be saved both from the attempt to enter a career in which he would almost certainly fail, and from the idle acceptance of a level beneath his capacities. Employment psychology, recognizing the same principles, rejects applicants whose intelligence predicts failure in the position sought, and in some cases discourages applicants whose intelligence is so high as to render it improbable that they would long remain in a given position. Vocational and employment psychology, however, have taken into consideration not only intelligence but a wide variety of special abilities. Standard laboratory methods (such as reaction-time, tests of motor co-ordination, etc.) are being supplemented more and more by special tests devised for special purposes.

The psychology of criminalism has also been profoundly affected by the testing movement. Early data collected by Goddard[1] and others indicated an extraordinary percentage of mental defectives among criminals, while more recent work, such as that of Healy,[2] has emphasized the fact that criminalism is in a large proportion of cases a definite product of social factors, requiring in many cases a fair level of intelligence, and demanding a course of training similar to that required for recognized callings. Mental deficiency has indeed been shown to play a large part in the causation of many crimes, particularly those of the " sporadic " type (such as " crimes of violence "), rather than of the " professional " type ; while those who commit " crimes of gain," such as forgery and burglary, seem on the whole to make test scores above the general average.[3]

---

[1] *The Criminal Imbecile* (1915).
[2] *E.g.*, Healy and Bronner, *Case Studies, Judge Baker Foundation* (1922).
[3] See, *e.g.*, Murchison, *Criminal Intelligence* (1926).

CHAPTER XXII

PERSONALITY

> After having established these proportions, I thought myself entering into port, but when I came to meditate on the union of the soul with the body I was as if cast back into the open sea.—*Leibnitz.*

WE must next attempt a brief survey of recent methods of measuring emotion and the more complex personality traits, and then give some attention to modern conceptions of the nature of personality.

The methods of measuring the emotions within recent years may be subdivided into three main categories : the physiological methods, the " behaviour " methods, and the " paper-and-pencil " methods of investigation. By physiological methods are meant studies of variation in the functions of different organs during emotion ; by behaviour methods, those in which the individual's total adjustment is expressed on some quantitative scale ; while " paper-and-pencil " methods are those in which the subject's reaction to printed or written material, or his manipulation of such material, is used as a criterion of emotional behaviour which is not conveniently observable by either of the first two methods.

One of the oldest and most widely exploited of the physiological methods is the " psychogalvanic reflex." Féré,[1] Tarchanoff,[2] and others studied late in the last century, the electrical phenomena associated with emotion ; Tarchanoff called attention to the current set up in the body of certain emotional states. But during emotional states there is also a decrease in the resistance of the body to an electrical current transmitted through it from an outside source ; the term " psychogalvanic reflex " has been generally used to designate the latter as well as the former electrical

---

[1] *C.R. de la Soc. de Biol.*, XL, 1888.
[2] *Pflüger's Archiv.*, XLVI, 1890.

phenomenon. Since, however, the two cannot be identified, some confusion has resulted ; we shall consider here only the changes in resistance to an outside current.

The galvanometer was early adopted by Jung and others of the Zürich School for use in conjunction with the association test. They have published much material illustrative of the way in which either conscious or unconscious emotional disturbance betrays itself through the galvanometric record, and regard the method as highly valuable in disclosing psychogenic factors unknown even to the patient. The introduction of the psychogalvanic method into normal psychology, with psychological rather than therapeutic purposes, was largely the work of Wells and Forbes.[1] They demonstrated a fairly close relation between the psychogalvanic reflex and the intensity of the emotion reported by their subjects. They did not use correlation methods, but defined four levels of emotionality, finding that these four levels corresponded in general to the degrees of electrical disturbance recorded. This strictly quantitative conception has stimulated much subsequent research, but the definiteness of the results has never been adequately confirmed. Some experimenters regard the reflex as a fairly precise measure ; others find but little relation between the record and the subject's report. Wells and Forbes also showed the possibility of employing the psychogalvanic method in conjunction with the association test, as Jung and others had done, using for this purpose both normal and psychotic subjects.[2] The sweat-glands appear to be responsible for the electrical disturbances. This accords with the current hypothesis that autonomic functions[3] are closely related to emotion.

Another fertile field of research upon the emotions is found in the vascular system. The behaviour of the pulse during emotion had always attracted attention,[4] and physiologists of the mid-nineteenth century naturally turned to it as a vital

[1] " On Certain Electrical Processes in the Human Body," etc. *Arch. of Psychol.* No. XVI, 1911.

[2] For recent work along these lines see W. W. Smith, *The Measurement of Emotion* (1922).

[3] Which are connected with the activities of glands and unstriped muscles.

[4] Galen, when asked to determine the cause of a young woman's nervousness, took her pulse while repeating to her a series of names. When a certain actor's name was pronounced the pulse betrayed her.

problem in "physiological psychology." That certain strong emotions do produce fairly consistent changes in pulse appears clear from recent evidence.[1] A kindred problem is the measurement of changes in the vascular system in such accessible parts as the hand and arm. Here we may distinguish measures of the quantity of blood present in a part of the body from measures of general blood pressure. The former problem is approached through the plethysmograph, a vessel of water so arranged that after the immersion of the hand the variations in the blood supply to that member cause a rise and fall in the water-level (an air chamber and a tambour making possible a smoked-drum record). This was used as an "instrument of precision" by the school of Wundt,[2] together with the study of the speed and strength of the pulse, and the rapidity and depth of breathing. Wundt reported certain regular variations in the functions thus measured, which depended upon the arousal of the various feelings described in his "tri-dimensional" theory. Most of the feeling states described by Wundt are generally regarded as emotions, and many attempts have been made to confirm the Leipzig data on the relation of such physiological changes to various affective states, simple and complex. Very discordant results have been obtained; neither plethysmograph, pulse, nor respiration has been clearly shown to bear any one-to-one relation to emotion or feeling as reported by the subject.[3] A recent attempt has, however, been made by Eng[4] to reinstate the plethysmograph as a means of measuring not only general tendencies but individual and group differences. Eng believes that the plethysmograph gives consistent and satisfactory results.

Great confusion exists as regards the significance of the large quantity of material published on the relation of blood pressure to emotion. A point upon which the evidence seems clear is the increase of blood pressure in most fear and rage responses; the work of Cannon[5] in 1915 appears to stand

---

[1] See e.g., Blatz, "The Cardiac, Respiratory and Electrical Phenomena Involved in the Emotion of Fear," *J. Exp. Psychol.*, VIII, 1925.

[2] See his *Physiological Psychology*, 6th ed., II (1910), p. 310.

[3] See e.g., Landis, "Studies of Emotional Reactions: V. Severe Emotional Upset," *J. Comp. Psychol*, VI, 1926.

[4] *Experimental Investigations into the Emotional Life of the Child Compared with that of the Adult* (1922).

[5] *Bodily Changes in Pain, Hunger, Fear and Rage.*

secure.   Measurements of both systolic and diastolic blood pressure, in these and other emotions, have frequently been published in recent years in connection with a host of "theories of the emotions." We cannot here do justice to any of these theories, and must content ourselves with the comment that in many cases blood-pressure records fail to bear any consistent and definable relation to the subject's verbal reports of his various emotions.

Similar confusion prevails with regard to certain physiological methods which have arisen in connection with the recent development of endocrinology.   Cannon[1] has reported that in animals and human beings emotional tension causes the liver to give up glycogen, which produces an increase in blood sugar to the point of glycosuria.   The best known, however, of the various endocrine methods is the measure of the "basal metabolism" (the rate at which body fuel is consumed), which is a fairly good index of the individual's thyroid activity.   While the method is not a gauge of emotion experienced at the time (the subject necessarily being quiet if the metabolism is to be basal), such a measure of the thyroid make-up has been assumed by many to be closely related to general emotionality.

It has frequently been assumed that these and other "physiological methods" are the most satisfactory key to the emotions.   It becomes increasingly apparent, however, that they are confronted with difficulties of great magnitude. Emotions appear to be complex patterns, whose nature can scarcely be described, much less accurately measured, through reference to one or even to three or four physiological changes.   Furthermore, even when the pattern is plotted with fair accuracy, this pattern may appear in one individual in states which he reports as "fear," and in another subject in states reported as "rage," or under some other caption. To reject the subject's report is simply to reject a group of factors, which, though elusive, are to the subject highly important.   It may be, of course, that, through the vagaries of experience, what one person calls "fear" may be identical with what another calls "rage," but it would appear at least more likely that existing physiological methods have not determined all the crucial elements in emotional response.

---

[1] *Op. cit.*, and elsewhere.

Whereas much of the work with " physiological methods " has been a sheer gift from physiologists to their psychological confrères, the " behaviour methods " of studying and measuring emotion have emanated almost without exception from psychological laboratories. A leader in this field is H. T. Moore, several of whose methods are most engaging. His " distraction " method[1] consists of putting the subject through a series of complicated mental tasks,[2] introducing during the series a stimulus provocative of emotion ; the amount of interference which the emotion causes in the prosecution of the task is an index to the intensity of the emotion. The subject's performance without distraction having been measured, it is measured again during and after the introduction, for example, of fear-producing stimuli. He is shown an instrument which will, he is informed, give him an electric shock, whenever the experimenter throws a switch. He must, nevertheless, work along as best he can, even when the shock is administered. During the work period the investigator constantly tinkers with the apparatus, pretending that he is repairing a slight defect, which will shortly permit the introduction of a shock. The subject's performance, while disturbed by this fear stimulus, can be compared both with a work period free from distraction and with periods in which " rage " stimuli (such as insults) and other emotional distractions are introduced. Moore's method does not, of course, involve such terminology as " units of emotion," but compares each subject with other subjects in respect to the amount of distraction which each kind of stimulus causes.

The work of Moore and Gilliland[3] upon " aggressiveness " is also illustrative of recent method. The subjects for this test were college students, each of whom had been ranked by his fellows in respect to his aggressiveness. The subject's " aggressiveness " was then compared with the number of times he permitted his gaze to wander from the experimenter before him. It was found that those who had

[1] " Laboratory Tests of Anger, Fear, and Sex Interest," *Am. J. Psychol.*, XXVIII, 1917.
[2] Such as constant increment addition.
[3] " The Measurement of Aggressiveness," *J. Appl. Psych.*, V, 1921. Here, as elsewhere, the distinction between an " emotional " trait and a " personality " trait is arbitrary ; aggressiveness is considered here merely for convenience.

been rated the most aggressive scarcely allowed the eyes to wander from the experimenter at all, whereas those near the foot of the " aggressiveness " scale did so a great many times during the experimental period. What the term " aggressiveness " involves is not, of course, clear. The value of the method consists in the attempt, however crude, to define quantitatively an emotional trait which ratings show to be fairly definitely recognizable. Moore's method illustrates a general characteristic of all such measures ; the test takes account of only a few aspects of trait-patterns which are highly complex. The isolation of measurable aspects of such patterns is, however, an important step.

Animal experimentation has yielded significant measurements of impulses or " drives," such as hunger and sex, notably by Moss's[1] " resistance " method and the Columbia " obstruction method."[2] The former finds how much electric shock an animal will take in striving towards an end ; the latter measures persistence by the frequency with which an animal crosses an electric grid in pursuit of its goal.

A vast quantity of experimental work has been done with association tests. Among their many uses with normal and psychopathic subjects none has been exploited more fully than their application as a test for emotional response to words, and thereby a test of emotional patterns to which the word may be a key. The commonest of their uses is the study of words which indicate simply the *quality* of the emotion aroused, pointing to the nature rather than to the extent of the emotional disturbance. But the classification and tabulation of words of a given emotional colouring, and, more especially, the study of variations in the association time, have offered possibilities for quantitative analysis. The number of reactions in which a stimulus is followed by a word indicating a personal experience, or placing a certain value upon the stimulus idea (as in *sky-beautiful*) has, for example, been used as a measure of an " egocentric "[3] tendency. Variability in

---

[1] " Study of Animal Drives," *J. Exp. Psychol.*, VII, 1924.

[2] Jenkins, Warner, and Warden, " Standard Apparatus for the Study of Animal Motivation," *J. Comp. Psychol.*, VI, 1926 ; Holden, " A Study of the Effect of Starvation upon Behavior by Means of the Obstruction Method," *Comp. Psychol. Monogr.*, III, 1925–6 (serial No. 17). Warner, " A Study of Sex Behavior in the White Rat by Means of the Obstruction Method," *Comp. Psychol. Monogr.*, IV, 1926–7 (serial No. 22).

[3] See F. L. Wells, " The Question of Association Types," *Psychol. Rev.*, XIX, 1912.

association time has also been regarded as a quantitative index to emotional unrest.

An extraordinary number of paper-and-pencil methods of measuring emotion have recently been published.   The first to attract wide attention was Woodworth's " Personal Data Sheet,"[1] used in the United States Army in the study of psychoneurotic patients.   The test consisted of a long series of questions to be answered by " yes " or " no."   The questions aimed to detect certain characteristic psycho-neurotic dispositions, e.g., " Do you make friends easily ? " or " Are you afraid of responsibility ? "   The questions are so framed that some " yes " and some " no " answers are " neurotic."   Only a few " neurotic " answers were written by most normal subjects, while psychoneurotic patients in military hospitals frequently gave such answers to as many as thirty per cent. of the questions.[2]   Several revisions of the Personal Data Sheet have appeared, and have been used in educational and clinical work.

In 1919 appeared the much more elaborate Pressey " cross-out " (X-O) test for investigating the emotions.[3]   The test consists of several major divisions, in each of which there are twenty-five lists of five words each.   In the first division the subject is instructed to draw a line through every word that is unpleasant.   Having completed this test, he must then draw a circle around the *most* unpleasant word in each group of five.   In other divisions of the test, the subject indicates in a similar way his feelings as to the wrongness of certain acts, and his tendency towards certain common worries.   The results of the entire test are scored in two ways : the number of words crossed out represents the subject's " affectivity," while his " idiosyncrasy " is the number of cases in which he draws a circle around a word other than the word most commonly circled by normal persons.   Broadly viewed, the idiosyncrasy score is an indication of the subject's tendency to unusual emotional responses.   Chambers[4] has shown that test-performance is related to college success, and by comparing children's with adults' records finds it

---

[1] See Franz, *Handbook of Mental Examination Methods*, 2nded.(1919).
[2] H. L. Hollingworth, *The Psychology of Functional Neuroses* (1920).
[3] S. L. Pressey and L. W. Pressey, " ' Cross-out ' Tests, with Sugges-tions as to a Group Scale of the Emotions," *J. Appl. Psychol.*, III.
[4] " Character Trait Tests and the Prognosis of College Achieve-ment," *J. Abn. and Soc. Psychol.*, XX, 1925–6.

possible to construct a "maturity" scale, by which the attainment of emotional maturity may be gauged.[1] While Pressey's method has been used chiefly for practical rather than scientific purposes, the maturity scale is an instance of the way in which such applications unearth significant psychological principles ; a quantitative determination of the change from the emotional reactions of childhood to those of adolescence and maturity gives promise of a substantial contribution to genetic psychology.

Experimental æsthetics, founded by Fechner (see p. 93) and developed in German and American laboratories, has also proved to be a fertile field for the study and measure- ment of individual differences. Washburn and her pupils[2] have published several such studies. She compared, for example, students specializing in literature with other students specializing in science. To both groups a series of stimuli was presented (auditory, olfactory, etc.), the subject's affective responses being rated on a scale from extremely pleasant to extremely unpleasant. A tabulation was made of the number of extremely strong affects reported by each group. The literary group displayed a much larger number of strong affects than the scientific group. The method is typical of many current investigations which seek to reduce to quantitative form a generalization suggested by everyday experience. Such research appears to be a neces- sary step in charting the way for experimental analysis of more complex æsthetic reactions.

It is natural to ask, in connection with all such measure- ments of the affective life, whether it is possible to distinguish innate emotional dispositions from those which are the results of past experience. Those methods which undertake to measure a specific emotion at the time of its occurrence would seem in general preferable to those which presuppose some stable and continuous emotional constituent in per- sonality. In practice, the results of specific conditionings have proved so difficult to exclude that it may well be doubted whether any test has as yet succeeded in measuring the emotional constitution of individuals with success equal

---

[1] "A Method of Measuring the Emotional Maturity of Children," *Ped. Sem.*, XXXII, 1925.
[2] Washburn, Hatt, and Holt, "Affective Sensitiveness in Poets and in Scientific Students," *Am. J. Psychol.*, XXXIV, 1923.

to that which has been obtained in the measurement of intelligence.

The rapid development of more complex "personality measurements" has been highly characteristic of recent quantitative psychology. It is, of course, arbitrary to draw any line between "emotional" and "personality" traits. Such lines are, however, sometimes drawn on the supposition that emotions are relatively simple entities, while personalities are complexes of many ; and this distinction may serve well enough for convenience.

The first extensive work on personality traits is that of Heymans and Wiersma.[1] Rating scales, already used by Fechner,[2] Galton,[3] Pearson,[4] and Cattell,[5] were employed in a wide survey of human traits, in which differences between individuals and groups were explored. Men and women in many walks of life were rated in respect to their interests, aptitudes, temperaments, etc. This method soon came into general use, and was subjected to various forms of statistical analysis, such as the correlations of the ratings of different judges, the intensive study of probable errors of such judgments, and the like. The results of such studies may be very briefly summarized. We may say that the attempt to derive a clear and comprehensive list of personality traits has proved hopelessly complicated. The list of traits named by Heymans and Wiersma has been followed by a long succession of similar lists in which both the terminology and the guiding concepts seem to lack solid foundation. One of the most painstaking of such lists is Yerkes and La Rue's *Outline of a Study of the Self* (1913), which presents a scheme for recording the details of growth and experience. The lists used for rating-scale work are usually much simpler and shorter.

A very elaborate application of rating-scale methods to the study of the interrelation of personality traits has been offered by Webb.[6] His work includes a study of such complicated traits as trustworthiness, eagerness for admira-

[1] *Zeitschr f. Psychol.*, XLII, 1906 (*et seq.*).
[2] *Vorschule der Aesthetik* (1876).
[3] *Inquiries into Human Faculty* (1883).
[4] " *On the Laws of Inheritance in Man*," E.g., *Biometrika*, III, 1904.
[5] E.g., *A Statistical Study of American Men of Science* (1906).
[6] " Character and Intelligence," *Brit. J. Psychol.*, *Monogr.* 3, 1915.
CC

tion, and originality of ideas. In this he used two groups of subjects, one made up of university students, the other of schoolboys ; only the data from the former will be noted here. The students were divided into groups of ten, and to each group were assigned two judges, who independently rated each individual. From the material obtained Webb concluded that there is, among character traits, a " general factor " comparable to Spearman's general factor in mental ability. This general factor is related to " persistence of motives " ; it enters, with different " saturation," into many complex traits. The statistical uncertainties attaching to Spearman's " G " appear necessarily to attach to this character-factor discovered by Webb.

Rating scales were also widely used in the United States Army in 1917–18 (under the direction of W. D. Scott) for the study of the abilities of officers.[1] The results confirmed existing suspicions as to flaws inherent in the rating-scale method, wherever the personal relation of subject and rater may be disposed toward bias. One of the most serious of these flaws, emphasized by Thorndike,[2] was the tendency to allow a high (or low) rating on one trait to draw the rater into the tendency to estimate other traits too high (or too low) ; this unwarranted tendency to lump all traits together has been dubbed the " halo " error. The rating scale seems to be tending to be crowded out by more objective methods, but it continues in many studies as an adjunct to such methods. The fact that so much attention is now being given to the rectification of methodological defects may perhaps mean that the rating scale has already passed through the most serious crisis in its existence, and is still capable of contributing useful data in cases where objective methods are not available.

Wide popularity has been enjoyed by Downey's " will-temperament " tests.[3] These have been made available both as " individual " and as " group " tests. In one test the subject must write a given phrase as rapidly as possible, and in another as slowly as possible ; his behaviour is regarded

[1] Adjutant General's Department, U.S. Army, *The Personnel System of the United States Army*, II (1919).
[2] " A Constant Error in Psychological Ratings," *J. Appl. Psychol.*, IV, 1920.
[3] *The Will-Temperament and its Testing* (1923).

as a key to his energy, his persistence, etc. When a variety of such tests has been given, the results are plotted on a " will-profile," which shows at a glance the interrelation between the traits measured. The " reliability " (self-correlation) of these tests has been found to be quite low.[1] This very fact has contributed much to the recognition of the discrepancy between complex " personality traits " and the simple functions necessarily selected for the first analysis through testing methods.

An illustration of many recent attempts to measure " social attitudes " is G. B. Watson's study of " fair-mindedness "[2] on certain economic, political, and religious issues. The subject's " bias " is measured by the number of instances in which, for example, a complex and controversial question is regarded by him as having one obviously true answer, and by the alteration of his logic as he moves from the region of his sympathies to the region of his antagonisms.

Another main division of " personality measurement " has been the attempt to trace relations between physical and mental traits, to diagnose personality through physiological or morphological characteristics. Though such correlations have long been assumed,[3] it is only with the parallel development of biometric and statistical methods within the last thirty years that such studies have appeared to merit serious attention. Nineteenth-century criminal anthropology, especially in the hands of Lombroso, had made much of the supposed relation between criminalism and physical type. The Italian school of anthropologists, though in general abandoning this position, has recently given much attention to the relations between body-form and personality. Some have suggested, for example, that those whose length of limb bears a certain relation to the volume of the trunk have certain distinguishing personality traits. Kretschmer's *Physique and Character* (1925) also indicates some close connections between psychiatric types and physical types ; the contemporary German literature on Kretschmer's methods is voluminous.

[1] May, " The Present Status of the Will-Temperament Tests," *J. Appl. Psychol.*, IX, 1925.
[2] *The Measurement of Fair-mindedness* (1925).
[3] Dessoir's *Outlines of the History of Psychology* (p. xiii f.) traces such " psychognostic " methods from the Greeks. Phrenology is, of course, such a method.

A good deal of interesting work has been reported regarding the relation of the face and of facial expression to personality. Pioneer work by Feleky[1] upon the ability of subjects to determine what was portrayed in the experimenter's face has been followed by a series of studies in which the ability to recognize different emotions under varying conditions has been measured.   The work of Langfeld,[2] for example, showed that some emotions could be much more easily recognized than others.   Though much thorough work on physiognomy has been published in Germany, it is only in the very recent work of Landis[3] that a histrionic " pose " has been replaced by the close and detailed study of photographs of individuals actually undergoing real and intense emotion.   Landis's work seems to show that at least a part of the success in interpreting facial expression is due to the existence of conventionalized patterns ; at least, the experiments found no emotion associated with a definite and uniform expression.

Another field in which some relation between physical traits and personality is frequently assumed is that of handwriting. Binet[4] reported considerable ability among " graphologists " to distinguish eminent men from humbler folk, and criminals from law-abiding citizens.   The possibility that the " graphologists " were already familiar with many of the handwriting specimens was, however, not excluded ; and more recent studies such as those of Hull and Montgomery[5] suggest little if any relation between personality and handwriting.

It is natural that the whole technique of personality study should be turned to practical account. One of the most interesting of such practical uses lies in the measurement of moral attitudes and conduct.   Voelker[6] devised for the Boy Scouts a series of practical tests for honesty, trustworthiness, etc.   In one of the honesty tests, for example, a boy is sent

---

[1] " The Expression of the Emotions," Psychol. Rev., XXI, 1914.
[2] " The Judgment of Emotions from Facial Expressions," J. Abn. Psychol., XIII, 1918-9.
[3] " Studies of Emotional Reaction. IV, General Behavior and Facial Expression," J. Comp. Psychol., IV, 1924.
[4] Les révélations de l'écriture d'après un contrôle scientifique (1906).
[5] " An Experimental Investigation of Certain Alleged Relations between Character and Handwriting," Psychol. Rev., XXVI, 1919.
[6] The Function of Ideals and Attitudes in Social Education, An Experimental Study (1921).

to a near-by shop, with the necessary money for a small purchase. The store-keeper, by previous arrangement with the experimenter, makes an apparent mistake in counting the change, and hands the boy a little more than the amount actually due to him. If the boy returns the overchange, the fact is entered on his "honesty" score. A systematic examination of the problem of character measurement has been recently undertaken by May and Hartshorne.[1] They have not only devised many tests of ethical information, ethical attitudes, the ability to foresee consequences of an act, etc., but have devised a definite scale for the measurement of honesty. This scale has been used with great numbers of school children, and is undergoing standardization. After giving children an arithmetic test, the experimenters make exact copies of the finished test-papers. The children are later given an opportunity to score their own papers. In some cases, the child need only erase a pencil check mark, in order to make his answer correct ; in other cases, the erasure of an ink mark encircling a given answer would be necessary. The special aspect of honesty involved is the resistance of the temptation to cheat; this resistance has been measured on a scale containing six steps. In practice, cheating at *any one* of these steps has been found to mean that children will with few exceptions cheat at every point *lower* (easier) on the scale. The study of honesty in a great variety of situations shows that in general the child's behaviour is (from the adult's point of view) extremely inconsistent ; yet as children grow older a " general " honesty factor becomes more prominent. Adult standards, especially in the favoured socio-economic group, are making for consistent conformity to the ethical code.

It is evident that the publication of methods of personality study has far outstripped their standardization and the study of their statistical reliability. The last few years have, however, witnessed such a rapid dissemination of statistical knowledge that these defects are already being amended. Together with such improvements in procedure has come the demand for a closer relation between qualitative clinical findings and the quantitative results from these personality

---

[1] " First Steps toward a Scale for Measuring Attitudes," *J. Ed. Psychol.*, XVII, 1926 ; *Studies in Deceit* (1928). See also Hartshorne, May, and Shuttleworth, *Studies in the Organization of Character* (1930).

measurements. The "clinical" study of normal persons (through case history methods), and on the other hand the study of psychopathic cases through the new testing methods, seem to offer a necessary corrective for the inadequacies of each procedure.[1]

Those who have occupied themselves with the measurement of personality traits have in general been even less concerned with the theory of personality than most intelligence testers have been with theories of intelligence. Nevertheless, despite their unconcern, they have materially contributed towards a view of personality which has gained headway in recent years. Personality, it is assumed, is simply a name for the *sum of all of an individual's traits*. The very isolation and measurement of traits involves such an analytical view, while the study of the intercorrelation of traits, far from balancing the analytic tendency, serves to accentuate the idea of the separateness of an individual's various characteristics. Correlation implies the presence of common *elements* entering into the composition of complex entities, suggesting that a more accurate and more detailed analysis would present personality simply as the answer to a complicated arithmetical problem.

But those who have measured personality have merely contributed to the popularity of a conception which has been gaining in prominence for several decades. Physiological and experimental psychology, at one time identified by some of the ablest leaders with the earnest attempt to separate the simpler empirical problems from the more profound problems of personality, have pressed forward with the acquisition of factual material to a point where such a separation no longer enjoys favour. Among psychologists whose interest is chiefly empirical, personality has therefore come to mean simply the *aggregate* of the organism's capacities.

The notion of such an aggregate nevertheless varies widely. For certain psychologists the term "sum" would be roughly a correct description of the relation of the whole personality to its constituent parts. For the *Gestalt* School and the behaviourists such arithmetical summation is not

---

[1] See, *e.g.*, G. B. Watson, "Character Tests of 1926," *Vocational Guidance Magazine*, V, 1927.

sufficient. Personality depends upon the organization and structure of the components. This conception is very characteristic of the outlook and method of Kantor[1] and the " organismic " school.

Psychiatry, however, has found it necessary to deal with personality as a whole to an extent usually greater than that demanded of the experimentalist, and it is therefore natural that psychiatric conceptions have added much to the richness of the term " personality." Pierre Janet (as was noted above, p. 184 f.) has occupied himself with the theoretical implications of " dissociation," that process by which certain functions may be split off from the conscious self, although still capable of manifesting their activity in other ways. For Janet, personality is the synthesis of many states and processes ; partial sundering of these tendencies gives the " psychasthenic personality," while a more complete dissociation produces hysterical phenomena. Janet has spoken of ideas, memories, impulses, even large segments of the structure of personality, as thus capable of dissociation. This study of dissociation inevitably led (as it did independently in the case of Freud) to the raising of questions about " unconscious " or " subconscious " mental processes. James, greatly interested in Janet's clinical data, found room, as we have seen (p. 209), both for " personal " and " impersonal " interpretations of these dissociated states. But that they were truly *mental* he did not doubt. Together with Starbuck, F. W. H. Myers, and many others familiar with contemporary psychiatric conceptions, he helped to systematize the idea of a " subconscious " or an " unconscious " self to which von Hartmann had already devoted attention. Early in the present century, however, many psychologists began to be disturbed by the wide currency of the notion of the subconscious, which was being used not only by psychiatrists and psychologists but by educated people generally. The idea of the " subconscious mind " had become for the reading public almost a matter of course. Against this, many psychologists have protested in vigorous language. They insist that what is conscious is conscious ; what is not conscious is simply outside the domain of psychology. Alleged " subconscious " processes are simply physiological processes.

[1] *The Principles of Psychology*, (1924–6).

Nevertheless, the direct experimental study of subconscious and unconscious mental states has been attempted by Morton Prince, Sidis, and many others. In one instance, for example, Prince[1] closely questioned his subject as to the clothing of an individual with whom she had just been talking. She could say only that he wore dark clothes. But when asked to write a description automatically, a full and correct description was given. The items, Prince believed, had been assimilated by a subconscious part of the self. A dissociated fragment of consciousness continued to function and to express itself, even though it could not make its way into personal awareness. Insisting on clear terminology, Prince differentiated between such dissociated or " co-conscious " fragments on the one hand and genuine secondary personalities or subconscious selves on the other.

While the view that dissociated states may be genuinely psychic and that mental work may be done outside the field of introspection has been vigorously defended by Prince,[2] Sidis,[3] Mühl[4] and many others, it has, in the nature of the case, been difficult to *prove* that such phenomena are not simply automatic. In the endeavour to refute this interpretation, believers in subconscious processes have laid special emphasis on the capacity of the subconscious to do *original creative work*, but even this has not satisfied their critics.

Quite aside from all questions of theory, a chief method of investigating the less easily accessible parts of personality has continued to be the use of hypnosis. The gradual ascendancy, however, of the Nancy over the Paris conceptions has given currency to the habit of thinking of hypnosis as simply a condition of extreme suggestibility in which dissociation is induced with relative ease. In the recent work of Wingfield[5] the whole notion of hypnotic " sleep " has been for most purposes dispensed with. Suggestion is given in the waking state, and nearly all the hypnotic phenomena (paralysis, contracture, anæsthesia, amnesia, dissociation

---

[1] *The Unconscious* (1914), p. 53.
[2] *Op. cit.*
[3] *Foundations of Normal and Abnormal Psychology* (1914).
[4] " Automatic Writing as an Indicator of the Fundamental Factors Underlying the Personality," *J. Abn. and Soc., Psychol.*, XVII, 1922-3 ; "Automatic Writing Combined with Crystal Gazing as a Means of Recalling Forgotten Incidents," *ibid.*, XIX, 1924-5.
[5] *Introduction to the Study of Hypnotism* (2nd ed., 1920).

with automatic writing, post-hypnotic suggestion) are produced without any appearance of sleep. W. R. Wells,[1] employing similar methods, has confirmed Wingfield's assertions, and has called attention to the special advantages which the method has for experimental psychology, in permitting the subject to witness the phenomena of dissociation and suggestion while in a waking state, and capable of observing, remembering, and reporting much that goes on.

Our knowledge of double and multiple personality, which thirty years ago rested chiefly upon the work of the Charcot-Janet school, has been greatly extended by Morton Prince's *Dissociation of a Personality* (1905), W. F. Prince's " The Doris Case of Multiple Personality,"[2] and several other studies. The fact has been abundantly confirmed that " alternating personalities " may by proper treatment be " fused," the reconstructed self retaining the memories of both. Another important element in Janet's description of multiple personality has been confirmed with special clearness in the " Doris Case." Janet had classified cases of alternating personality under two captions, which we may for convenience call " type A " and " type B." In the former, each of the alternating personalities is in ignorance of all that is done by the other ; when a personality " appears " it recalls only what last occurred before its disappearance, just as a man, awakening, may forget his dreams. In the second group, the " type B " cases, one personality is ignorant of all that is done by the other, but the second is nevertheless fully aware not only of its own previous activities but of all those carried out by the first. The Doris case presented several clear examples of the " type B " organization. " Real Doris " was ignorant of the doings of " Margaret," though Margaret knew of Doris's doings. Neither Doris nor Margaret knew anything of the life of another personality, " Sleeping Margaret," who was nevertheless thoroughly familiar with the activities of both.

T. W. Mitchell[3] has concluded from the work of Janet, Morton Prince, W. F. Prince, and others, that in alternating personalities of " type A " (where the two selves are mutually

---

[1] " Experiments in Waking Hypnosis for Instructional Purposes," *J. Abn. Psychol. and Soc. Psychol.*, XVIII, 1923–4.
[2] *Proc. Am. Soc. for Psychical Res.*, IX, 1915, and X, 1916.
[3] *The Psychology of Medicine* (1921).

exclusive) the personality disclosed in hypnosis is neither
the one nor the other, but possesses the memories of both.
When, on the contrary, an alternating personality of " type
B " is studied, the hypnotic personality turns out to be simply
the *more inclusive* of the two selves.   We might say, in other
words, that in " type B " one self is a fragment of the whole
personality, but the other is simply the whole personality,
which can be reached through hypnosis.   From these considerations Mitchell concludes that there never is really more
than one *personality*, namely, the inclusive one, which,
however difficult it may be to reach, includes all the materials,
so to speak, of which the rest are made.

The assumptions regarding the unconscious or subconscious,
implicit in this theory, present for many psychologists insuperable obstacles to the acceptance of such a view.   One illustration of a somewhat simpler approach is the personality
theory of Rosanoff.[1]   The various types of constitutional
mental disease are, Rosanoff suggests, definite hereditary
patterns.   These   patterns   may,   however,   appear   in
incomplete form.   The depressed, though not positively
psychotic, individual may be intermediate in constitution
between the normal and the full-fledged psychotic who suffers
from " depression."   Similarly, other personality types may
be incomplete manifestations of familiar clinical entities.
This is but one of a host of views which have pictured personality in terms of variation away from a norm towards any
one of various distinct types of maladjustment.   We may
thus have epileptoid, hysteroid, schizoid, neurasthenic,
psychasthenic personalities, etc., a given individual lying
anywhere between the normal and the definite clinical picture.
Similarly, the endocrine types familiar to the clinician have
been regarded merely as extremes of very common forms of
imperfect glandular balance.   All personality, in fact, may
be regarded as deriving from such chemical factors.   Further
consideration will be given to this view in Chapter XXIII.
Attention is given elsewhere[2] to the important contributions
of Stern and Jung to the theory of personality.

In answer to James's question whether all mental states are
intrinsically " personal," no very definite evidence is yet

---

[1] " A Theory of Personality Based Mainly on Psychiatric Experience,"
Psychol. Bull., XVII, 1920.
[2] P. 422 and p. 331.

available. In Freud's system, it is supposed that during dissociation each tendency continues to strive, with an effort which is truly *personal*, despite the fact that the dissociated fragments are at war with another. The view that mental states and processes are never merely mental states and processes, but always the manifestation of a self, has been defended with especial vigour by Calkins.[1] The unit of mental life is for her neither a sensation, such as red, nor an act, such as seeing red ; it is nothing less than such a totality as the *self, seeing red*. Such a " self, seeing red " is always, though in varying degrees, self-conscious. Such a self-psychology cannot permit any corner of psychological existence to call itself impersonal.

Just as the problem of the subconscious is interwoven with the problem of personality, so the latter is interwoven with the problem of the relation of mind and body. Perhaps the most prevalent attitude of contemporary psychologists is to regard the problem as outside the scope of psychology as at present defined. This attitude, however, very naturally means in practice a refusal to admit that any such problem exists. This again turns out upon closer examination to mean among many psychologists that the answer to the problem is quite simple, and that philosophy has made itself much trouble over many unproductive and unreal problems. When we turn to ask what this simple and obvious answer is, we find persisting, without great alteration, a variety of answers prevalent in the nineteenth century, indeed, a number of them prevalent in the ancient world. Many of them have, however, taken on special colouring as a result of the scientific and philosophical events of the last few decades, and we may attempt a brief characterization of a few of their contemporary forms.

Interactionism is still alive, though its adherents appear to be frankly in the position of defending it against difficult odds. One of the most comprehensive statements of the claims of interactionism is McDougall's[2] " animistic " doctrine, a justification of the *a priori* and common-sense opinion that " things " and " selves " are ultimately and absolutely distinct. An organism is no mere mechanism, but a body with a constantly governing and integrating " anima "

[1] *E.g., A First Book in Psychology* (1910).
[2] *Body and Mind* (1911).

or spirit. Without such a regulating principle, mind could have no being. Bergson's[1] insistence that some aspects of memory are independent of any basis in brain physiology is another prominent form of psychophysical " dualism."

Nineteenth-century physiological psychology, as a part of its task of keeping free from metaphysical problems, allowed great weight to the claims of " psychophysical parallelism," the view that mental events and physiological events go on side by side, neither one being the cause of the other. This became, in fact, the "orthodox" view for experimental psychologists, and it is still prevalent. Its difficulties, however, have led to increasing impatience. The statement that the thrust of a pin does not cause pain, or that a hasty decision bears no causal relation to a hasty act, seems not only an injury to common sense, but an interference with experimental procedure.[2] The view has consequently tended to lose ground in the face of various forms of " monism " which may be very briefly indicated.

It may be said that " materialism," as Cabanis stated it, has undergone a number of modifications necessarily incident to recent changes in the concept of " matter." Matter is no longer the obvious bulky moving tangible thing which it was in the time of Cabanis. Matter itself turns into energy under known conditions. Its electronic constitution and the laws which govern the change of matter into energy have made mathematical conceptions more and more important, while " substances " have become less and less tangible. And energy itself is so difficult either to describe or to use as a conceptual tool, except through mathematical symbols, that matter has naturally suffered the same fate. Materialism, then, while clinging to its traditional presuppositions, has no longer taken for granted the possibility of our directly comprehending just what matter is. The essential postulate of materialism, however, appears to be the conviction that conscious life is ultimately made up of particles which are

---

[1] *Matter and Memory* (1896).
[2] Its practical difficulties are suggested in Pillsbury's words : " For convenience we shall often seem to imply that activity in sensory neurones produces changes in consciousness and that ideas start motor discharges that lead to action. This is not to be regarded as committing the author to any theory of the real connection between body and mind, but as a lapse into popular speech." (*Essentials of Psychology*, 1911, p. 48.)

entirely devoid of all conscious quality ; the synthesis of
non-mental units gives an aggregate to which the name
" experience " or " mind " or " consciousness " is applied.
Loeb's *Mechanistic Conception of Life* (1912) is perhaps the
most popular of the many volumes which have kept the
fundamental principles of materialism alive among psychologists.

A view which has also the advantage of avoiding every
sort of dualism is the doctrine that the particles of which the
physical universe is composed are similar to those of which
experience is composed. Instead of proceeding from unconscious bits to conscious aggregates, this view proceeds from
" experience " as a datum, and contends that every real
entity in the universe is of like nature. The theory that
" matter " is simply a way in which conscious reality may be
apprehended by another consciousness has undergone many
refinements. Physico-chemical processes are themselves
regarded as ultimately psychic ; subdivisions of physical
structure are in reality the elementary forms of psychic
existence. The philosophic implications of the view were
elaborated by C. A. Strong[1] twenty-five years ago, while
Troland[2] has recently done much to justify such a position
in terms of our contemporary knowledge of physics and
chemistry. This modern " panpsychism" permits no
dualism between physical events and mental events. That
which is in itself mental is known to the physical scientist
under the form of a mathematical symbol. When we observe
a " physical" change, there are, to be sure, two events, but
both are psychic. A *genuinely psychic* event is going on, let
us say, in the test-tube, and in addition to this there is going
on a series of experiences in the observer. What the observer
calls an external event is the experience through which he is
passing, while outside his experience another experience is in
progress. If now it be asked what is going on in the brain
of the observer, the reply is that the physico-chemical changes
of the observer's brain are simply the same events which he,
as a conscious individual, undergoes. The term " physico-
chemical" is the kind of term that we use when we try to
describe an experience without entering into it. This is, of
course, not idealism of the Berkeleyan form. All the data

[1] *Why the Mind Has a Body* (1903).
[2] *E.g., The Mystery of Mind* (1926).

of the sciences are real, not only for the observer, but for the entities observed.

Neo-realism, since the days of Mach and James, has enjoyed a lively growth, and, especially through the writings of Holt, Montague, and Perry,[1] has undergone modifications which have made it acceptable to psychologists who demand a monistic theory. Consciousness is not an entity added to the organism. It is, on the contrary, a special relation between the organism and the object. Originally adapted for the explanation of cognitive processes, it has been developed also to cover emotional and volitional events. The problem of hallucinations and other apparently disturbing instances of incongruity between object and percept have engaged serious attention. Neo-realism appears to be competing, not unsuccessfully, with other contemporary forms of monism.

[1] See, for example, their contributions as three of the six authors of *The New Realism* (1912).

CHAPTER XXIII

CONTEMPORARY PHYSIOLOGICAL PSYCHOLOGY

The nature of the mind and soul is bodily.—*Lucretius.*

THE term " physiological psychology " has gradually undergone a delimitation since the age dominated by Helmholtz and Wundt. Much, for example, of contemporary introspective psychology, though pursuing problems discussed by Wundt, would scarcely be called " physiological." Many of the fields, moreover, once included under the term, have yielded such a rich harvest of experimental results that they have become almost separate provinces. Studies of optics and acoustics, for example, may be annually numbered by the hundreds; the lower senses have been studied almost as vigorously; reaction-time and psychophysics have been the subject of such extensive labours that many volumes would be needed to summarize the results. These fields now have their own bibliographies and historical treatments, and we cannot here do them justice.[1] We must, however, remind the reader of the extraordinary importance for the history of psychology which attaches to these departments of inquiry; quite aside from the volume of factual material which they have yielded, they have played a major rôle in revealing the way toward an experimental psychology.

Our concern in this chapter is with the development of research upon the functions of the central and autonomic nervous systems and the glands of internal secretion, in relation to important advances in psychological theory which have attended such research.

A profound alteration in the conception of cortical localization has followed from the clinical and, more especially, from the experimental studies of the last twenty years. In

[1] The reader will find Titchener's *Experimental Psychology* (1901–5), and Fröbes's *Lehrbuch der experimentellen Psychologie* (1920) of special value; though neither is expressly historical, each contains much historical material on special problems.

the first years of the century fairly definite and precise localization of sensory and motor functions was accepted for both man and other mammals, and the view was current that each stimulus-response connection in the central nervous system resided in some specific neurone-pathway, the low resistance of whose synapses predetermined the course of the neural impulse. Such definite connections were supposed to exist not only between sensory and motor regions, but within regions adjacent to these, which, as we have seen (p. 202), were regarded as co-ordinating centres, controlling the pattern of motor responses and making possible the " interpretation " of complex sensory impressions under the form of percepts. No conviction in this field was more definite than the belief that each form of aphasia always resulted from injury in a specific region. As early as 1906, however, Marie[1] protested vigorously against such an interpretation, insisting that aphasia was simply one aspect of general intellectual disorganization attending gross cortical injury. He and others pointed to the numerous instances in which aphasia is not found despite the predisposing lesions appearing later in post-mortem examinations. While failing in their purpose of forcing neurologists to give up the whole concept of cortical localization in relation to aphasia, they have induced much skepticism and agnosticism on the subject. It is noteworthy that the recent classification of aphasic types by Head[2] is based simply upon psychological patterns and not upon cortical localization.[3] These psychological patterns do not conform to traditional notions of " faculties." The use of given *grammatical categories*, for example, may be affected. The whole question of ultimate categories or forms of mental process is under discussion (see p. 434, footnote 2).

In the meantime the experimental work of Franz[4] upon the frontal and occipital lobes of monkeys included the study of areas not known to have sensory and motor functions, that is (to borrow a term from human psychology), the associa-

[1] Marie's data and conclusions are obtainable in Moutier, *L'aphasie de Broca* (1908).
[2] *E.g.*, " Disorders of Symbolic Thinking and Expression," *Brit. J. Psychol.*, XI, 1920–1, *Aphasia and Kindred Disorders of Speech* (1926).
[3] For a synthesis of work on human cerebral functions, see Piéron, *Thought and the Brain* (1923). See also Child, *The Origin and Development of the Nervous System* (1921).
[4] *E.g.*, " On the Functions of the Cerebrum : The Frontal Lobes," *Arch. of Psychol.*, No. II, 1907.

tion areas. He showed that certain habits recently learned by the animals were completely lost after removal of large parts of the brain, and that such removal also greatly increased the difficulty of acquiring new habits. In view of the fact that the material removed, in the case of the frontal lobes, was of considerable bulk, it was not surprising that the frontal lobes appeared to be of special importance, in relation both to retention and to the learning of new habits.

The work of Lashley and Franz[1], however, soon unearthed serious difficulties in even such a vague statement of localization as the foregoing. It became difficult to establish any specific locus within which habits resided. The many researches of Lashley have in recent years suggested the necessity of profound alteration in the theory of localization. Monkeys in which the *entire* pre-Rolandic motor area was removed recovered all the lost capacities for movement, this fact apparently indicating that other centres may suffice for motor control.[2] Similarly, paradoxical as the result appears, the visual area of the rat was shown to be unnecessary for visual discrimination. To be sure, the removal of the visual cortex destroyed an already formed visual discrimination habit, but the animals very quickly regained the lost habit.[3] It appeared that other centres in the nervous system were capable of carrying out even such complex functions.[4]

As regards the matter of specific localization of the pathways for habit, Lashley has shown that a variety of motor habits are unaffected by the removal of small areas in the cortex. In a large group of animals which had learned the same habit, individual rats were subjected to a variety of operations ; in some animals one region, in other animals another region, was removed, so that every part of the cortex was studied. Strangely enough, none of the animals completely lost the habit. The cutting out of a small region did not *obliterate* a habit pathway. Yet the whole cortex was thus examined. Very large injuries to the cortex did, how-

---

[1] *E.g.*, " The Effects of Cerebral Destruction upon Habit Formation and Retention in the Albino Rat," *Psychobiology*, I, 1917.

[2] " The Retention of Motor Habits after Destruction of the So-called Motor Areas in Primates," *Arch. of Neurol. and Psychiatry*, XII, 1924.

[3] Studies of Cerebral Function in Learning, I, *Psychobiology*, II 1920.

[4] The general fact that several centres may co-operate in the carrying out of a function had long been known.

DD

ever, destroy established habits, though the differential significance of the specific regions was not apparent.[1]

Very similar results have been obtained in connection with the functions of the cortex in relation to *new* learning. Gross injury to the cortex appeared to impede learning, while slight injuries appeared to exercise no such effect, no matter what their localization. From these and a great many other studies, Lashley has continued to urge the hypothesis that points in the cortex are " equipotential " in relation to learning. The implications of all this for human psychology are far from clear. It is, indeed, probable that the specialization of function in the mammalian brain becomes more definite as we proceed to higher forms, and that localization in the human cortex is considerably more definite than that found in the rat. Nevertheless, the effect of Lashley's work has been to introduce much uncertainty where confidence had begun to reign. And the interpretation of human habit in terms of specific pathways, though by no means dislodged, has encountered a difficulty which seems scarcely likely to be removed, except perhaps through much more direct clinical and experimental evidence. If, in the rat, habits must be construed as general behaviour patterns depending upon cortical patterns, rather than simple " pathways," how can human habits be reasonably stated in terms of such pathways?[2] It may well be, of course, that many pathways are simultaneously established and simultaneously utilized in the case of all habit, so that, though no local injury can destroy the habit, it may nevertheless be quite correctly described in terms of the traditional pathways with lowered synaptic resistance. But this is sheer conjecture—one of many possible conjectures. At this writing psychology has not found its way out from this forest of interrogation points.

Early in the present century, the work of J. N. Langley[3] helped to clarify the functions of the " autonomic " nervous

[1] A bibliography and critique of many localization studies by Lashley and others appears in Herrick, *Brains of Rats and Men* (1926).

[2] Lashley's work has also called in question the alleged effect of practice in lowering synaptic resistance (see p. 205). It seems doubtful, in fact, whether the whole conception of specific neural pathways can be said to have helped toward more accurate statement of any psychological problem.

[3] Schäfer's *Textbook of Physiology*, II (1900), p. 616 f.

system.   While " sympathetic " fibres had long been known to be connected with visceral disturbances and therefore presumably with emotion, Langley's demonstration that unstriped muscles and glands are controlled by nerve fibres lying outside of, and to some extent functionally independent of, the central system, was fraught with psychological implications.   It soon became natural to think of the emotional life as dependent on the autonomic system, just as cognitive functions were thought of as aspects of central nervous functions.   The central nervous system has been regarded as the seat of intelligence, much clinical evidence pointing to the close relation between brain degeneration and intellectual degeneration ; while the autonomic system has come to be looked upon as the seat both of simple affects (pleasantness and unpleasantness) and of emotion.   Nevertheless, Head and Holmes[1] have brought forward important evidence to show that lesions of the *thalamus* are associated with profound affective disturbances.   From this, as well as from more recent clinical material on epidemic encephalitis, it appears probable that affective functions are to a large degree dependent upon the mid-brain.   The separation between " cognitive " and " affective " seems, in fact, to be far from simple. An experiment indicating the difficulties of the problem is the study, by Head and his collaborators[2], of the regeneration of injured cutaneous nerve.   The investigation of its functions during recovery seemed to indicate that " touch " is by no means a unitary process.   It was necessary to distinguish at least a " protopathic " function, which gave but the vague awareness of the location of points stimulated, and an " epicritic " function, which enabled the subject to localize a stimulus much more accurately.   This distinction, though supported by some subsequent investigations, has been challenged by Boring[3] and others, and much investigation and discussion have followed.   In Head's work, protopathic functions had a definitely affective character—they were unpleasant—while epicritic functions appeared to be purely cognitive.   The distinction between pain and unpleasantness,

[1] " Sensory Disturbances from Cerebral Lesions," *Brain*, XXXIV 1911-2.
[2] *E.g.*, Head and Sherren, "The Consequences of Injury to the Peripheral Nerves in Man." *Brain*, XXVIII, 1905.
[3] " Cutaneous Sensation after Nerve-division," *Q. J. Exp. Physiol.*, X, 1916.

which, since the work of Blix and Goldscheider, had been regarded as clear-cut, has again become confused. The fact that some painful stimuli may actually be pleasant appears to stand secure. All that can safely be said is that present evidence makes difficult not only a sharp antithesis between central and autonomic functions, but any clear line of separation between cognitive and affective processes.

Closely bound up with such studies of autonomic functions is the recent growth of endocrinology, in such fashion as to exert great influence upon psychology. The nineteenth century had witnessed remarkable advances in the understanding of the functions of the ductless glands. Addison's[1] study of tuberculosis of the adrenal glands, Brown-Séquard's[2] study of the secretions of sex, and Baumann's[3] demonstration of the importance of iodine in the thyroid secretion, are instances of clinical and experimental progress to which many scores of physicians made substantial contributions. These contributions, despite their significance for psychiatry, were not generally recognized to be of psychological importance until very recently. A desultory account of cretinism is all that the psychologist seemed concerned to offer. Even Kendall's[4] epoch-making discovery of the chemical constitution of thyroxin, the active principle of the thyroid gland, attracted very little attention among psychologists.

The chief factor precipitating a radical change in the attitude of the psychologist was the publication, in 1915, of Cannon's[5] studies upon the functions of the adrenal glands. Cannon reported that fear and rage, experimentally excited in dogs and in cats, led to active secretion of adrenalin, with the result that blood pressure was raised, glycogen liberated from the liver, and the striped muscles stimulated to heightened activity. These emotions, then, directly involved a great variety of physiological changes, in the production of which the endocrines, and of course the "sympathetic" fibres leading to them, were all-important. Crile's[6] study of thyroid

---

[1] On the Constitutional and Local Effects of the Disease of the Suprarenal Capsules (1855).

[2] C. R. de la Soc. de Biol., XLI, 1889.

[3] E.g., Münch. Med. Wochenschr., XLIII, 1896.

[4] The Isolation in Crystalline Form of the Compound Containing Iodin, which Occurs in the Thyroid (1915).

[5] Bodily Changes in Pain, Hunger, Fear and Rage. (Cannon's work on the endocrines had already been in progress for several years.)

[6] E.g., The Origin and Nature of the Emotions (1915)

functions also became well known to psychologists during and immediately after the war. These and many other contributions from physiologists and clinicians have not only awakened the interest of psychologists in the anomalies of personality which attend disordered glandular systems, but have offered the hope that many aspects of normal personality can be stated in terms of glandular constitution.

The rapid advances in the understanding of autonomic and endocrine functions has in fact engendered much discussion among physiologists and psychologists as to the physical basis of " personality." The central nervous system had been regarded, since the seventeenth century, as the substrate of mental life. But the work of such men as Langley, Crile, and Cannon has suggested various competing theories. One is to the effect that the autonomic nervous system is the core of physical selfhood, both the central system and the endocrines serving as instruments through which autonomic strivings exercise their control of the body.[1] Or, central and autonomic systems may be held to enjoy a co-operative control—a " consular " authority, so to speak. In sharp contrast to such views is the recently popular belief in the " chemical " nature of personality. The glands of internal secretion are regarded as the prime movers both in the growth and in the exercise of personal traits, each personality depending upon the emotional and volitional aspects of a " glandular balance." The over-rapid and uncritical acceptance of some aspects of the glandular theory has produced a marked reaction,[2] and compromise positions appear to enjoy distinctly greater favour, while the collection of pertinent data on the significance of the endocrines for personality continues.

Waldeyer's " neurone theory " has done much to help psychologists to think in definite neurological terms. The work of Sherrington during the opening years of the century, described in his *Integrative Action of the Nervous System*

---

[1] *E.g.*, Kempf, " The Autonomic Functions and the Personality," *Nerv. and Ment. Dis. Monogr. Ser. No.* 28, 1918.

[2] " ..... certain handbooks of misinformation which enable the laity to diagnose glandular balance with the finality of a palmist or a phrenologist."—H. E. Starr, before the *American Psychological Association*, 1926.

(1906), did even more. Fundamental conceptions for neurophysiology were defined and in many cases experimentally verified, frequently with reference to psychological implications.

The experimental study of the reflex arc in normal and decerebrate mammals underwent a series of refinements. When a single stimulus was too weak to elicit a motor response, the repeated application of the same weak stimulus was found to be capable, by " summation," of traversing the threshold, throwing the reflex into full swing. But simultaneous, as well as successive, stimuli might co-operate with or " facilitate " one another. When a stimulus at one point was too weak to set the reflex going, a stimulus at another point might, although itself too weak, join forces with the first, evoking the response. In other cases, a stimulus which would ordinarily evoke a reflex response was found to be " inhibited " by another stimulus. Such " facilitation " and " inhibition," already familiar to physiologists,[1] were elaborately analysed, and definite evidence was offered to show their relation to the functions of the synapse. Both processes seemed to be effected by synapses intermediate between receptor and organ of response ; two pathways, reaching a synapse, might either aid or interfere with one another. " Reciprocal inhibition " was demonstrated in numerous instances ; the innervation of extensor muscles involved not only the inactivity but the *lowered tonus* of the flexor muscles of the same limbs. The process by which one pathway was opened served also to block pathways leading to opposed action.[2] The supposition that facilitation and inhibition are synaptic functions was greatly strengthened by Sherrington's study of the effect of fatigue and drugs. A bit of nerve tissue containing no synapses proved very insusceptible to fatigue, whereas regions containing synapses could conduct only for a brief period without the occurrence of fatigue. Certain drugs were found to block off an impulse quite effectively if applied to a region containing synapses,

---

[1] Especially through the work of Exner, *Pflüger's Archiv.*, XXVIII, 1882.

[2] McDougall's " drainage theory " of reciprocal inhibition (*Physiological Psychology*, 1905) held that when A-B and C-D are antagonistic reflexes, A-B, while functioning, draws off the energy of C, so that the response D is inhibited ; fatigue in the pathway A-B makes possible the sudden activity of C-D, draining the energy from A.

while regions containing none were practically unaffected. Other drugs, instead of increasing, greatly reduced synaptic resistance.

All this work, then, confirmed for psychologists the extraordinary importance of the synapse for facilitation and inhibition in higher processes. The nature of synaptic function, however, was not disclosed by Sherrington's methods, and to this problem more than two decades of active research have still failed to give any definite answer. The most fruitful inquiry, however, seems to be that associated with the names of Nernst,[1] Lillie,[2] and Lucas.[3] Theoretical and experimental conditions alike suggest that the nerve current is a " wave of depolarization " which passes along the nerve fibre whenever a stimulus disturbs the delicate balance of positive and negative ions produced in the metabolism of the nerve. An instant after the depolarization of a given point that point is in " refractory phase," another instant later it is in a condition of " hyper-excitability," and again it returns to its normal state ; thus the wave has a definite frequency. Now each synapse is conceived to have its own refractory phase and period of hyper-excitability. When the frequency of two nerve-impulses is so timed that the depolarization wave from one arrives at the synapse while it is in refractory phase from the other, inhibition occurs. Similarly, when the wave strikes at a moment of hyper-excitability, facilitation occurs. The hypothesis presents difficulties, the problem being highly complex. Such a view is illustrative, however, of the advances of physiological chemistry, and the growing insistence that the synapse should be conceived in such terms as to throw genuine light upon the phenomena of facilitation and inhibition. The " chronaxy " theory of Lapicque[4] employs similar quantitative concepts, defining the functions of the synapse in terms of the time it takes to excite a neurone. " Every tissue has, as it were, its own private time-value."[5] Only when the time-value of one neurone is equal to that of

---

[1] *Arch. f. d. ges. Physiol.*, CXXII, 1908.
[2] " The Relation of Stimulation and Conduction in Irritable Tissues to Changes in the Permeability of the Limiting Membranes," *Am. J. Physiol.*, XXVIII, 1911, *Protoplasmic Action and Nervous Action* (1923).
[3] *The Conduction of the Nervous Impulse* (1917).
[4] *L'excitabilité en fonction du temps* (1926).
[5] C. K. Ogden, *The Meaning of Psychology* (1926), p. 52 f.

another, or longer *by an integral number of times*, can conduction occur.

We may here refer very briefly to the study of nervous and mental phenomena connected with work, fatigue, and sleep. The phenomena of the " curve of work," especially the increasing or decreasing efficiency which attends continued application to a task, were investigated late in the nineteenth century by Cattell,[1] Mosso,[2] Kraepelin,[3] and others. Studies of fatigue have been very numerous in recent years, especially in connection with industrial problems. The study of the curve of work during the day, and of the effect of rest-periods, has apparently yielded results of immediate practical value.

Interwoven with such concerns is the attempt to clarify the problem of " mental fatigue." Mosso,[4] Sherrington,[5] and others have made it clear that there is such a thing as nervous fatigue aside from muscular fatigue, but this has not proved to be a solution of the problem. Nor has Sherrington's demonstration that nervous fatigue is chiefly a matter of the synapse proved sufficient. To be sure, physical work may, as in Dockeray's[6] experiments, make subsequent mental work more difficult. But evidence that mental work causes, within a short time, a marked decrease in the efficiency in the mental task involved, has been hard to find. The gruelling twelve-hour mental-multiplication task of Arai,[7] and many studies with periods of two to four hours, suggest that profound fatigue in mental functions is at best a phenomenon much rarer than had been supposed. The studies of Dodge,[8] Muscio,[9] and others, make it doubtful, in fact, whether there is any single entity underlying the term " fatigue."

The influence of humidity, temperature, illumination, and other factors bearing upon efficiency, has been examined in

[1] *Philos. Stud.*, III, 1886.
[2] *E.g., Arch. ital. de biol.*, XIII, 1890.
[3] *E.g., Philos. Stud.*, XIX, 1902.
[4] *Arch. ital. de biol.*, XIII, 1890.
[5] *Integrative Action of the Nervous System* (1906).
[6] " The Effects of Physical Fatigue on Mental Efficiency," *Kansas Univ. Sci. Bull.*, IX, 1915.
[7] *Mental Fatigue* (1912).
[8] " The Laws of Relative Fatigue," *Psychol. Rev.*, XXIV, 1917.
[9] *E.g.,* " Is a Fatigue Test Possible ? " *Brit. J. Psychol,*, XII, 1921-2.

Great Britain, Germany, and the United States, especially during the last fifteen years.[1] However, the most intensive as well as the most satisfactory work in this department, is the study of the influence of drugs. The many investigations of Kraepelin[2] have been supplemented by the work of Rivers,[3] Dodge and Benedict,[4] and others, on the effects of alcohol ; of Hollingworth[5] on the effects of caffein ; of Hull[6] on the effects of tobacco ; and by many other studies.

" Theories of sleep "[7] have become abundant. While the results of experimentation are far from clear, fatigue poisons evidently do help to induce sleep, but posture, freedom from disturbance, and habit clearly play an important rôle. Freedom from disturbance has been especially emphasized by Sidis,[8] whose experimental induction in both animals and human beings of quasi-sleeping or " hypnoidal " states has served to justify this emphasis. Postural and other muscular factors have been stressed by H. M. Johnson.[9] Between the rival assertions that the brain during sleep is over-supplied with blood and that it is under-supplied, the former appears through the work of J. F. Shepard[10] to have gained the ascendancy. Evidently the fragments of evidence available serve only to make the nature of sleep as obscure as that of " fatigue."

---

[1] For an account of research upon these and allied problems, see Poffenberger, *Applied Psychology* (1927).

[2] *E.g., Münch. Med. Wochenschr.*, XLVI, 1899.

[3] *The Influence of Alcohol and Other Drugs on Fatigue* (1908).

[4] *The Psychological Effects of Alcohol* (1915).

[5] " The Influence of Caffein on Mental and Motor Efficiency," *Arch. of Psychol.*, No. XXII, 1912.

[6] " The Influence of Tobacco Smoking on Mental and Motor Efficiency," *Psychol. Monogr.*, XXXIII, 1924.

[7] A summary is given in Howell's *Text Book of Physiology*, 7th ed. (1918).

[8] " An Experimental Study of Sleep," *J. Abn. Psychol.*, III, 1908–9.

[9] " An Essay toward an Adequate Explanation of Sleep," *Psychol. Bull.*, XXIII, 1926.

[10] *The Circulation and Sleep* (1914).

CHAPTER XXIV

A SUMMARY AND AN INTERPRETATION

The order and connection of ideas is the same as the order and connection of things.—Spinoza.

A BRIEF review of the major movements which have been considered may take the form of examining the changes in interest which have constantly marked new fields for intensive study, as well as that of outlining a few general characteristics of the whole period under consideration. The former task is the simpler, and may best be undertaken first.

The introduction of experimental method into the study of sensory functions had already brought promise, in the days of Bell and Goethe, that psychology as well as physiology was to be profoundly affected. In the hands of Weber such a hope was carried much nearer to fulfilment ; not only were many sensory and perceptual functions experimentally studied, but a great generalization regarding " just noticeable differences " was offered, which led, in the hands of Fechner, to the establishment of those " psychophysical methods " which did so much to teach psychologists to think in quantitative and in experimental terms. During the middle of the century came also the epoch-making investigations of Helmholtz, in the physiology of eye and ear, and in the measurement of reaction-time. The first fruits of the evolutionary theory appeared in Galton's study of individual differences, with special reference to heredity. His research on imagery and association marked further fields for experimental examination. The movement led by Wundt, and having its headquarters in the Leipzig laboratory for psychology, led, in the work of Ebbinghaus, Cattell, and many others, to the remarkably rapid conquest of many complicated problems in memory, perception, and association. The end of the nineteenth century, and the first years of the twentieth, witnessed not only the extension of experimental methods to include some of the most complex processes of thinking and willing, but the delimitation of several new branches of psychology

406

which aimed to be empirical even though a thorough-going
experimental technique was not yet available. The psychology of childhood, social psychology, and the psychology of
religion became recognized fields, each with its empirical
technique. In the same period the experimental study of
learning took on new forms in the analysis of motor skill,
and in the founding of an experimental animal psychology.
The data upon learning and memory, together with new
materials from neurology and physiology, made possible the
fusion of the traditional problems of learning, memory, association, perception, and reasoning; the " neurone theory "
and the " conditioned reflex " served as clues in the simplification of these problems. The " behaviourism " which
appeared as one consequence of these events had soon
to contend with another psychological system, psychoanalysis, which, arising from clinical studies, began in the
second decade of the present century to alter in many ways
the outlines traced by laboratory psychology. Perhaps the
two greatest interests of the last decade of psychological
history are the analysis of the affective life and the development of instruments to measure intelligence and other
complex functions.

The picture thus rudely drawn, exaggerating, even more
than has the preceding text, the dominance of special problems
and the sharpness of transitions, is subject to some geographical qualifications. German psychology, so long the vanguard
of experimentalism, has tended, in recent years, to emphasize
philosophical problems, in some of which experimental methods
are gladly used at crucial points, while in others most
students are quite content to dispense with them. French
psychology has, for several generations, had its centre in
psychiatric conceptions, but has, in the work of Binet, contributed powerfully to the testing movement. The two foci
around which American psychology has revolved are experimental method and the technique of testing. British psychology, while until very recently much less cordial to experimental research, has, since Galton, continued to make
important contributions to statistical method. The influence
of Austria has been felt in the psychoanalytic movement,
while Switzerland, long renowned in education, has continued
to do much for the science of pedagogy. The chief Italian
contributions have come by way of neurology. Russian

work upon the "conditioned response" has leavened psychology everywhere.

Throughout the last few decades certain general tendencies seem to be fairly consistently at work, serving to make contemporary psychology a creature quite unlike the psychology of Helmholtz's day, not only in respect to a greater store of knowledge, but in respect to its fundamental purposes.

First, as regards the transition from structural to functional problems. The hope of analysing the ultimate constituents of mental life and of stating their interrelations has slowly waned, partly because of the immense difficulties encountered, and partly because of a biological interest, which, following the evolutionary theory, has made *functions* and *adjustments* the matters of most absorbing interest. The desire to make psychology a biological science has constantly impelled psychologists to find in their subject matter instances of general biological laws. The practical demands of education and industry have contributed their quota to the tendency.

Secondly, the habit of thinking of mental life as an aggregate of parts has tended to give way to the notion of the organism as a whole. The evolutionary theory has played its part here also. But the experimental problems of physiology and psychology have themselves frequently proved refractory to a purely analytic method. The necessity of understanding the interrelation of functions has made it necessary to look for larger patterns of experience and behaviour, patterns comprising, in many cases, the whole life of the individual. Psychoanalysis and the *Gestalt* psychology appear to be not the cause, but simply two important expressions of this trend.

Thirdly, in consequence of the first two movements, and of the constant emphasis of science upon the mathematical method, psychology has moved from qualitative to quantitative problems. The dream of Herbart and Fechner, of stating the inner recesses of experience in quantitative terms, has not been fulfilled ; but the analysis of processes and functions has, since Helmholtz, yielded a richer and richer harvest of quantitative laws. Such laws, whether pertaining to the time-relations of mental processes, or to the phenomena of learning and forgetting, or to the growth of intelligence, or to other complex statistical problems, give to students of contemporary psychology the sense of speaking in the "universal language of science." Long baffled by the inability to cite verifiable laws relating to the world of mental qualities, they have found themselves, in many cases, enabled through mathematical methods to generalize, to predict, and to control.

Fourthly, there has come about, in consequence of all these tendencies, an unexpected change of emphasis : experimental methods have in many fields been displaced by genetic and statistical methods. The hope of success in an experiment depends upon the possibility of isolating distinct factors, and treating separately the influence of each experimental variable upon the phenomenon whose nature is under examination. Experimentation, in this sense of the term, was a fruitful—in fact, the only fruitful—method in the analysis of many of those problems of physiological psychology which dominated the latter part of the nineteenth century. As more complicated problems have been approached, and as the raising of new problems has more and more outstripped the experimenter's ingenuity in devising suitable methods, diffidence or even despair has in many cases tended to replace the enthusiasm of a generation ago. Not, indeed, that experimental methods have ceased to gain in variety and in reliability ; but they have been hopelessly unable to keep pace with the imperative demand for more factual material upon the emotional and volitional life, the nature of suggestibility and imitation, the relative importance of heredity and environment in the causation of individual differences, the manner in which social likes and dislikes, ambitions and ideals, are acquired, and a host of equally pressing questions.

But another method of analysing complex phenomena has been gaining headway, one which the biologist has employed with profit for a century. Complicated things are apt, most of the time, to have relatively simple origins, and this holds good for the study of individuals, of species, and even in many cases of social groups. The importance of embryology for anatomy and histology can scarcely be exaggerated. Just such a genetic approach is now demanded by students of nearly every branch of psychology. The meagre data now furnished by the psychology of childhood and adolescence are eagerly caught up by all who seek to understand the intricacies of adult life. The origin of attitudes and purposes is, however, not the only type of problem which has thus undergone metamorphosis. Even such time-honoured questions as those relating to reasoning and perception are coming to be seen as essentially developmental problems.

The growth of statistical methods is no less striking. Pearson's correlation method has been in use only a third of a century, yet nearly every problem in which quantities are handled now witnesses its use, or the use of the much more complicated mathematical methods which have developed from it. The relation between two variables has actually been found to be statable in other terms than those of experiment. The intelligent use of correlation methods permits the detection of relations in many situations which defy experimental analysis. Even the degree of dependence may be indicated, or, more strictly, the relative importance of one causal factor in comparison with others. From this emerges a fact fraught with remarkable possibilities. Yule's[1] method of "partial correlation" has made possible the mathematical "isolation" of variables which cannot be isolated experimentally. The computation of the correlation between any two factors in a complex situation was previously impossible, because the many unknowns might be related to one or to both of the variables under consideration. Partial correlations remove any or all desired variables from a complex; the correlation of any two may then be worked.

But correlation methods necessitate in general large numbers of cases, besides involving many other difficulties and dangers, and it is too early to tell whither they are leading. What they have already yielded and what they are likely to yield to psychology through constant statistical advances is nevertheless of such major importance as to lead the writer to the opinion that the only twentieth-century discovery comparable in importance to the conditioned-response method is the method of partial correlations.

There is, of course, no opposition between genetic and statistical methods on the one hand and experimental methods on the other. All three are, in fact, used together

---

[1] *An Introduction to the Theory of Statistics* (1911).

in many studies. Further, experimental methods, having the longest history and having attained a more thorough testing in the hands of many generations of scientists, are likely to remain the most direct and satisfactory method for many problems, and the court of last appeal whenever they are available.

The development of quantitative methods in the psychology of the past three generations, whether as an adjunct to experimental, to genetic, or to other inquiries, seems, however, to have certain profound implications for the subject matter of psychology as a science. These implications have already become apparent for many subdivisions of psychology, and appear to be in a fair way to attain equal significance for the entire field.

The first mathematical generalization yielded by nineteenth-century psychology was " Weber's Law." It became apparent in the course of time that the law held only in a " middle range " of intensities, and that many other difficulties attended not only the attempt to give it metaphysical significance, but even its verification as a law of " just noticeable differences."

The studies of Ebbinghaus yielded a mathematical generalization of radically different character. He demonstrated clearly, in his own case, that beyond a given point learning ceased to increase in even pace with the time expended on the task. Arithmetically increasing units of time brought, to be sure, increasing achievement, but achievement which followed the principle of " diminishing returns." The type of curve thus plotted was duplicated by Ebbinghaus's " curve of forgetting," except, of course, that it was inverted. In forgetting, as in learning, the effect of constant additional units of time was to produce less and less change in the organism. Cattell's study of the effect of practice upon reaction-time gave similar results ; in other words, a different form of learning exhibited the same principle of diminishing returns. The work of Bryan and Harter further confirmed the principle in quite another sort of learning. And whatever complexities are introduced by other variables or constants, Ebbinghaus's general quantitative conception of the form of learning and forgetting curves has been very solidly established.[1] Thurstone,[2] utilizing this principle, has recently offered a formula to cover all the phenomena of learning, account being taken of difficulties in the material and of many other factors. Another instance of this principle of " diminishing returns " appears in the phenomena of intellectual growth. To compare the intellectual gain during a given year with that occurring during another year presents difficulties ; but it is clear from recent work that, if not at birth, at least somewhere in the growth-curve the increase of intelligence begins to " taper off." Diminishing returns from time are evident.

The "normal frequency curve " of intelligence and of many other abilities presents another mathematical generalization of wide significance. The fact that normal frequency curves are found at each age-level during intellectual growth makes it possible to construct, so to speak, a poly-dimensional statement of mental functions ; three or more dimensions are already employed in some formulæ for individual abilities. The extensive statistical work of Spearman and his school, whatever the final position assigned to the theory of " general " and " special " factors, offers another highly important " two-dimensional " or " poly-dimensional " approach to psychological data. The quantitative laws already discovered in the fields of optics, acoustics, reaction-time, fatigue, and pharmaco-psychology, to mention only a few departments, have already become very numerous. Applied psychology has been enabled, in many cases, to predict successfully the output of work to be expected from given conditions of illumination, ventilation, climate, diet, etc. The great complexity of the factors entering into any mental activity make difficult, however, the establishment of laws of wide general validity. They are, moreover, subject to a fundamental qualification. Apparently, individual differences of three major types must be taken into account in all general laws. Individuals differ in maturity, in experience, and in hereditary constitution. At least these three variables appear

---

[1] At the " physiological limit " learning curves seem to become straight lines. Actually we are dealing with a new and confusing factor. The subject's benefit from practice balances against his losses from disuse ; the beginnings of the curve of forgetting are masked by the effects of continued effort.

[2] " The Learning Curve Equation," *Psychol. Monogr.*, XXVI, 1918-9.

to be necessary in addition to all those pertaining to any special problem.

The reader will have noticed, however, that not one of the laws indicated is a law pertaining to mental states in relation to other such states. The great majority of them, in fact, look suspiciously like *physiological* laws, and nothing more. To this point we must give closer attention.

The principle of diminishing returns, so important in the study of learning and forgetting, is apparent in many relatively simple nervous and muscular changes. Even the modification of non-living objects as a result of physical agencies, obeys, in many cases, such a law. There is every reason to believe that the law of diminishing returns in learning and forgetting is no mere " parallel " to laws which hold for the modification of the nervous system. They appear to be, quite simply, the *same* laws. The quantitative advances of physiology are in the mean time leading physiologists to speak, as physicists do, largely in terms of numbers, letters, cosines, and integrals. Physiology, in other words, is undergoing a metamorphosis identical with that which characterizes psychology. Every new quantitative generalization in either science brings nearer the discovery, by both groups, of a system of laws which hold for the phenomena of the other science in exactly the same sense in which they hold for their own.

Quite aside from all theories as to the relation of mind and body, the subject matter of psychology and the subject matter of physiology are already merging, and seem likely before long to become simply one subject matter—the quantitative laws of the organism. It is perhaps not entirely fanciful to suggest that as our knowledge and our language become more precise, the answer to the question, " How much does it hurt ? " may be " $42xy^3cosA$."

Of course, all physical and mathematical research into the nature of quantities must affect such a quantitative psychology. In particular the " quantum theory " makes it probable that integers rather than continua will be the chief conceptual tools. Something not unlike the dream of the Pythagoreans may, in fact, be fulfilled. " This solid, solid universe " may turn out to be, as far as science can know it, simply a pattern of numbers.

And belief in the finality of science seems to be the first

EE

element in the credo of contemporary psychology, all other finalities being abandoned to the claims of relativism. A brief attempt to describe what "science" currently means may therefore be ventured. At least four steps in scientific method seem generally recognized : observation; classification of observations; hypotheses as to relations present among data ; isolation of separate factors in the situation, in order to verify or refute such hypotheses. None of these steps needs to be defined in rigidly quantitative terms ; yet, historically, all have tended, and continue to tend, in the direction of such definition. "Science" means, then, if this summary is not essentially incorrect, one special method of handling the world quantitatively ; and, among quantitative methods, the one which has in most cases proved most effective.

The procedure just described involves certain presuppositions as to the possibilities of "analytic" method ; it is based upon the axiom that the whole is the sum of its parts. For most purposes this procedure has justified itself. Not only psychology, but physical science, is at present in the throes of the complex problem as to the possibility, through the analytic method, of understanding the structure or constitution of real things. At this writing it appears probable, however, that quantitative methods are applicable to the study of relations and structures, as well as to that of constituent parts, and that the various steps in scientific method are equally suitable for the analysis of constituent parts and for the determination of types of organization. The possibility of confirming through experimental and mathematical methods even such relational systems as "relativity" itself is illuminating.

There remain, however, not only vast possibilities for the discovery of more adequate intellectual instruments than those known to contemporary "science," but at least a reasonable possibility that our whole conception of quantities may, as we have long been told so earnestly, turn out to be just as relative as "knowledge" itself. Moreover, men are scarcely likely to lose interest in their own experiences and those of their fellows, and their desire to understand those experiences is scarcely likely to be satisfied by any of the rich treasures which quantitative methods may yield. The direct examination of much of our own experience is admittedly difficult, and the establishment of even the roughest working principles regarding the nature and interrelations of such experience is more than baffling. But, when the laws of physiology and ot quantitative psychology have merged, a century hence, psychology will, I think, still be struggling, and with some measure of success, to devise reliable methods for the direct study of experience, methods which we cannot at present even dimly outline. The study of our own selves is an occupation so absorbing that neither the inadequacy of existing methods nor our despair of finding new ones may be allowed to survive. It may well be that psychology, precisely because of its concern with problems refractory to existing methods, will be the means of wresting from nature new methods and realities which will in time become indispensable to every effort to understand our world.

BIBLIOGRAPHICAL NOTE

Though the bibliography of a volume like the present really consists of the titles of all the books and articles mentioned in text or footnotes, it is appropriate to name here a few books to which I owe special obligation.

BARNES et al., *The History and Prospects of the Social Sciences.*

BRETT, *A History of Psychology,* volumes II and III.

HALL, *The Founders of Modern Psychology.*

HENMON et al., " The Psychological Researches of J. McK. Cattell," *Arch. of Psychol.,* No. 30.

LADD and WOODWORTH, *Elements of Physiological Psychology.*

MERZ, *History of European Thought in the Nineteenth Century.*

RAND, *The Classical Psychologists.*

TITCHENER, *The Experimental Psychology of the Thought-Processes.*

SUPPLEMENT

Contemporary German Psychology

BY

HEINRICH KLUVER

CHAPTER XXV

CONTEMPORARY GERMAN PSYCHOLOGY AS A "NATURAL
SCIENCE"

IN the following the attempt will be made to consider some
aspects of contemporary German psychology in more detail.
Examining the different fields of research and the different
methods used, the attempt at mere enumeration of these
aspects with regard to research material and method may not
present serious difficulties. Difficulties of this kind, however,
arise at once if the historian wishes to sketch the dominant
features in modern Germany psychology. The determination of the dominant trends is more than a mere recording of
such trends ; it is an historical *interpretation* of these trends.

Viewed historically, it seems, at least so far as German
psychology is concerned, that the chief trend is toward a
qualitative psychology and that Hans Henning[1] characterizes
this trend adequately when he writes, " Until the turn of the
century it was believed that one could grasp the mind with
number and measure . . . since 1900 there has developed a
qualitative psychology which concerns itself less with numbers and more with kinds of experience and qualitative
analysis." It would undoubtedly be incorrect to characterize
all trends of modern German psychology as qualitative, as
it would be inadequate to say that the tendency to quantification dominated all fields of psychology before 1900. But

---

[1] *Cf*. Ogden, R.M., " Are there any sensations ? " *Am. J. Psychol.*,
XXXIII, 1922.

it seems to be true that from the turn of the century on, the qualitative trend has become more and more dominant, a trend which, as could easily be shown, originated in the nineteenth century. It is also fair to say that before 1900 physiological psychology, with its emphasis on " measure " and " number," and with its close relation to natural science, was in the foreground, so that Ziehen[1] could write, " Empirical psychology has become physiological psychology." As regards *quæstiones facti* this " empirical " psychology was satisfied with determining the " facts " in a rather limited field, and—owing to its dependence on the methods of natural science—with recording them as real " facts," especially when they permitted of quantitative treatment. A strong positivistic trend is easily recognizable in the field of scientific psychology in Germany before 1900, but then, at first hard to recognize, " the voice of a mild scepticism "— to use Felix Krueger's term—was heard when the results of all this painstaking work were examined. The " hopelessness " of such a psychology, to employ one of Moebius' phrases, was emphasized, and psychologists became less and less inclined to teach what Dunlap has called a " pseudofinal system of facts."

Thus the historian may consider the turning away from the positivistic trend as the dominant feature of contemporary German psychology. If we inquire into the " why " of this change—we shall not attempt here to give an exhaustive answer—it will be necessary to view the history of modern German psychology not as an isolated phenomenon but as a development which is closely related to the history of other fields of scientific and non-scientific endeavour. Here the theory of the historian Karl Lamprecht, Wundt's colleague at Leipzig, is of considerable interest. For Lamprecht, history is " social psychological science," in fact nothing but " applied psychology."[2] For him, German history in its political, social, economic, and scientific aspects—and not only German history—is a sequence of periods of " psychic dissociation " and of " synthesis." He believes that it is characteristic of the periods of dissociation and transition that men are overwhelmed by a vast amount of hitherto unknown, or at

---

[1] Ziehen, T., *Leitfaden der physiologischen Psychologie* (1891).
[2] Lamprecht, K., *Moderne Geschichtswissenschaft* (1905).

least unusual stimuli, by thousands of new impressions which cannot be synthesized. Consequently, a naturalistic attitude, a state of dissociation arises. Lamprecht views the last decades of the nineteenth century as such a transitional epoch, in which not only radical socio-political and economic changes took place, but in which natural science underwent most important revolutions. In such an era of transition both the natural scientist and the psychologist " make their investigations under the pressure of an unheard-of nervous tension . . . under these circumstances sciences exhibit a tendency to a minute division of labour." Whether or not the positivistic trend during the last decades of the nineteenth and at the beginning of the twentieth century can be explained by Lamprecht's very attractive theory as due to the " dissociating " influence of new stimuli which are said to destroy the synthesis of psychic life is an unsettled matter. It is clear that this theory itself is open to many objections, especially on account of its close relation to " cyclic " interpretations of history.

We assume, however, that Lamprecht is right in bringing out the fact that in the period in question the chief interest, not only in psychology but in most sciences, was directed towards the *quæstiones facti* and very often towards *savoir pour prévoir*. Moreover, it seems fair to say that present-day psychology testifies to the fact that it is concerned more with " synthesis " in Lamprecht's sense than with " facts."

Furthermore, to explain the " empirical," " positivistic " and " quantitative " trend before the rise of a qualitative psychology in Germany, it is necessary to recall the fact that psychology in Germany was and still is closely related to philosophy. Considering this close alliance of psychology and philosophy, the attempt might be made to trace the change in psychology back to certain developments in philosophy. Having obtained clarity as to the nature of the developments in philosophy, it might not be difficult, then, to account for the dominant trend in modern psychology.

First, the alleged alliance of psychology and philosophy is to be considered. A psychologist, for instance, in America, where psychology has " freed " itself from philosophy, may be somewhat surprised at the fact that work in physiological psychology or in experimental psychology in general should necessarily develop great interest in philosophy. He might well understand that those aiming at a " psychological psychology," as Arthur Stein calls it, need a philosophical basis ; but why this philosophical basis should be necessary for someone who is interested in experimentation and collection of facts will be less clear to him.   It is not our task here to discuss the relation between philosophy and psychology, but we must simply record the fact that in general even the " biologically- " or " experimentally-minded " psychologist in Germany up to the present day resorts to philosophy. Even if he wishes to reduce psychological work to the careful collection of " facts," he tries philosophically to justify this endeavour on theoretical grounds.   Even if he considers philosophy as incompatible with biological psychology, he seeks by the very use of philosophical methods to justify this aversion.   This point is illustrated by glancing over a list of German psychologists belonging to different " schools." Their close relation to philosophy becomes apparent, no matter whether they are contemporaries or not.   Adopting provisionally Messer's classification,[1] we have on the one hand a group of psychologists who chiefly depend on experimental methods and emphasize the physiological aspects, and on the other hand " pure " psychologists whose chief method is introspection and whose chief interest is centred in " higher " mental processes.   In the first group we may name men like Wundt, Ziehen, Ebbinghaus and G. E. Müller, in the second group Lipps, Cornelius, Brentano, Ehrenfels, Meinong, Witasek, Stumpf, Pfänder, Brunswig, Scheler, and Twardowski.   Messer places himself and the representatives and adherents of the Würzburg School, as Külpe, Marbe, Bühler, Lindworsky, Hönigswald, Selz, and Girgensohn, between the " experimental " and " pure " psychologists.   The perusal of such a list brings home to us that most of these men have contributed work or have been interested in epistemology, logic, ethics, æsthetics, *Wissenschaftstheorie* or other fields of philosophy.   The connection between philosophy and psychology has been and still is a very close one in Germany.

The question remains : in what way does the student of contemporary philosophical thought account for the main tendencies of current psychology ?   To put the inquiry in

---

[1] Messer, A., *Psychologie* (1914).

this form seems to beg the question. As regards the relation of psychology to philosophy, it is more often a case of mutual dependence than a dependence of psychology on philosophy ; it seems, furthermore, that sometimes the main conceptions of present-day psychology assume a striking similarity to concepts developed in fields of philosophical thought which are far from being closely related to psychology. To prove such a statement would require a rather detailed analysis which cannot be undertaken here. It may suffice to call attention to the dominant conceptions of contemporary philosophy by referring to the outstanding philosophical movements, the influence of which makes itself felt in psychology as well as in other sciences. Here we may mention the different Neo-Kantian schools (Riehl ; H. Cohen, Natorp, Cassirer ; Windelband, Rickert, Lask ; L. Nelson) ; Husserl's phenomenology; and the group of " *Lebensphilosophen*," who represent a certain anti-intellectualistic point of view. We can readily see how the Neo-Kantian emphasis on " acts " which posit " phenomena " and on " functions " which make " experience " possible has been instrumental in shaping the concepts of current psychology. A similar importance must be attached to the " descriptive analysis " in the field of " phenomenology " and the rejection of quantification in the case of the " *Lebensphilosophen*." There is no doubt that present-day psychology emphasizes " functions " and " acts " more than " phenomena," the dynamic more than the static, the synthetic view and the description of the various aspects of a phenomenon more than the analysis, and the inadequate, though quantitative, consideration of only one aspect of the phenomenon ; it emphasizes the " whole " more than the " elements." In short, the main conceptions developed stand in rather close relation to present-day philosophical formulations.

We may say that the rise of a " qualitative " psychology finds, if not its explanation, at least its counterpart in certain dominant trends of German philosophy. The fact that this qualitative trend in psychology is closely related to similar trends not only in various fields of social science, but also of " natural science," does not need any further elaboration. This close relation is not surprising, since the line of demarcation between " scientific philosophy " and the different sciences has always been a fluctuating one.

In the following we shall undertake a brief characterization of the main " schools " in contemporary German psychology. Such an analysis should show that the attempt to epitomize this psychology by referring to it as a " qualitative " one seems to be historically justifiable, but it will also show that there are other trends which are not to be overlooked. In attempting a characterization, we shall not begin by reviewing the developments in different fields of research. A survey of this kind would perhaps lead us to the conclusion that the development of " psychotechnics " (industrial psychology and related fields) in recent years is the most conspicuous phenomenon in German psychology. From such an angle it would be necessary to record for instance that the " German State Railway " has established hundreds of psychotechnical testing stations. Of course, it is an interesting problem for the historian to show the ramifications of recent psychological research in different fields : from psychophysical investigations (Wirth) to " psycho- " and " electrodiagnosis " (Moede, Piorkowski, Giese), from the social psychology of chicks to " geopsychology " (Hellpach) ; but there is no doubt that a deeper historical understanding will be arrived at by reviewing the principles rather than the fields of research, the hypotheses directing research rather than the " facts " found in starting from one of these hypotheses.

We shall consider first the " personalistic psychology " of William Stern.[1] It is not necessary to summarize his work in experimental, " differential," and applied psychology, in child psychology, in the psychology of testimony and of language, though this work abundantly illustrates many of the theses of " personalistic psychology."

This psychology is closely related to Stern's philosophical system, his " critical personalism " set forth in three volumes. It is Stern's belief that " scientific psychology and personalistic philosophy " belong necessarily together. Many of the conceptions of personalistic psychology, therefore, can only

[1] Cf. the three volumes of Person und Sache : Vol. I, Ableitung und Grundlehre, 2nd ed. 1923 ; Vol. II, Die menschliche Persönlichkeit, 3rd ed. 1923 ; Vol. III, Wertphilosophie, 1924. Die Psychologie und der Personalismus (1917). " Die menschliche Persönlichkeit und ihr psychisches Leben," Zeitschr. f.päd. Psychol., XXI, 1920. Cf. William Stern, vol. 6 of Die Philosophie der Gegenwart in Selbstdarstellungen.

be fully appreciated through recourse to personalism. The basic concepts of this philosophical system throw light on Stern's psychology. From the point of view of philosophical analysis it may be said that " critical personalism " is opposed to positivism and apriorism as well as to all varieties of what Stern calls " naïve personalism." From a psychological standpoint it is of considerable interest to point out that here neither " conscious processes " nor " behaviour," but the undivided totality of " person " is made the point of departure for a system of philosophy and, of course, for psychology. The recourse to " wholeness " and the rejection of an " atomistic " point of view which seems to be characteristic of German psychology nowadays finds a *systematic* foundation in Stern's personalistic philosophy. In defining " person," *unitas multiplex*, purposiveness and singularity are named as chief characteristics. It is obvious that here the teleological aspect is emphasized. The " person " is viewed as a " purposive individual unity " striving toward certain ends. Stern admits that the psychic as well as the physical side of the " person " can be subjected to a rigid mechanistic interpretation ; in fact the starting point of his whole system is the antagonism of the teleological and the mechanistic principles of " person " and " object," of the " personalistic " and the " impersonalistic " view. But his assumption is that this antagonism disappears on the basis of a " teleomechanical parallelism " ; furthermore that this antagonism is not identical with the mind-body dualism. In fact, it is possible to interpret bodily phenomena teleologically or—to use his term—" personalistically," and mental phenomena mechanistically. The " person," however, is " psychophysically neutral," and the undeniable fact that persons whose characteristics are psychophysically neutral exist must be the point of departure for any psychological system. The facts of " consciousness " or of the " organism " cannot serve as a starting point. It is not difficult to see that the characteristics of " person," purposive activity, integration of parts and individualization, are those characteristics which the psychic and the physical side have in common. But physical as well as psychic life is to be considered as a secondary phenomenon ; the undivided totality of the person is of prime importance.

That the individual is *in-divisibile* is a fundamental fact frequently lost sight of by introspectionists and behaviourists. This fact, however, is basic for personalistic psychology. From the point of view of this psychology it is pertinent to ask why a behaviourist takes the trouble to " prove " the non-existence or non-importance of consciousness, whereas one would expect from him a positive interest in what the chief characteristics of the " behaviour " of a human being really are, as compared, for instance, with a stone. Why, one may ask as a " personalist," bother about the alleged processes of consciousness, and why not go ahead with the description of the behaviour irrespective of its mental or organic components ? But returning from " the youthful theoretical phenomenon of behaviourism," as Anathon Aall calls it, to personalistic theory, some further implications of the " psychophysical neutrality " of " person " should be considered. It is Stern's view that this concept is especially illuminating, in fact is basic for the understanding of problems like " constitution," " temperament " and " character," " self-preservation " and " development," " types " and " Gestalten," " disposition " and " heredity," " expression," " action " and " reaction." It is, for instance, not the outstanding feature of a so-called volitional act that we have on the one hand a sequence of bodily movements, on the other hand concomitant conscious processes, but that the objective environmental constellation is changed by an undivided psychophysical act of a purposive nature. (It is, perhaps, unnecessary to remark that purposiveness does not always imply consciousness ; it is " beyond " psychic and physical.) That scientific analysis may justify an artificial isolation of the psychic and the physical component of such an act may be admitted ; but it also must be admitted that psychology cannot leave out of account those characteristics which present themselves before such a separation. In general Stern holds that the relation of the " person " to the " environment " is not satisfactorily explained by nativistic or empiristic theories. He points to the psychophysically neutral fact of " convergence," i.e., to the fact that every action and reaction, every temporary and permanent characteristic is to be interpreted as the product of an " inner " tendency and an " external " factor. Psychologically, one must realize an interdependence, a constant convergence of " person " and " environment," in the sense that on the one

hand the tendencies directed towards certain ends " pre-
dispose " the person to select a limited part of the objective
world as " environment " and that on the other hand the
objective factors in the environmental constellation decide
whether or not the teleological activity of the person reaches
its ends.

In this connection it is best made clear that the S–R
(stimulus-response) formula is not applicable in personalistic
psychology when the relation of " person " to " environment " is under consideration. Stern writes $\dfrac{S-P,}{R}$
emphasizing the teleological relation. The isolated stimulus
is not directly related to the isolated response of the person as
expressed in the " mechanistic " S–R formula, but to the
person (P). A certain light-stimulus, then, does not call
forth an optical perception, but causes the person to respond
with a perceptive act on the basis of his " auto-teleological "
tendencies.

It is easy to see why for a personalistic psychology
consciousness is not of primary importance, and why the
function and meaning of consciousness is determined by
recourse to the " person." The attempt to ascribe a special
" substance " to the psychic or consider it as an aggregate
of conscious elements is rejected. It would be of some interest to show in what way Stern shows that " psychic phenomena " or " psychic elements " presuppose the existence of
acts; again, how these acts presuppose " dispositions," etc.;
but we are only concerned here with the rôle of the whole
psychic life within the psychophysically neutral person.
May it suffice to state that a study of Stern's works makes
clear that with regard to the psychic life, the author is interested in its causal " explanation " as well as in the interpretation of its " meaning." The physical and the psychic are
yoked together in the purposive behaviour of the person,
which implies that a " bit " of mental behaviour cannot
have a constant relation to a " bit " of organic behaviour.
This conclusion is of far-reaching importance for the " science
of expression," to use Klages' term,[1] and for characterology.
The attempt to relate " facial expressions " or " hand move-

---

[1] *Cf.* Klages, L., *Ausdrucksbewegung und Gestaltungskraft, Grundlegung der Wissenschaft vom Ausdruck* (1923).

ments in writing " to definite mental states or processes must necessarily be futile. The teleological activity of the total person does not permit of such an isolation of mind-body elements. It is not possible here to consider how Stern determines the function of conscious processes by recourse to " conflicts " in the convergence of " person " and " environment," and how he, in spite of his anti-psychoanalytical polemic, justifies the subconscious as a " necessary supplement " to the conscious with its fragmentary and discontinuous character ; it may be said at least that the conscious processes elicited in the contact between " environment " and " person," between " object " and " subject," necessarily misinform us about the " object "—" illusions " of perception, memory and thinking are very frequent—but also with regard to the " subject," since conscious states and processes deceive us, as brought out for instance in psychoanalytical studies. It is not only a fact that conscious processes represent the " objective " and " subjective " world inadequately or incorrectly, but it also is a necessity understood only in the light of " personalistic psychology," for which consciousness is a phenomenon of secondary importance. It is, perhaps, unnecessary to add that Stern, whose earlier work stressed the causal " explanation " of phenomena more than the interpretation of their " meaning," not only emphasizes the " wholeness " and the " Struktur "[1] of the person, but— aiming at a " teleomathematics "—develops definite views on " measurement." The various changes which his system has undergone have not been mentioned, but it should at least be brought out that not only in philosophy, but also in biology and medicine (F. Kraus[2]), " personalistic " conceptions have proved to be extremely valuable.

In turning to *Gestalt* psychology, it becomes apparent in the work of Wertheimer, Köhler and Koffka that the emphasis on qualitative aspects does not exclude painstaking experimentation. The insistence on the " wholeness " character of psychic phenomena does not mean, as becomes evident from an examination of the publications of this

---

[1] Krueger, F., " Der Strukturbegriff in der Psychologie," *Ber. üb. d. VIII. Kong. f. exp. Psychol.*, 1923.
[2] Kraus, F., *Allgemeine und spezielle Pathologie der Person* (1919).

school,[1] that productive experimental work is impossible. It is possible even in the overworked field of perception. But *Gestalt* psychology favours an "*unbefangenes Sehen*" (unbiassed seeing) of the phenomena in the sense of Goethe, Purkinje, Joh. Müller, and Mach, rejecting analysis which destroys the characteristic wholeness properties. Observation does not lead us to " elements " or " molecules " like sensation. The fact that observation does not force us to admit the existence of " sensation molecules " should be taken into consideration as a point of fundamental importance for psychological work. To quote Köhler: " I look up to the homogeneous blue sky of to-day and find it continuous. Not the slightest indication of its being composed of real units, nothing of limits or of any discontinuities. One may answer that my simple observation is not the method to decide this point, but I cannot agree with this argument, since we need, first of all, concepts for the understanding of our immediate experience ; and the sensation loses a considerable share of its importance as a fundamental concept, if, taking it as something of the molecule type, we find nothing to substantiate this idea in direct observation. The continuity of that region of the sky or of any homogeneous field is a positive property of it. And we see that our fundamental theoretical concept in this form does nothing to make this property understood. On the contrary, a special hypothesis would be needed in order to explain how, in spite of the existence of sensation molecules the homogeneous field becomes a continuum. Therefore the only thing produced by this useless assumption is a complication of theory. And I lay the more stress on this fact, as we shall see very soon that there do occur parts in sensory fields which are real objective units though they certainly are not ' sensations.' The concept of sensation tends to hide for us the importance of these other realities and has done so for a considerable time. . . . "[2] Simple observation informs us that " real objective units " as part of the sensory field exist ; observation shows us that the phenomena are "*gestaltet*"[3], that seeing a house and a tree

[1] See the bibliography in Helson, H., " The psychology of *Gestalt*," *Am. J. Psychol.*, XXXVI, 1925, 342, 494 ; XXXVII, 1926, 25, 189.
[2] Köhler, W., " An Aspect of Gestalt Psychology," *Psychologies of 1925*.
[3] *Cf.* Wertheimer, " Untersuchungen zur Lehre von der Gestalt. II," *Psychol. Forsch.*, IV, 1923, 301.

does not give us x sensations corresponding to the house and y sensations corresponding to the tree—for instance, 189 house and 124 tree sensations. Observation merely shows us a house and a tree. Even if we admit·that we have exactly 189 house and 124 tree sensations, the fact still remains that phenomenally we have the characteristic *Gestalt* of a tree and of a house. The fact remains that we cannot have $x-a$, for instance, 170, sensations and $y+a$, 143, sensations. The phenomenal world represents certain characteristic groupings and configurations ; it has a certain order which cannot be accounted for on a " summative " basis. To quote Koffka, " The sum of sensations is not equal to our phenomenal world."[1] A report on a sum of sensations, referring to hue, brightness, saturation, locality, etc., must necessarily leave out of account many aspects of the phenomenal world with its attractive or repulsive, beautiful or ugly, stimulating or indifferent objects. One might say that the aspects not considered in a sensationalistic account serve as a starting point for *Gestalt* psychology.

The above example is taken from the field of optical perception. It is assumed, however, that work in other fields would also demonstrate the fact that the phenomena of mental life are always more or less " *gestaltet*," are always determined by certain " wholeness-laws " (Wertheimer). Wertheimer is interested in the formulation of " laws." It is not quite to the point to criticize the *Gestalt* school for rejecting the method of analysis as the " chief instrument of scientific psychology." To reject, or to show the limited importance of, the " analytical attitude "[2] in psychological experimentation does not imply the abolition of scientific analysis. The fact that mental phenomena are " *gestaltet* " and have certain characteristic wholeness-properties and wholeness-tendencies does not necessarily imply that they fail to obey definite laws. To reject the " analysis " of the introspectionist who isolates contents from their own connections, and to disagree with the " analytical attitude " of the behaviourist who observes behaviour " bit by bit," keeping down to the facts that can be registered or measured,

[1] Koffka, K., " Psychologie der Wahrnehmung," *VIIIth Intern. Cong. of Psychol.*, 1926 (Pub. 1927).
[2] *Cf.* especially Koffka, " Introspection and the Method of Psychology," *Brit. J. Psychol.*, XV, 1924.

is not at all identical with rejecting scientific analysis. This view can be easily confirmed by examining the experimental work done by the *Gestalt* school. We need not attempt such an examination, but it is desirable to call attention to these experiments in general. Some of the phenomena studied from the *Gestalt* angle are perception of movement, contrast phenomena, after-images, stereoscopic vision, the perception of colours, the influence of form on colour, various optical "illusions" and the relation of "figure" to "ground." Problems in other sense fields have also been attacked, and work has been done in animal psychology, child psychology, psychology of thinking and of language.[1] *Gestalt* theory, though it was formulated in connection with studies in the field of optical perception, aims to be more than a theory of perception, even more than a psychological theory.

In 1912 Wertheimer,[2] in his study of apparent movement, reached the conclusion that the perception of movement is a perception *per se*, a phenomenon *sui generis*. If two stationary stimuli are exposed in quick succession, as can be easily done in a stroboscope, a single moving object may be perceived. Apparent movement may possess all the attributes of real movement. Wertheimer advanced a physiological hypothesis, that it is not the excitation process of separate cortical cells nor the sum of the single excitations which is important in phenomenal movement, but that we have to assume "cross-processes" and total processes which result as specific wholes from the excitation of the single cells. We may mention here that Koffka, Hartmann and Köhler[3] have modified Wertheimer's "short-circuit theory," and that much experimental work has been done on the various phenomena of movement and fusion since 1912. Such work shows *in concreto* what is meant by the *Gestalt* point of view, although it would be quite impossible to derive the full meaning of this hypothesis from a study of this work. Phenomena like "movement," "form," etc., receive no

---

[1] *Cf.* for example, Köhler, *The Mentality of Apes* (1925) ; Koffka, *The Growth of the Mind* (1925).

[2] Wertheimer, "Experimentelle Studien über das Sehen von Bewegungen," *Zeitschr. f. Psychol.*, LXI, 1912. See also, *Drei Abhandlungen zur Gestalttheorie* (1925).

[3] Hartmann, "Neue Verschmelzungsprobleme," *Psychol. Forsch.*, III, 1923, 319 ; Köhler, "Zur Theorie der stroboskopischen Bewegung," *Psychol. Forsch.*, III, 1923, 397.

FF

explanation through reference to purely psychological principles. Such an explanation is attempted for instance by Linke,[1] who contends that the " simultaneous," " optimal " and " successive " stages in Wertheimer's movement can be accounted for in terms of the psychological phenomena themselves without recourse to physiology. But " the main thesis of *Gestalt* theory may be said to be that physical *Gestalten* of the nervous system possess properties parallel to their phenomenal correlates." We cannot accuse the *Gestalt* psychologists of neglecting the description of the properties of the phenomenal world, since they have stressed —as has been shown above—many hitherto neglected aspects of the phenomena. Aiming at " wholeness-laws," they have demonstrated in different studies in perception that conditions in one place influence conditions in another place, that we always deal with a set of stimuli rather than a totally isolated stimulus, that not the local properties of the stimuli, but the relations of those properties to each other are decisive. Nevertheless, *Gestalt* psychologists are not satisfied with such a phenomenological account. Köhler[2] demands that the organic processes, that processes in the central nervous system, should share the essential functional characteristics of mental processes. Now psychology, as the science which deals with mental processes, finds—to follow Köhler's definition—*Gestalten* as states or processes whose characteristic properties and effects are not capable of being compounded from the properties and effects of their so-called parts. Spatial forms and melodies are more than a summation of colour points or of tones, etc. (Mach, v. Ehrenfels[3]). Hypotheses concerning physiological action cannot neglect such psychic *Gestalten*. Psychologically, we do not find independent elements, but " dependent differentials " ; we find *Gestalten* which are more than the sum of their parts, and which are transposable, since they do not depend on any given set of elements (the two " criteria " of v. Ehrenfels). " Evidently only a kind of process which cannot be split up into independent local elements would be acceptable as

---

[1] Linke, *Grundfragen der Wahrnehmungslehre* (1919).
[2] Köhler, *Die physischen Gestalten in Ruhe und im stationären Zustand* (1924).
[3] Mach, *Analysis of Sensations* (1886). Ehrenfels, C. von., " Ueber Gestaltqualitäten," *Vierteljahrsch. f. wiss. Philos.*, XIV, 1890, 249.

a correlate of real form." Physiologically, we must assume, therefore, that the processes in the central nervous system are not summations of separate excitations or " and-connections," to use Wertheimer's term, but *Gestalt* processes. Physiological *Gestalten* then correspond to psychic *Gestalten*. If it could be demonstrated that in the realm of physics we have also *Gestalten* possessing properties not compoundable from their parts, a deeper understanding of physiological and, of course, of psychic *Gestalten*, could be obtained. Now Köhler tries to prove the existence of physical *Gestalten* and to show the importance of such an approach for psychology. We cannot state his views on this subject, but it is made clear that *Gestalt* theory is more than a psychological theory. It is brought out at the same time that the work previously done on *Gestaltqualitäten* is not basic for this theory. To mention only a few names : v. Ehrenfels, Höfler, Meinong, Cornelius, Witasek, Benussi, Marty, Mach, Stout, Titchener, Lipps, Bühler, Stumpf, Schumann and Gelb have been interested in this concept of *Gestaltqualität*. Gelb, dealing with this concept, traces it back to Plato ; most students of the Graz school have been concerned with " shapes," " wholes," " relations," " founded contents " and " objects of higher order." We may say that the study of the literature on these problems exhibits a striking contrast to the views of *Gestalt* psychology. It is of interest to see how Cassirer,[1] for whom the concept of " invariance " has become of outstanding importance in the logical analysis of natural science, comments on the work which is concerned with *Gestaltqualitäten*. He says : " The possibility of retaining an *invariant* in its meaning, while the members of the relation undergo the most various transformations, is only illumined and established from a new side in purely psychological considerations." This interpretation written by a Neo-Kantian brings home to us that *Gestalt* psychology and psychology of *Gestaltqualitäten* are different fields.

It is wrong to assume that the *Gestalt* school hypostatizes " wholeness," as it would be wrong to think that personalistic psychology hypostatizes the " teleology " of the person. A closer study shows at once that in either case we have to do with a carefully worked out hypothesis which, as is claimed,

---

[1] Cassirer, *Substance and Function and Einstein's Theory of Relativity* (1923).

accounts satisfactorily for the facts available. To admit that " associative " processes occur—in a bad cold perhaps (Wertheimer)—is one thing ; to reject the " association-hypothesis " is another thing. Wertheimer's " wholeness-hypothesis " is compatible with the fact that associations *exist*, but not with the association-*hypothesis*. Both the " bundle-hypothesis," which assumes that mental life can be reduced to the summation of elements, and the " association-hypothesis " imply " summation-concepts." But why employ such concepts—this is Wertheimer's question—since it can be shown that a " summation ," that a mere mechanical " addition " takes place only exceptionally and only under special conditions and only within narrow limits ? Why consider such an atypical case as characteristic of the whole of mental life ? Observation, as has been shown above, forces us to work with " wholeness-concepts."

It is clear that the views of *Gestalt* psychology can only be adequately appreciated in a system of psychology written from this angle. This system does not exist. It is obviously difficult to show the value of the *Gestalt* hypothesis, not only for the fields of psychology and physiology, but also if a reinterpretation of Kantian " categories " or of " causality " in physics is undertaken. It is the difficulty of the task which we wish to emphasize. There is no question about the desirability of such a system. We cannot properly speak of a new system of psychology unless the theory takes into account the findings in the different fields of natural and social science ; unless, to put it differently, the psychologist takes a definite " philosophical " stand. It is in the field of *natural* philosophy most of all that Köhler and Wertheimer have advanced a number of definite views. In general, their position may be characterized as decidedly anti-Humian. " Experience " is not considered as the all-determining factor. " The *Gestalt* problem in perception does not admit of an empiristic interpretation."[1] Empiristic interpretations are not favoured in the field of perception ; they are also rejected when it comes to formulating a philosophical theory. It may in fact be true that " association psychology is really *dead* now," as Hans Driesch asserts, in *The Crisis in Psychology*.[2] In

[1] Köhler, W., " Gestaltprobleme und Anfänge einer Gestalttheorie," *Jahresber. üb. d. ges. Physiol. u. exp. Pharmak.*, 1922, 512.
[2] Driesch, H., *The Crisis in Psychology* (1925).

Germany it seems to be dead, at least in the works on psychological *theory*—but it is not true, of course, that philosophy has done away with empiristic views. We can understand, therefore, the attempt at a destructive criticism of Hume's philosophy. It goes without saying that the influence of " past experience " cannot be neglected. To turn to optical perception : the grouping, the order, in the field of vision, is determined (1) by a complex of external stimuli ; (2) by a " *Gestalt* disposition " which is the resultant of previous perceptive processes ; (3) by the conditions of the " somatic field," in which the physiological processes corresponding to the perceived *Gestalten* take place and which may be influenced by conditions in other cortical areas. In some processes the psychic correlate has the character of " inner activity." This account shows that the *Gestalt* psychologist is aware of the influence of " past experience " ; nevertheless the " qualitative and topographical aspects of the stimulus configuration " are his chief concern. Examining these qualitative and topographical aspects, he finds that it is not " past experience," frequency, exercise, etc., which is responsible for the appearance of *Gestalten*, but that *Gestalten* are presupposed in the acquisition of experiences, in learning. To refer to optical perception, " this influence of previous life, instead of showing how experience *makes* units out of something else, *presupposes* the existence of the unit as such in previous seeing."

The emphasis on the qualitative and topographical aspects of the phenomena makes it also clear that " elements " of any kind must be considered as derivatives and that the *prius* is a phenomenal world which calls forth perceptive, affective, evaluative and æsthetic " experiences," a world with meaningful objects in a certain order, an environment with good, bad, beautiful, repulsive, simple, symmetrical, hard, soft, well- and ill-defined objects.

It is not surprising, furthermore, that the *Gestalt* psychologist rejects the " constancy hypothesis," the direct point-for-point correlation between sensation and stimulus, and the S-R (stimulus-response) formula in its mechanistic sense. It often seems as if for the " empirical " worker who is concerned with " finding " stimulus-response relationships nothing is left to do but to improve his " technique." *Gestalt* psychology points out the questionable value of such a procedure, and calls attention to the fundamental difficulties involved.

It appears that such skepticism, or, to express it positively, the insistence on "*phänomenale Analyse*"[1] and on the "meaning" of organic processes has led to extremely valuable results in questions of cerebral localization, in a field in which the endeavour to establish "point-for-point representations" has led, as Edinger thinks, to a certain barrenness.[2] But, if we consider it a "biological necessity," as Goldstein and Fuchs do, that in complete hemianopsia the "reorganization" of the visual field must produce conditions similar to normal ones, we understand for instance why the function of the anatomical fovea is taken over by a more eccentric part of the retina situated in the intact area, by a "pseudofovea," a fovea in the functional sense. Such biologically orientated views do not lead to "barrenness," but are the starting point for productive experimental work.

It seems to the present writer that the work on cerebral cases in Frankfurt illustrates very well the two features which appear to be the outstanding and most characteristic features of *Gestalt* psychology, the insistence on "phenomenal analysis" and on a non-mechanical account of organic processes and of the organism. A further remark is necessary. Some of the views which we have ascribed to *Gestalt* psychology can also be found in the works of other German psychologists. Similar statements must be made about the other "schools." We are not here concerned with tracing such interrelations, but wish to emphasize merely the main conceptions of the current schools.

Turning to the "developmental psychology" of Felix Krueger,[3] it becomes obvious that the approach to psychological problems in his school is in many ways related to an approach from the *Gestalt* angle. In fact, Sander[4] recently

[1] Goldstein, K., "Die Topik der Grosshirnrinde in ihrer klinischen Bedeutung," *Dtsch. Zeitschr. f. Nervenhk.*, LXXVII, 1923.
   Gelb and Goldstein, *Psychologische Analysen hirnpathologischer Fälle auf Grund von Untersuchungen Hirnverletzter* (1920).
[2] *Cf.* Klüver, H., "Visual Disturbances after Cerebral Lesions," *Psychol. Bull.*, XXIV, 1927.
[3] Krueger, *Ueber Entwicklungspsychologie* (1915). *Cf.* also the volumes of the *Arbeiten zur Entwicklungspsychologie.*
[4] Sander, "Ueber Gestaltqualitäten," *VIIIth Intern. Cong. of Psychol.*

pointed out that the work on *Gestaltqualitäten* in the Leipzig laboratory confirmed the findings especially of Koffka, Köhler and Wertheimer. Originally, the concept of *Gestaltqualität* testified to the fact that many investigators had rediscovered wholeness-characteristics in mental life where " exact " work seemed to demonstrate nothing but " elements " and combinations of elements. In developing the concept of *Gestaltqualität*, justice was done to certain wholeness properties of the phenomena, but in explaining these properties they were considered as secondary products dependent on the properties of the " parts " or " elements," *i.e.*, as derivatives. Krueger and his followers are inclined to reject the view that " *Gestaltqualitäten* " are the result of " collective attention," or of " creative synthesis," or of " production processes " on the basis of certain unalterable " parts." They assert that it can be shown experimentally that the relation of the " whole " to the " parts " is a different one. Dealing specifically with *Gestalten*, the experiments demonstrate that the " total quality " of the *Gestalt* dominates the qualities of the parts—that these parts, the subwholes, have different " weight," that they participate to a different degree in the total quality of the " *Gestalt*." Genetically this total quality is prior to the " part properties." We first become conscious of the whole, and then of the parts. It is assumed, furthermore, that *Gestalten*, as well-defined and articulated experiences, have developed from a complete, fused, undifferentiated and unarticulated experience.

It is the emphasis on the developmental aspects which seems to distinguish the *Gestalt* school from the Leipzig school. " Developmental " psychology, which is, according to H. Werner,[1] different from " genetic " psychology in America, has certainly not been neglected by Köhler, Koffka and Wertheimer, but there is no doubt that the developmental point of view stands more in the foreground of the work of Krueger and others in the Leipzig laboratory. Here the different fields of perception have been attacked from this point of view ; in addition, Krueger demands that developmental psychology obtain results which can be utilized by philology, pedagogy, ethnology, political economy, and history. In short, it is necessary, he thinks, to establish a

[1] *Cf.* Werner, *Einführung in die Entwicklungspsychologie* (1926).

close correlation with the social sciences. After the passing of the pre-experimental period, psychologists lost sight of the fact that " scientific " psychology was chiefly based on results obtained from normal and educated adults belonging to the social circle of the experimenter. This one-sidedness, of course, may be remedied by taking animals, children and " primitives " as subjects. The fact that most of the results of Stumpf's " tone psychology " are primarily based on " statistical findings in unmusical Germans and on physiological hypotheses " may be remedied by studying the " musical consciousness " of " primitive " individuals, and by recording their music phonographically.

But more has to be done, so Krueger believes, than merely to extend the fields of research. The psychologist has to take into account cultural facts. Problems of the development of the individual can only be adequately dealt with through the consideration of social conditions. The problem of the position of psychology in relation to the different sciences and fields of research becomes important for Krueger. The problem of " historical causality " arises. History does not deal with the individual in the sense in which a biologically orientated psychology deals with the individual. Neither the problems of history nor of " developmental psychology " can be solved by taking subjects to the laboratory. At least, a developmental psychology which aims at a psychological understanding of the different cultural manifestations, such as law, religion, etc., or the " historical structure " of the individual mind cannot proceed in such a way. This indicates that many questions raised in modern sociology, history, and philosophy of history are of great interest for " developmental psychology " as conceived by Krueger. It may be added, with regard to the psychological development of " objective " cultural manifestations, that the " organic " point of view is stressed. To give an example : an enumeration of " objective " legal norms, the presentation of a " system of law " which in its objectivity is detached from other cultural manifestations, does not make clear the psychological development of these norms. Wundt's approach in *Das Recht* is inadequate. It is necessary to bring out the organic connection of law with religious, social, political and economic conditions, to show in *concrete cases* in what way these various factors constitute

special features in the " cultural whole." The phenomenology of this *Kulturganze* is a prerequisite for the appreciation
of the *one* aspect, *e.g.*, of the legal norms.

From Krueger's " developmental psychology " we turn to
the work of the Marburg school on the " eidetic type." In
this school genetic questions are dominant. The studies
published during the last few years by the Marburg Institute
of Psychology seek to determine the psychological characteristics of the eidetic type. These researches are more than
contributions to various " problems of the classical theory
of perception " ; the attempt is made to substantiate a genetic
interpretation of mental life. Although social phenomena are
also viewed from this angle, E. R. Jaensch's work on the
eidetic type can only be appreciated as a contribution to
biological psychology.

According to Jaensch, " eidetic " individuals are persons
who possess *Anschauungsbilder* (percept-images, eidetic
images).[1] " The eidetic image is a subjective visual phenomenon which is found in many young people, but not so
often among adults ; if, for instance, a person with eidetic
imagery is asked to look attentively at an object—regardless
whether it be of two or three dimensions—this person sees
the object again when he closes his eyes or looks at a ground
which serves as a background for the image." Thus one may
speak of " certain images of an hallucinatory clearness, in
other words, special forms of perception-like images "
(Kroh) or as Urbantschitsch[2]—who in his book of 1907 first
dealt extensively with these phenomena—of " perceptual
memory-images." Urbantschitsch contrasted these perceptual memory-images with the " ordinary visual memory-
image." In the first case, an object is really " seen," in the
second case, it is merely " imagined." The fact is stressed

---

[1] *Cf.* especially Jaensch, E. R., *Ueber den Aufbau der Wahrnehmungs-
welt und ihre Struktur im Jugendalter* (1923) ; Jaensch, W., *Grundzüge
einer Physiologie und Klinik der psychophysischen Persönlichkeit* (1926) ;
Kroh, O., *Subjektive Anschauungsbilder bei Jugendlichen.   Eine psycho-
logisch-pädagogische Untersuchung* (1922) ; Klüver, H., " An Experimental Study of the Eidetic Type," *Gen. Psychol. Monogr.*, 1, 2, 1926 ;
Klüver, H., " Studies on the Eidetic Type and on Eidetic Imagery,"
Psychol. Bull., XXV, 1928.
[2] Urbantschitsch, V., *Ueber subjektive optische Anschauungsbilder*
(1907).

that an eidetic individual is able to *see* an object—" in the real sense of the word "—either immediately after the exposure or after a considerable lapse of time. Phenomenologically, one may illustrate these subjective visual phenomena by referring to positive or negative after-images. Eidetic images may arise "spontaneously" or " at will," without a preceding exposure; they may be almost photographic in fidelity, or deviate from the stimulus object in certain characteristic ways. Eidetic images differ from hallucinations in that the eidetic person generally does not believe in the objective reality of the phenomena. Eidetic images, therefore, have been called pseudohallucinations. It is clear that for the study of these phenomena all investigations dealing with hallucinations, pseudohallucinations in the clinical sense, illusions, the different kinds of subjective visual phenomena and of sensory after-effects are of great importance. E. R. Jaensch, unable to accept the view that eidetic images are necessarily of pathological nature, stimulated his assistants and students to look for individuals with images of this kind. It happened that Kroh in 1917 discovered that eidetic images are frequently found in normal children. Since that time much research has been done on the eidetic disposition, and eidetic phenomena have been subjected to systematic experimentation.

The Marburg investigators assert on the basis of this work that these phenomena are not pathological, but that they represent quite normal and common phenomena in childhood. It is maintained that we have also eidetic images in the auditory, tactual and olfactory fields. In fact, Hans Henning[1] states that in the field of " lower senses " a revival of sensory impressions does not take place in the form of " representations " or " memory-images," but in the form of eidetic images. Imagery in the field of the lower senses means for him eidetic imagery.

Subjective visual phenomena similar to those investigated by the Marburg school have, of course, been observed before Urbantschitsch and Jaensch. Here the reports of Goethe, Purkinje, J. Müller, Henle, G. H. Meyer, Wigan, Brodie, Fechner, Galton, Ebbecke, Staudenmaier, and others should be mentioned. The various characteristics of eidetic images

---

[1] Henning, H., *Der Geruch* (1924) ; Henning, H. *Psychologie der Gegenwart* (1925).

in children, as determined experimentally by Jaensch and his collaborators, cannot be described here, but we shall outline the general views developed on the basis of these investigations.

It is maintained that "the eidetic stage is to a certain extent a normal stage of development." Herwig[1] reports that among 205 boys in Marburg, age 10 to 14.6 years, 76 boys, 37 per cent., were eidetic. Krellenberg[2] refers to school classes with 32, 26, 28, 46, 17, 34, 67 per cent. respectively. In Breslau, Fischer and Hirschberg[3] found 99·3 per cent. (139 eidetic individuals among 140). H. Zeman[4] found 88 per cent. (176 among 200) in Vienna. In Breslau, as well as in Vienna, the figures for the female sex are higher. The Breslau and Vienna figures include those weak cases in which only slight traces of the eidetic disposition can be demonstrated. Kroh in Marburg reports 61 per cent. among children and 7 per cent. among adults. Since the eidetic stage is therefore to a certain extent a "normal" stage, and since the investigations have shown that certain permanent characteristics of the fully developed consciousness of the adult are more distinct in their preceding developmental stage, genetic psychology must pay special attention to the eidetic stage. It is also maintained that in the Marburg subjects the same laws hold for eidetic phenomena and for the phenomena of normal perception. The laws for eidetic phenomena are only "quantitatively different." The interpretation, for instance, of localization, horopter, contrast, etc., in the eidetic image is applied to the corresponding phenomena in normal perception. It is obvious, however, that the irregular ("apsychonomic") eidetic images observed by Urbantschitsch cannot be utilized for the solution of problems of normal perception.

The genetic point of view is also emphasized when it comes

[1] Herwig, B., "Ueber den inneren Farbensinn der Jugendlichen und seine Beziehung zu den allgemeinen Fragen des Lichtsinns," *Zeitschr. f. Psychol.* LXXXVII, 1921.

[2] Krellenberg, P., "Ueber die Herausdifferenzierung der Wahrnehmungs-und Vorstellungswelt aus der originären eidetischen Einheit," *Zeitschr. f. Psychol.*, LXXXVIII, 1922.

[3] Fischer, S., and Hirschberg, H., "Die Verbreitung der eidetischen Anlage im Jugendalter und ihre Beziehungen zu körperlichen Merkmalen," *Zeitschr. d. f. ges. Neurol. u. Psychiat.*, LXXXVIII, 1924.

[4] Zeman, H., "Verbreitung und Grad der eidetischen Anlage." *Zeitschr. f. Psychol.*, XCVI, 1924.

to comparing eidetic images (E I), after-images (A I) and memory-images (M I). Since E I are apparently in some respects similar to A I and at the same time show a certain relation to M I, it becomes important to draw a line of demarcation between A I, E I, and M I. The determination of E I concerning colour, size, intensity, " weight," richness in detail, relation to background, the degree of " plasticity " and flexibility, the degree of " coherence," the degree of " invariance," the relation to distracting stimuli, is made *with reference to* A I and M I. Jaensch arrives at the conclusion that A I, E I, and M I are three " levels of memory." He speaks of a hierarchy of memory levels, the lowest of which is the A I and the highest the M I. Memory which teleologically may be viewed as a unity must be psychologically considered as consisting of a number of " memories " : a memory of A I, a memory of E I and a memory of M I. Krellenberg states on the basis of his experiments that in many cases the eidetic stage is preceded by a " unitary phase " in which A I, E I, and M I are hardly differentiated. It is believed that this—which may be called an undifferentiated E I—is the ontogenetic source of our perceptions, and that many characteristics of these perceptions (for instance, " stability " of colours, etc.) can be adequately explained through recourse to the " unitary phase."

For a genetic interpretation of mind as a whole an investigation of visual eidetic imagery can hardly furnish sufficient material. But Jaensch points out that research on eidetic imagery and research on the eidetic type are two different things. The eidetic individual, that is in general the individual before and up to puberty, and the non-eidetic individual, which means in general the adult, are not only quantitatively, but also qualitatively, different. Jaensch and his co-workers seek to show that the presence of eidetic imagery in an individual implies that the after-images, the memory-images, the perceptions, the intellectual, emotional and volitional life, as well as the bodily make-up of this individual, show certain " typical " characteristics. The eidetic " type," therefore, really refers to a biotype with certain psychophysical characteristics.

Experimental results show that aside from differences in the " degree " of eidetic imagery—" weak " and " strong " cases, five degrees being distinguished—differences in " type " arise. E. R. Jaensch and W. Jaensch describe two types. In the case of the *first type*, for instance, the eidetic image may be nothing but a visualized idea ; the person " sees " what he is thinking of. He can, without effort—frequently without preceding exposure—call up eidetic images and banish them " at will " ; he can change the form, colour localization, etc., of the image, if such changes are " meaningful"; spontaneous eidetic images are viewed as "natural" and normal ; the phenomena have in most cases the colour of the stimulus object ; they are rich in detail and very plastic ; the values for Emmert's law are about the same as found for memory-images ; " fluxion " is very pronounced ; the phenomena may last indefinitely, the duration depending on the person ; the person's after-images are generally " normal," his memory-images fluctuating and unstable. In the case of the *second type* the eidetic image has more the character of an after-image ; to " see " phenomena at will is in most cases impossible ; the eidetic image perseveres in spite of the intention to banish it ; the person is often unable to change the form and colour; the process of changing seems very strenuous and proceeds very slowly ; spontaneous eidetic images do not occur very often ; they are frequently considered unpleasant or even " uncanny " ; the phenomena show in most cases the complementary colour ; they are often not very distinct ; Emmert's law is in most cases confirmed ; in general there is no fluxion ; the duration is independent of the " will " of the person ; the after-images last longer and the memory-images display a certain perseverating character. This enumeration of the distinguishing characteristics of the two types does not take into account the somatic side of the two eidetic types. The first is called the B-type (referring to the Basedow syndrome), the second the T-type (referring to tetany). W. Jaensch, on the basis of his clinical investigations, tries to substantiate the view that the eidetic image of the B-type is only one symptom in the complex of B-symptoms as they have been ascertained clinically and psychologically. The same holds for the eidetic image of the T-type. Theoretically, W. Jaensch assumes two distinct " psychophysical reaction systems," the empirical study of which—as could be shown so far—can be profitably guided by starting from the " optical symptoms," *i.e.*, from the eidetic images. To start from cases with distinctly different eidetic imagery has, as we learn, the further advantage that light is thrown on cases with " mixed " imagery. It is asserted that, empirically, beside the pure B- and T-type, a BT- and TB-type, a TE (epileptoid component)- and BH (hysterical component)-type, and other pathological subtypes, have to be distinguished.

In our discussion we have chiefly stressed the genetic aspects in the field of eidetic research, as set forth by E. R. Jaensch. We may add that he believes that eidetic research from a genetic point of view is of far-reaching importance for certain problems of biology, sociology, mythology, pedagogy, art and even philology. Jaensch's studies have stimulated research on the eidetic disposition, not only in the psychological laboratories of Germany and Austria, but also in America, England, France and Italy. So far, many of the findings of Jaensch have been confirmed. Some points of great theoretical importance, however, are as yet not established, as, for instance, the assumption that the eidetic stage is a " normal " stage, and that the laws for normal and eidetic vision differ only quantitatively ; furthermore, that the presence of eidetic imagery points to other " typical " characteristics of the individual.

CHAPTER XXVI

CONTEMPORARY GERMAN PSYCHOLOGY AS A " CULTURAL
SCIENCE "

At the International Congress of Psychology in 1926 one of
the symposia was concerned with the problems of " understanding and explaining in psychology " (L. Binswanger,
Th. Erismann, G. Ewald, E. Spranger). In this last chapter
we shall deal with these problems, that is, with certain aspects
of " *geisteswissenschaftliche Psychologie* "[1] (cultural science
psychology). Only a few of the views developed in this
field can be discussed here. In this field, more than anywhere else, the historian has to record controversial matters.
The discussion of " understanding " and " explaining,"
which involves a radical reconsideration of the " foundations " of psychology, convinces us more than anything else
that there may be some justification in speaking of a " crisis
in psychology."

We may succeed in clarifying some of the " critical "
issues involved by starting with certain writings in modern
logic. The Southwest German School has attempted to
define the logical and epistemological implications in the
work of those sciences which do not belong to natural science.
It is believed that a certain clarity has been attained with
regard to the premises and methods of natural science ; that
similar clarity, however, is to be desired for those sciences
which are vaguely called " *Geisteswissenschaften.*" The
analysis carried out in this school has sought to bring out the
fact that there exists a certain antagonism between these

---

[1] The word " Geisteswissenschaften " appears for the first time, as
Rothacker points out, in J. Schiel's translation (1849) of Mill's *Logic*.
Schiel uses this term for the English " moral sciences." At present,
the terms " *Geisteswissenschaften* " and " *Kulturwissenschaften* " are
used interchangeably. We shall, therefore, translate " geisteswissen-
schaftliche Psychologie " as " cultural science psychology." *Cf.*
Rothacker, " Logik und Systematik der Geisteswissenschaften," in
Handbuch der Philosophie, ed. by Baeumker and Schröder.

sciences and natural sciences. Rickert,[1] for example, in contrasting cultural and natural sciences, finds that it is the concept of value which is of outstanding importance in the field of cultural sciences. Causal laws and historical " laws " are different. Windelband[2] finds that the methods used in natural science are by no means the only ones which are to be considered " scientific."˙ The methods of history have the same scientific dignity. Natural sciences are " nomothetic," cultural sciences " idiographic." Whether we proceed " nomothetically " or " idiographically," whether we try to see causal connection or the uniqueness, the individual character, of the phenomena, depends on the object of our research. There is no reason for calling the first procedure " scientific " and the second non-scientific. If psychology uses the " individualizing " method of the historian, it must be considered a cultural science ; if it uses the " generalizing " (aiming at laws) procedure of the physicist, it is to be regarded as one of the natural sciences. As it happens, Rickert considers psychology to belong to the same logical type as physics. He asserts that every psychology which aims at an investigation of the inner necessities of cultural events is impossible.

But in the meantime, a cultural science psychology has developed which regards itself as antagonistic to, or at least, different from, a " natural science psychology." It is claimed that psychology does not belong to the same logical type as physics, that it is not evident at all that psychology, in order to proceed " scientifically," should aim at " laws " in the way the different natural sciences do. There is no doubt that in the development of cultural science psychology this work of the Southwest German School, in which the distinctiveness of the methodology of cultural science has been emphasized, has been of great importance.

Of even greater importance is the work of Wilhelm Dilthey, who was, as James remarks, a man " overflowing with information with regard to everything knowable and unknowable."[3] It is not surprising that Dilthey (1833–1911), living in a

---

[1] *Ueber die Grenzen der naturwissenschaftlichen Begriffsbildung,* 2nd ed. (1913) ; *Kulturwissenschaft und Naturwissenschaft,* 2nd ed. (1910).
[2] *Cf.* especially *Präludien,* 6th ed. (1919). Also *Geschichte und Naturwissenschaft* (1894).
[3] *Cf. The Letters of William James.*

period in which, after the breakdown of Hegel's metaphysical
speculations, empirical research was flourishing, was of the
opinion that "metaphysicians are fools." This dictum,
reported by Paul Natorp, and the remark of Benno Erdmann[1]
that Dilthey was vehemently opposed to both the traditional
philosophy of history and the " new " psychology, may bring
home to us that Dilthey's work[2] contains many heterogeneous
elements. It is a very difficult task to give a succinct statement of his psychological views. The " new " psychology
mentioned above was the psychology represented by H.
Ebbinghaus. Many of the arguments advanced at present
in the discussion of "understanding" and "explaining"
were formulated for the first time in the Dilthey-Ebbinghaus
controversy.[3] Dilthey attacks the "explanatory" psychology of Ebbinghaus, which, as he thinks, is modelled after the
ideal of "atomistic" physics, and consists chiefly of
hypotheses. To do justice to the special character of
cultural sciences this explanatory psychology has to be
replaced by a "descriptive" psychology. (Here Dilthey
recalls the fact that a distinction between an " explanatory "
and a " descriptive " psychology was made by Ch. Wolff
—" *psychologia rationalis* " and " *psychologia empirica* "—
and by Drobisch and Waitz). Psychology as conceived
by Dilthey is the foundation of all cultural sciences. It
is the process of *understanding* which becomes of fundamental importance. This process is in the last analysis
an " artistic process," a process in which we are constantly
aware of the reference of the parts to a totality. Somehow,
we experience that a sentence, a gesture, an action, briefly,
that a part, is always embedded in an articulated whole,
in a *Strukturzusammenhang*. The fact that such a *Strukturzusammenhang* is experienced must be the starting point
for psychology. " The *Strukturzusammenhang* is experi-

---

[1] Gedächtnisrede auf Wilhelm Dilthey, *Abh. d. Kgl. Pr. Akad. d.
Wiss.* (1910).
   [2] *Ideen über eine beschreibende und zergliedernde Psychologie* (1894).
Beiträge zum Studium der Individualität (1896). *Sitz. d. Kgl. Pr. Akad.
d. Wiss. z.* Berlin, 1894. " *Ueber den Aufbau der geschichtlichen Welt
in den Geisteswissenschaften.*"   *Abh. d. Kgl. Pr. Akad, d. Wiss.* (1916),
Philos.-Hist. Kl. " Die Typen der Weltanschauung und ihre Ausbildung
in den metaphysischen Systemen." *Weltanschauung,* edited by M.
Frischeisen-Köhler (1911).
   [3] Ebbinghaus, H., " Ueber erklärende und beschreibende Psychologie," *Zeitschr. f. Psychol.,* IX, 161.

GG

enced." This is Dilthey's concise formula. These inner experiences in which we " understand " a sentence, a gesture, an action, passion and suffering, human life and history, are by no means hypothetical processes, but represent the firm basis for a descriptive psychology. Such a psychology does not begin with " elements "—as natural science and explanatory psychology do—in order to " construct " causal connections, but it begins with the experienced, inner connections. It starts from the experienced *Strukturzusammenhang* in order to describe its various aspects " analytically." As subtle as such an analysis may be, it never arrives at " the construction of the entire causal nexus of psychic processes." To contrast these two aspects : " *Die Natur erklären wir, das Seelenleben verstehen wir.*" Natural science and natural science psychology " explain," cultural science psychology " understands." We call attention to the fact that this simple statement is the result of a very elaborate and painstaking analysis. It has greatly stimulated modern thought from Simmel to Spranger, and the logical and psychological complexity of the concept of " understanding " has been illuminated during the decades since the Ebbinghaus-Dilthey controversy. There is an enormous difference, however, between " understanding," as formulated by Dilthey, and the concept of " understanding " as it is elaborated with dozens of distinct meanings in modern discussions.

It is easy to grasp why during the last two decades the dissatisfaction with " explanatory " psychology has grown considerably. It became apparent that empirical psychology, starting with " elements " of some kind in the laboratory, could not attain the promised insight into the higher processes of the mind, nor could it do justice to the fact that man is an historical being as well as a mammal. Lamprecht, with his view that history is applied psychology, had to rely on a psychology which was interested in the ultimately distinguishable elements. He had to rely on the work of the generation of Ebbinghaus, Lipps, Wundt, etc. It is not surprising, therefore, that he again and again demanded a " psychic mechanics " as the foundation of history. Of course, such a psychic mechanics, working with the conceptions of a " natural science psychology " involves tremendous difficulties. What Lamprecht needed was a psychology which should change the point of departure and relate the totality of personality to the various manifestations of an historically conditioned environment. A cultural science psychology, worthy of its name, Spranger believes, is able to meet such demands.

Since Spranger is undoubtedly one of the leaders in the field of modern cultural science psychology,we shall characterize here some of the views set forth in his *Lebensformen*.[1] This book brings to light elements closely related to Dilthey's work, and represents, Spranger thinks, the first attempt at the *construction*, not merely the methodological foundation, of cultural science psychology. The result is a *type* psychology, a discussion of the "fundamental types of individuality." The author portrays (1) the theoretical man, (2) the economic man, (3) the æsthetic man, (4) the social man, (5) the man of power, (6) the religious man. The question arises immediately, why does cultural science psychology assume the form of a *type* psychology?[2] Spranger outlines a psychology which he calls *Struktur*[3] psychology in opposition to the "atomistic" psychology which includes nearly all contemporary psychological schools. For him, meaning is of prime importance. Psychologically, we have to start from totalities characterized by "meaning relations." A relationship is called meaningful when all its constituent parts and processes become intelligible with respect to a total performance of *value* import. From this point of view a machine as well as an organism may be meaningful. Spranger believes that he goes beyond Dilthey in assuming that mind is more than a teleological structure which is regulated by tendencies to self-preservation. His main point is that we must start from the personality as a whole as it stands in intimate contact with an historically developed cultural environment. To isolate the individual artificially from this environment would be a fruitless task. There exist definite connections. In the "religious" or the "cognitive" attitude, for example, we impart meaning to this environment. In cultural science psychology we have to start from facts of this kind. The significance of such an approach becomes apparent when we recall that representations, feelings, and drives play a rôle

[1] See also Spranger, "Psychologie und Verstehen," *Histor. Zeitschr.*, CIII, 1909.
[2] *Cf.* Klüver, H., "The problem of type in 'cultural science psychology,'" *J. Philos.*, XXII, 1925.
[3] For the meaning of the term, see Krueger, "Der Strukturbegriff in der Psychologie," *Ber. üb. d.* VIII. *Kong. f. exp. Psychol.*, 1923.

in the cognitive as well as in the religious attitude. In themselves, representations, feelings and drives are *meaningless* material; they remain subjective states, " ego-conditions," and are inexplicable to other individuals. But one individual can explain to another the *meaning* of his subjective experiences. With regard to the *meaning* we may point in the same direction ; in fact, we can have in common only the *meaning* of our subjective experiences, not the processes themselves. In certain " acts " we objectify our meaning and call the result science, technology, art, religion, society, law, etc. An understanding of these " objectifications," of such cultural provinces, is only to be arrived at through the *acts* and the meaning intended in them. Considering the large number of " acts," we must " isolate," " idealize," and separate wherever we find a difference in meaning. Thus Spranger characterizes as individual *Geistesakte* scientific, economic, æsthetic and religious acts. Just how he defines the *meaning* intended in each of these act-classes cannot be discussed here. The " sympathy " and " mastery " acts have to be added as acts concerned with other individuals. Thus we have six different classes of " acts " through which meaning is objectified or expressed in science, economic organization, religion, etc. If we consider one of the six " meaning-tendencies " as dominant in an individual—for instance, the " æsthetic acts "—we have to speak of an " æsthetic man," although it is apparent that all the other five " meaning-tendencies " are present to a certain extent.

That is the method by which Spranger arrives at the above-mentioned six " ideal fundamental types." It is necessary to consider his procedure in some detail, though many important points in his theory cannot be presented.[1] It is clear at least that this type psychology is a rather complicated affair and not simply a matter of classifying human beings as theoretical, æsthetic men, etc. Spranger's types are " schemata of understanding." The six fundamental types cannot be identified empirically. Reality presents nothing but complex types, but these can be understood by reference to the " ideal " types. These " pure " types are not psychologically empirical types, nor even historical types, but are conceptual instruments for the understanding of

---

[1] We are leaving out of account those points with regard to which Spranger has recently changed his views.

historical reality. Spranger starts, as does Dilthey's opponent, Ebbinghaus, from the individual. But his next step is away from "explanatory," empirical psychology. The detailed analysis of sensations and representations and of the emotional and volitional life of the individual is the chief concern of "explanatory psychology." Spranger, without concerning himself with such analyses, directly considers the relation of the total individual to the historical environment. The individual with whom Spranger is concerned does not stand in an environment in which certain " stimuli " elicit, for example, sensory responses. It is the historical *milieu* which interests Spranger ; it is the individual as an historical being which is the chief concern of his cultural science psychology. The acts of the individual are viewed in their relation to art, to science, etc., and to other " trans-subjective " manifestations of cultural life. Each of these " spheres of meaning " has certain distinct features. Nevertheless, if we consider the complexity of historical life, the distinction between different spheres is not easily made. However, when, instead of the manifestations of the cultural life, we take the individual as a starting point, we find relatively few " meaning-tendencies." We find, so Spranger asserts, the above six " types." Now these schemata really enable us to understand man in his relations to the historical environment, to the " trans-subjective " phenomena of " art," " science," " social life," etc. Let us imagine, for example, an individual for whom *one* meaning-tendency, *one* value, appears as dominant ; for example, the value of science. On the basis of this assumption we can conceive the *Lebensform* of the " theoretical " man, the theoretical type. The fact that empirically " the fundamental principle of science," objectivity, cannot dominate a *Lebensform* entirely, does not matter in this connection. The " ideal " theoretical man is a construction. To understand the empirical individual we need such devices. It is, therefore, the problem of understanding which is basic for Spranger's psychology, a problem which was considered by B. Erdmann to be *the* problem for the foundation of *Geisteswissenschaften*. Spranger points out that he arrived at his fundamental types by " the study of history and faithful daily observation." He thinks it necessary, however, to do more work on these " typical categories " ; such work may eventually change them. One may object, as Stern does, for instance, to giving the type theory the name of psychology. But the problem of " understanding " and " explaining," the question whether or not there are two kinds of psychology—an " understanding " and an " explanatory " psychology ; a " cultural science psychology " and a " natural science psychology "—is more than a terminological matter. Obviously, the " types " established by Jung, Rorschach, Jaensch, Kretschmer, Ewald and Birnbaum are of a different nature from Spranger's " ideal types." These investigators are interested in the empirical determination of types. It must be said that this work constitutes one of the outstanding features of current German psychology.[1] Different as the empirical approach may be, theoretically the type concept is used to denote individuals who are in some way comparable with respect to their essential characteristics (Kronfeld). Certainly this type concept has nothing in common with the " types " of a " cultural science psychology." If one encounters the statement that the type problem is the most fundamental problem of contemporary psychology it is clear that reference is made to the problem of " understanding." Our representation of Spranger's views may have left the impression that this question is chiefly of interest to philosophers ; but at the same time it is true that it has been a subject of dispute for about fifteen years in psychopathology. We refer here to the discussion concerning the distinction between " causal relations " and " relations to be appreciated by understanding " (" kausale " and " verständliche Zusammenhänge "). In brief, it is the distinction between " causal explanation " and " psychological understanding " introduced into psychopathology by K. Jaspers. Jaspers[2] speaks of a " static " understanding, in which we realize and apprehend the mental states of " other egos " and on the other hand a " genetic " understanding in which we conceive of the way one mental state arises from another. We explain causally by establishing objective relations between a number of elements on the basis of many observations. Again and again Jaspers points out that the fact that we have found

---

[1] Cf. Klüver, H., "An Analysis of Recent Work on the Problem of Psychological Types," J. Nerv. and Ment. Dis., LXII, 1925.
[2] Jaspers, K., Allgemeine Psychopathologie (1913). See also "Kausale und verständliche Zusammenhänge zwischen Schicksal und Psychose bei der Dementia præcox," Zeitschr. f. d. ges. Neurol. u. Psychiat, XIV, 1913.

a certain relation through " understanding " proves nothing with regard to the frequency of the real occurrence of this relation.

These remarks show that the problem of " understanding " is attacked here from an angle very different from that of Spranger. To appreciate this difference we must point to two facts. The one is Jaspers's relation to phenomenology. The work of Husserl and Scheler, as well as Brentano's work, have not only been stimulating for psychological theory but also for empirical work in normal and abnormal psychology. An analysis of Husserl's investigations is out of the question here, since they deal with some of the most difficult questions of philosophy. Brief mention may be made of some of his conceptions.[1]

Husserl contrasts the " phenomenological attitude " with the " natural attitude " (*natürliche Einstellung*). Naturally the individual takes the world in which he thinks, hates and loves as " actually given " and is interested in the happenings, the objects, the theories, the truths of this world as phenomena to be accepted or rejected, to be believed or disbelieved, in short, he is interested in them for the sake of something else, " for the sake of consequences." In the " phenomenological attitude " we eliminate these consequences, we put them " into parentheses." We may be aware that an object is *existent*, but we do not make any use of this existence, *i.e.*, we do not prove or disprove anything by referring to the fact of existence. " I eliminate all sciences which are related to the natural world ; although I do not intend to object to them, I make absolutely no use of their validity. Not a single proposition that belongs to the natural context, and is perfectly evident to me, is now admitted as valid or invalid ; not one is actually accepted, not one serves me as a foundation." Thus Husserl eliminates the " validity " which an object or proposition may have, and its " systematic " importance. " Any object whatsoever—it may be real or unreal, logical, alogical, or even illogical—may be phenomenologically approached or *purified; i.e.*, deprived of its natural or

---

[1] *Cf.* especially Husserl, *Logische Untersuchungen*, and *Ideen zu einer reinen Phänomenologie und phänomenologischen Philosophie. Allgemeine Einführung in die reine Phänomenologie.* Scheler, M., *Der Formalismus in der Ethik und die materiale Wertethik. Cf.* also Appendix D in Ogden and Richards, *The Meaning of Meaning.*

systematic connections."¹ Such a theoretically "disconnected" object, called the "phenomenon," is obtained by elimination of "natural or systematic connections," by "phenomenological reduction." Thus phenomenology—to give the formulation of Lanz—defines itself as a "*study of objects in their relation to consciousness in a state of supreme impartiality, when the face-value and systematic significance of the objects concerned does not come into consideration.*" We "bracket" the "natural" connections of the object, we suspend our judgment in order not to lose sight of the actually given phenomenon, which is frequently covered with "traditions," "theories," "explanations." The method of phenomenological reduction may be applied to phenomena like "red," "blue," "truth," "beauty," "meaning," "sign," "symbol," "object," etc. "A definite shade of red may be determined in many different ways. For example, as the colour that is enunciated by the word ' red ' (colour itself being already a substitution, a reduction) ; as the colour of this thing or this particular surface ; as the colour that ' I see ' ; as the colour of this particular number and length of vibrations. It appears here as an x of an equation. The phenomenological experience alone can give us the ' red ' itself, in which the totality of those determinations, and signs and symbols find their ultimate fulfillment. It transforms the x into a fact of *Anschauung*." (Scheler). Phenomenologically, red is not a "sensation" or "vibration" or a "cortical process" or an "illusion," etc. "Being even an illusion, it cannot get rid of its ' essence ' even by pronouncing it illusory." Phenomenology deals with the "*essentia*," with *Wesenheiten ;* it is not a "science of facts" (*Tatsachenwissenschaft*). It examines the "essence" of "red," or "truth," or "Jupiter." We find, for instance, that it is inadequate to say that "Jupiter" has only a psychological existence in our imagination ; for imaginary processes "are real occurrences, and Jupiter is not a real occurrence : he

¹ Lanz, "The New Phenomenology," *Monist*, XXXIV, 1924. In general we shall follow Lanz's presentation, although it does not take into account the recent developments in phenomenology, nor does it pay attention to many fundamental distinctions made by Husserl, as for instance between "phänomenologisch," "deskriptiv," and "reell," or between the different kinds of "Ich," etc. It seems as if phenomenology can be profitably approached through the study of Brentano.

does not exist anywhere." The object of our imagination or, in general, of consciousness, is different from the state of consciousness in which it appears. The " object " of intention is different from the " act " of intention. It is different not in an existential sense, " but merely as *a different centre of possible predication.*"

Just a few of the conceptions of phenomenology have been stated here, but it is easy to understand that under the influence of this school the problems involved in psychological concepts, as for instance, " function," " act," " intention," " phenomenon," and " sign," have found a concise formulation. Under the influence of the phenomenologists who rely on *Anschauung* (immanent inspection) the tendency to view phenomena in an unprejudiced way and, first of all, to describe without reference to preconceived notions, has received a strong impetus. Consequently, the demand for a " phenomenal analysis " has been voiced not only in psychology, but also in other fields of research. In psychology, and especially in psychopathology, the attempt has been made to appreciate and apprehend mental states and processes without reference to (frequently hypothetical) somatic processes. Results have been sought on the basis of an " immanent-psychological analysis." Finally, understanding has been introduced as a method. Whether or not such developments still have close relation to phenomenology is a different matter ; but the influence of this " philosophical " school cannot be denied. This school is unquestionably responsible to a remarkable extent for the shift from " explanation " to " meaning," which is so often apparent in current psychology. Its influence is easily recognized in the work of psychologists like Linke, Pfänder, Geiger, Schapp and Brunswig. In psychopathology phenomenological studies have been published by Schilder, Schneider, Kronfeld, Storch, Mayer-Gross and others. Most of these investigators have been greatly stimulated by Scheler's work.[1] To return to Jaspers, we may note that not only his work in psychopathology but also his attempt at a psychology of *Weltanschauungen*[2] shows the influence of phenomenological views.

But to appreciate fully Jaspers's position as regards an

---

[1] *Cf.* especially Scheler, M., *Wesen und Formen der Sympathie* (1923).
[2] Jaspers, *Psychologie der Weltanschauungen* (1922).

" understanding " psychology, it is also necessary to consider his relation to M. Weber.[1] It is Weber's concept of the " Idealtypus " (ideal type) to which Jaspers attributes a pre-eminent significance in psychology and psychopathology. Weber, emphasizing the special nature of cultural science, assumes that no system of laws, however perfect, can elucidate the meaning of a cultural manifestation because cultural events presuppose the value import ; that is, in cognizing a cultural event only a certain aspect of it becomes significant. Here the " ideal type " has a definite function. We begin with an " exaggeration of certain elements of experience," we stress certain features of the event disproportionately and efface others, we construct relations which on the basis of our knowledge seem possible. In short, we devise a sort of logical model, the ideal type, for the situation. It is, then, the object of special research to determine how reality differs from this ideal type. Only later investigations can settle the question whether this type is a fantastic product or a scientifically fruitful conception. Thus all representations of ideal types, for instance, of the *essence* of Christianity, are only of questionable value if they are viewed as historical representations of the empirically existent ; although they are of high heuristic importance for research and of great systematic value for representation if they are used as conceptual tools for " comparison " and for " measurement " of reality. The ideal type is not an evaluation but a construction for heuristic purposes. Jaspers takes over this concept. In the case of Weber, as well as of Jaspers, we cannot speak of a new " discovery." What happens is that a procedure which has been used before is given an explicit methodological formulation. Jaspers himself believes that perspicacious investigators have always made use " instinctively " of the ideal type. The " ideal type " of mania, for example, has been constructed (gaiety plus incoherence plus emotional pressure) ; so with the hysterical character. Such a method does not lead to enumerations *ad infinitum*, but discovers meaningful relationships, whether we have to do with ideal types of diseases or of *Weltanschauungen* or of other phenomena.

---

[1] Klüver, H., " M. Weber's ' ideal type ' in psychology," *J. Philos.*, XXIII, 1926. Weber, M., " Die ' Objektivität ' sozialwissenschaftlicher und sozialpolitischer Erkenntnis," *Arch. f. Sozialwiss. u. Sozialpolitik*, XIX, 1904.

Our presentation of Jaspers's views has shown that the concept of " understanding " is not clearly formulated in his system ; it is to be admitted, however, that the difficulties involved are great.

In contrasting " causal " and " understanding " psychology in this chapter we have tried to picture one of the most characteristic features of contemporary German psychology. So far nothing seems to be settled with regard to the questions raised.   Whether there is one scientific psychology or whether there are two kinds of psychology, whether there is a necessary antagonism between " causal " and " understanding " psychology or whether they supplement each other—these and kindred questions have not been answered with finality.

NAME INDEX

HH

SUBJECT INDEX